Surgical Oncology

Current Concepts and Practice

Surgical Oncology
Current Concepts and Practice

Edited by

C. S. McArdle MD, FRCS(Eng), FRCS(Ed), FRCS(Glas)
Consultant Surgeon and Honorary Clinical Lecturer,
University Department of Surgery, Royal Infirmary, Glasgow

Butterworths
London Boston Singapore Sydney Toronto Wellington

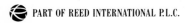 PART OF REED INTERNATIONAL P.L.C.

First published, 1990

© Butterworth & Co (Publishers) Ltd, 1990

British Library Cataloguing in Publication Data

Surgical oncology.
  1. Man. Cancer. Surgery
  I. McArdle, C. S. (Colin S)
  616.994059

ISBN 0-407-01700-3

Library of Congress Cataloging-in-Publication Data

Surgical oncology/edited by C.S. McArdle.
     p. cm.
  Includes bibliographical references.
  ISBN 0-407-01700-3 :
  1. Cancer – Surgery. I. McArdle, C.S. (Colin Stewart)
  [DNLM: 1. Neoplasms–surgery. QZ 268 S96112]
RD651.S9323 1990
616.99′4–dc20
DNLM/DLC
for Library of Congress   90-1706
                                         CIP

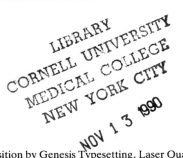
Composition by Genesis Typesetting, Laser Quay, Rochester, Kent
Printed and bound in Great Britain by Hartnolls Ltd, Bodmin, Cornwall

Preface

Approximately 250 000 new cancer patients are registered in the UK each year. It has been estimated that one in three people will develop some form of cancer during their lifetime.

With the exception of lung cancer most common solid tumours present initially to surgeons. The management of patients with cancer therefore forms an important part of most surgeons' workload.

Unfortunately many patients already have either obvious metastases or occult disseminated disease at the time of initial presentation. Increasingly there is evidence that these patients may benefit from a multidisciplinary approach. It is therefore important that individual surgeons are aware of the potential contribution made by radiotherapists and oncologists to patient care.

Some tumours however, do not appear to have the potential to metastasize; nevertheless, these patients may die of local recurrence. It is in these patients that the skills of the surgeon are paramount; better surgeons may achieve better results.

Some surgeons have a somewhat nihilistic attitude to cancer. Certainly there have been few dramatic surgical breakthroughs in the last few decades. There is little to be learned from the analysis of uncontrolled studies; unfortunately, the proportion of patients entered into randomized studies is relatively low. Perhaps if more surgeons were prepared to support these studies we would all learn more about the natural history and management of these diseases.

Surgical oncology has emerged as a new specialty and its future is as yet uncertain. Nevertheless it seems clear that the time has come for most patients with cancer to be treated by specialist surgeons or at a specialist centre.

Contributors

D. C. Carter MD FRCS(Glas) FRCS (Ed)
Regius Professor of Surgery, University of Edinburgh, Edinburgh Royal Infirmary

M. A. Cornbleet BSc MD FRCPE
Consultant Medical Oncologist, Department of Clinical Oncology, Western General Hospital, Edinburgh

G. D. Chisholm ChM PRCS(Ed) FRCS(Eng) Hon FRACS
Professor of Surgery, University Department of Surgery/Urology, Western General Hospital, Edinburgh

D. Cunningham MD FRCP
Senior Lecturer and Consultant Physician, Section of Medicine, Institute of Cancer Research, Royal Marsden Hospital, London and Surrey

J. R. Farndon BSc MD FRCS
Professor of Surgery, University of Bristol, Bristol Royal Infirmary

S. B. Kaye BSc MD FRCP
Professor of Medical Oncology, CRC Department of Medical Oncology, University of Glasgow

David J. Kerr MSc MD MRCP
Senior Lecturer and Honorary Consultant Physician, CRC Department of Medical Oncology, University of Glasgow

David Kirk DM FRCS(Eng) FRCS(Glas)
Consultant Urologist, Western Infirmary, Glasgow

C. S. McArdle MD FRCS(Eng) FRCS(Ed) FRCS(Glas)
Consultant Surgeon and Honorary Lecturer, University Department of Surgery, Royal Infirmary, Glasgow

Ian A. McGregor ChM DSc FRCS(Eng) FRCS(Glas) Hon FRACS Hon FRCSI Hon FRCS(Ed) Hon FACS
Consulting Plastic Surgeon, Royal Infirmary, Glasgow

Rona M. MacKie MD FRCP FRCPath
Professor of Dermatology, University of Glasgow, Western Infirmary, Glasgow

J. Pooley MD FRCS(Eng)
Consultant and Senior Lecturer, Department of Orthopaedic Surgery, University of Newcastle-upon-Tyne, Royal Victoria Infirmary, Newcastle-upon-Tyne

Alastair W. S. Ritchie MD FRCS(Ed)
Senior Lecturer, University Department of Surgery/Urology, Western General Hospital, Edinburgh

M. Soukop FRCP
Consultant Medical Oncologist, Department of Medical Oncology, Royal Infirmary, Glasgow

A. Watson MD FRCS(Ed) FRCS(Eng)
Professor of Surgery, Royal North Shore Hospital, Sydney, Australia

Contents

Chapter 1

Carcinoma of the oesophagus

A. Watson

Introduction

Carcinoma of the oesophagus is, fortunately, a relatively uncommon malignancy with a mean incidence in the UK of approximately 7.5 per 100 000 population. However, this translates into some 4000 deaths per annum in the UK from oesophageal cancer and its significance as a major therapeutic challenge arises firstly from the magnitude of surgery required to excise the tumours and secondly from the poor long-term survival figures following resection.

In the Western world, oesophageal tumours are almost invariably advanced at the time of presentation, as by the time dysphagia occurs, some two-thirds of the circumference of the oesophagus is involved by tumour (Edwards, 1974). It is hardly surprising, therefore, that inoperability rates up to 30% of those considered suitable for surgery have been reported, with 5-year survival rates as low as 4% (Earlam and Cunha-Melo, 1980a). More optimistic reports, however, emanate from the East, with 5-year survival rates of 34% being reported from Japan (Akiyama *et al.*, 1981) and even 96% from China in superficial lesions detected by screening (Huang, 1981). Much attention has been directed in recent years to earlier diagnosis, improved staging and careful selection with resulting improvement in operability rates and 5-year survival rates in the order of 15%.

Epidemiology

Oesophageal carcinoma is characterized by considerable variation in its incidence in different parts of the world. The highest incidence in Europe occurs in the provinces of Normandy and Brittany where it reaches 60 per 100 000 population. Higher incidence still occurs in Transkei and East Africa where it reaches 80 per 100 000 population, Northern China with over 100 per 100 000 population and the highest reported incidence is in the Caspian littoral of Iran where the incidence reaches 260 per 100 000 population (Joint Iran–International Agency for Research on Cancer Group Study, 1977). In these areas of extremely high incidence, a 50-fold decrease in incidence occurs within a distance of a few hundred miles, emphasizing the important role of environmental factors in aetiology.

1

Aetiological factors

Race

In most multiracial areas, carcinoma of the oesophagus is more prevalent in blacks than whites. This is particularly so in South Africa, especially in the Bantu, and in the USA the incidence is four times greater amongst the black population than whites. There are exceptions, however, particularly in Brazil where higher incidence occurs in whites than blacks. In the areas of high incidence in Northern China and Iran, the disease principally affects those of Mongolian extraction.

Sex

In most series, carcinoma of the oesophagus is more prevalent in males, the male preponderance in the UK being approximately 1.4:1. In Alaska and Sri Lanka, females are more commonly affected than males, but the difference is likely to be environmental due to locally differing ingestion habits in these areas.

Diet

Dietary deficiencies have been shown to be relevant in some epidemiological studies. Deficiencies of vitamins A, C and riboflavin were highlighted in high incidence areas by the Joint Iran/Iraq Study Group. Deficiency of trace elements such as zinc and molybdenum has also been highlighted in areas such as China and South Africa, where subsistence farming on soil deficient in these substances can increase nitrosamine concentration in plant growth (Yang, 1980). Yang found that in general terms, incidence of oesophageal cancer in China was higher amongst families with nutritionally inadequate diets, than in those with better diets in the same area.

Alcohol and tobacco

Alcohol and tobacco can be incriminated in many areas where the disease is prevalent, and it has been estimated that these factors account for at least 80% of oesophageal cancer in males in France, the United States and Japan (Day, Munoz and Ghadirian, 1982). In Brittany, the risk of developing oesophageal carcinoma in a male alcoholic who smokes is 44 times greater than that of a non-smoker and non-drinker from the same area (Lambert, Audigier and Tuyns, 1978). Alcohol and tobacco are felt to be relevant as they are both sources of nitrosamines and it has been suggested that alcohol may facilitate the penetration of carcinogenic agents into the oesophageal mucosa (Tuyns, Pequiqnot and Abbatucci, 1979).

Other ingested substances

The high incidence of oesophageal carcinoma in certain parts of the world reflects local habits and customs in relation to ingestion or inhalation of a wide variety of agents. In the areas of very high incidence in Iran and China, where neither alcohol nor tobacco is relevant, opium smoking has been shown to be an important factor (Cook-Mozaffari et al., 1979). The pyrolysis of opium yields carcinogenic agents, probably heterocyclic amino compounds, which predispose to a marked oesophagitis, distributed throughout the whole of the oesophagus, which is a premalignant lesion (Munoz and Crespi, 1984). Other ingested agents which have been found to be important are chillis and spices in India (Baruah, 1979), bracken fern in Japan (Hirayama, 1979), betel nuts in Sri Lanka (Stephen and Uragoda, 1970) and cereals contaminated by the Fusarium species in China and Transkei (Marasas, Van Rensburg and Mirocha, 1979). In China, pickled vegetables fermented until covered with mould have been incriminated as an important aetiological factor, the incidence varying directly with consumption. Experimental oesophageal cancer has been produced in chickens fed on the same substance (Yang, 1980).

The temperature of ingestion also seems to be a relevant factor in China, Singapore and Japan where tea and tea-gruel are drunk at very high temperatures (De Jong *et al.*, 1974). In areas of highest incidence, the aetiology is often multifactorial and possibly cumulative, parts of China and Iran having in common dietary deficiencies, the frequent drinking of hot tea and opium smoking.

Occupation

In view of the importance of environmental factors discussed above, it is perhaps surprising that few reports have associated oesophageal cancer with occupational exposure. In Sweden, vulcanization workers have a ten-fold increase in incidence of oesophageal cancer compared with matched controls (Norell *et al.*, 1983). Occupations related to production of alcoholic drinks have long been recognized to carry a higher than average incidence of oesophageal cancer (Young and Russell, 1926).

Genetic factors

There is little evidence of a strong genetic influence in the genesis of oesophageal carcinoma with the exception of sufferers from tylosis. This condition, associated with hyperkeratosis of the palms and soles, is inherited and transmitted by an autosomal dominant gene of high penetrance. Two families have been reported, with 95% of relatives exhibiting tylosis eventually developing oesophageal carcinoma, but there was no evidence of the disease in family members without tylosis (Harper, Harper and Howel-Evans, 1970).

Premalignant lesions

Corrosive strictures

There have been several reports of squamous-cell carcinoma developing many years after strictures caused by the ingestion of caustic agents (Bigelow, 1953; Lansing, Ferrante and Oschner, 1969). These carcinomas tend to occur between 20–40 years after ingestion of the corrosive agent (which is most common in childhood). The tumours, therefore, tend to occur at an earlier age than usual and the sex distribution is equal. It has been suggested that the presence of a corrosive stricture increases the likelihood of the development of oesophageal carcinoma by 1000-fold (Kiviranta, 1952).

Achalasia

There have been numerous reports implicating achalasia as a premalignant condition, chronic irritation due to stasis within the oesophagus being considered the relevant factor. The reported incidence varies between 2.8% (Postlethwait, 1979) to 29% (Ellis, 1960), the variation being felt to be associated with the duration of achalasia.

The tumours are almost invariably squamous carcinoma and can occur at all levels in the oesophagus. Early effective treatment of achalasia has therefore been advocated to reduce the incidence of carcinoma (Belsey, 1966), although carcinoma can occur after myotomy (Lortat-Jacob et al., 1969) because of the grossly impaired motility in such patients. Careful endoscopic surveillance of patients with achalasia, even following successful treatment, would therefore appear appropriate.

Barrett's oesophagus

When Barrett's oesophagus was originally described in 1950, the columnar-lined lower oesophagus was considered to be due to a congenitally short oesophagus (Barrett, 1950). However, subsequent clinical and experimental studies have clearly shown this to be an acquired condition, consequent on longstanding gastro-oesophageal reflux, in which damaged squamous epithelium becomes replaced by columnar epithelium (Bremner, 1984). That Barrett's oesophagus is associated with a high prevalence of oesophageal adenocarcinoma is established beyond doubt (Shafer, 1971; Naef, Savary and Ozello, 1975; Sjogren and Johnson, 1983). What is unclear is the true incidence of oesophageal carcinoma or indeed of Barrett's oesophagus itself, since only symptomatic patients present themselves for investigation. One of the largest studies of the prevalence of oesophageal adenocarcinoma in Barrett's epithelium was conducted by Naef, Savary and Ozello (1975) in which 1225 patients with reflux oesophagitis were endoscoped. Of these, 140 had Barrett's oesophagus and 12 had oesophageal adenocarcinoma arising from the columnar epithelium. However, most reports are of the coincidental finding of oesophageal adenocarcinoma and Barrett's oesophagus; few long-term prospective studies having been performed. Cameron and Payne (1983) followed up 77 patients who were still alive out of 104 having attended the Mayo Clinic with a diagnosis of Barrett's oesophagus, only two of whom developed adenocarcinoma after a mean follow-up period of 8.5 years, the risk being 1 per 441 years of patient follow-up. The inference was that the true incidence of adenocarcinoma in Barrett's oesophagus was so low as not to justify screening, but several subsequent series have placed the risk much higher at between 1 in 175 and 1 in 56 per year of patient follow-up (Spechler et al., 1984; Robertson et al., 1988; Van der Veen et al., 1989).

The management and surveillance requirements of patients with Barrett's oesophagus are controversial because of the low anticipated yield of screening programmes and absence of convincing evidence that regression of Barrett's epithelium occurs following successful anti-reflux treatment. Prospective studies by Wesdorp et al. (1981), Dooner and Cleator (1982) and Bremner (1984) showed no evidence of regression. Brand et al. (1980) showed a reversion of columnar-lined oesophagus to squamous epithelium in 4 of 14 patients undergoing anti-reflux surgery, but there was no correlation between the reported reversion and the successful correction of reflux, and this study has been criticized on account of inadequate histological data. Furthermore, the development of adenocarcinoma following successful anti-reflux surgery has been reported (Haggitt et al., 1978; Hamilton et al., 1984). It would appear reasonable in patients documented as having Barrett's columnar-lined oesophagus to treat the reflux effectively, either medically or surgically as appropriate, and keep the patient under endoscopic surveillance. The presence of severe dysplasia has been shown to be a particular risk factor, especially in males who smoke (Smith *et al.*, 1984), in patients who have 'extended Barrett's' with greater than 8 cm involvement and patients who have had previous gastric surgery (Van der Veen *et al.*, 1989).

High-grade dysplasia correlates well with early adenocarcinoma (Reid *et al.*, 1988) and there is some evidence to suggest that aneuploidy detected on flow cytometry may be a more sensitive indicator of malignant potential (Haggitt *et al.*, 1988).

While regular surveillance of all patients with Barrett's oesophagus may present a formidable logistic and economic task, there would appear to be some merit in surveillance of such high-risk patients, particularly those who are considered likely to withstand resection if a carcinoma is detected (Atkinson, 1989). Skinner *et al.*, (1983) have suggested prophylactic resection in patients with high-grade dysplasia who are considered fit for resection, and many of these patients are found to have an adjacent focus of invasive adenocarcinoma. Susequent survival of patients so treated is considerably greater than in patients who have undergone resection for symptomatic adenocarcinoma (Skinner, 1985), but the risk of operative morbidity and mortality has to be weighed against the risk of development of adenocarcinoma.

Reflux strictures of the oesophagus

Several series have alluded to the increased prevalence of oesophageal adenocarcinoma in patients with reflux strictures (Moghissi, 1979; Ogilvie, Ferguson and Atkinson, 1980; Watson, 1984a), the likely mechanism being the development of columnarization, as 76% of reflux strictures are associated with Barrett's oesophagus, the strictures occurring at the squamo-columnar junction (Hill, Gelfand and Bauermeister, 1970). Such carcinomas have, in our experience, only developed in elderly patients managed conservatively by intermittent dilatation and pharmacological reflux control and have not occurred in younger patients in whom surgical reflux control was employed (Watson, 1987a). If younger patients are managed by more conservative means, regular surveillance with endoscopic biopsy and cytology would appear appropriate, particularly where dilatation requirements are increasing.

Coeliac disease

Whilst not strictly a premalignant condition, several authors have reported an increased incidence of oesophageal carcinoma in patients with coeliac disease, reaching 1.6% (Holmes *et al.*, 1974; Cooper *et al.*, 1980). Several reasons have been postulated for this increased risk, including nutritional deficiencies, increased mucosal permeability to carcinogens and impaired immunological competence.

Experimental models

Spontaneous neoplasms of the oesophagus are extremely rare in laboratory animals and no special strain of laboratory animal with a high incidence of oesophageal cancer has been reported. However, a high incidence of spontaneous oesophageal tumours may occur in domestic animals from areas where the incidence of oesophageal cancer in man is high. Yang (1980) has reported an incidence of spontaneous oesophageal tumours in chickens from the Linxian province of China of 175.8 per 100 000, which is similar to the incidence in man in the same area. A similar phenomenon has been reported in cattle in Kenya, both these situations being believed to reflect environmental factors. There is no evidence available as to whether the incidence of oesophageal cancer in such animals is modified when they are transferred to other environments with a low incidence (Reuber, 1985).

With regard to artificial induction of oesophageal cancers in laboratory animals, most reported series relate to the ingestion of nitrosamines in mice, rats and rabbits (Napalkov and Pozharisski, 1969; Druckrey, 1972; Reuber, 1977). Such lesions progress from moderate to severe dysplasia, to carcinoma-in-situ and then frank malignancy and mirror the pathological picture in human carcinomas in areas such as China, where high concentrations of nitrosamines have been found in water and food samples (Yang, 1980).

Pathology

Site of tumours

The oesophagus has been traditionally divided into thirds: the upper lying above the arch of the aorta, the middle third between the arch of the aorta and the inferior pulmonary vein and the lower third between the latter and the gastro-oesophageal junction. The relative distribution of tumours within these segments of the oesophagus varies from series to series. Upper third lesions comprise 5–20%, but most authors are agreed that the remaining tumours are evenly distributed between the middle and lower thirds (McKeown, 1972; Kirk, 1987).

Macroscopic pathology

Oesophageal tumours are most commonly fungating and exophytic, this type representing some 60% of all tumours. Ulcerative tumours comprise 25% and the remaining 15% are diffuse infiltrative tumours (Troncoso and Riddell, 1985). The majority of tumours presenting with dysphagia are circumferential at the time of diagnosis, and approximately 70% of tumours are greater than 4 cm in length (DeMeester and Lafontaine, 1985). As one might expect, tumour length correlates with depth of invasion, tumour spread and hence survival.

A collective review by Rosenberg, Franklin and Steiger (1981) showed that in tumours 5 cm or less in length, 40% were localized to the oesophagus, 25% extended beyond the oesophagus and 35% were unresectable or had distant metastases. In tumours longer than 5 cm, only 10% were localized to the oesophageal wall, 55% extended beyond the oesophagus and 75% were unresectable or had distant metastases. In our own series, some of our 5-year survivors were in patients with tumours longer than 6 cm, and 1–2 year survival occurred in some patients with tumours 8–10 cm in length (Watson, 1990).

Microscopic pathology

The majority of oesophageal carcinomas are squamous in origin, and it is generally reported that these constitute approximately 90% of all oesophageal cancers (Troncoso and Riddell, 1985). The remainder are principally adenocarcinomas although there are rare variants of both squamous and adeno lesions which have been reported. However, there is growing evidence that the prevalence of adenocarcinoma is increasing, some series reporting over 40% of adenocarcinomas (Watson, 1982; Cameron, 1987; Wolfe et al., 1987).

Squamous tumours arise from the normal squamous epithelium covering the oesophagus, and may be of varying degrees of differentiation. Dysplasia and carcinoma-in-situ may precede the appearance of invasive carcinoma, and indeed such areas may be seen adjacent to such tumours. In our experience, squamous lesions are less advanced at the time of presentation than adenocarcinoma, 20% as opposed to 0% being superficial to the muscularis propria, with 54% having lymph node involvement as compared to 85% of adenocarcinomas. These factors are reflected in survival, mean survival for squamous lesions being 32.4 months in our series as opposed to 15.1 months for adenocarcinoma (Watson, 1987). Squamous tumours have the added advantage of being relatively more radiosensitive than adenocarcinomas.

Rare variants of squamous carcinoma which may occur include verrucous carcinoma, sometimes seen in association with achalasia and oesophageal diverticulum, and spindle-cell carcinomas which often achieve considerable size, both these variants being of low-grade malignancy and carrying a relatively favourable prognosis. Small-cell carcinoma on the other hand is a rare variant in which these tumours behave like oat-cell bronchial tumours arising from the argyrophil cells of the basal layer of the mucosa and may rarely secrete calcitonin and ACTH. These are extremely invasive tumours, metastasizing widely and consequently are associated with a very poor prognosis.

Adenocarcinoma of the oesophagus is most commonly seen in the lower third of the oesophagus, but pooled data show that 8% of adenocarcinomas occur in the upper and middle thirds (Giuli, 1984). They arise from mucosal or submucosal glands, heterotopic gastric mucosa or from Barrett's columnar-lined oesophagus, the latter accounting for approximately 86% of adenocarcinoma (Haggitt et al., 1978). These latter tumours show a microscopic spectrum similar to that seen in gastric carcinomas, but the 'intestinal' type predominates. Ultrastructural and histochemical differences between the oesophageal columnar epithelium, gastric fundal epithelium and small intestinal epithelium, have suggested a metaplastic origin for columnar epithelium in Barrett's oesophagus (Paull et al., 1976). The neoplastic change, most predominant in the intestinal metaplasia, is preceded by increasing dysplasia and carcinoma-in-situ. It has been estimated that of patients with high-grade dysplasia or carcinoma-in-situ, about 50% already have an infiltrating carcinoma (Troncoso and Riddell, 1985). Thus, there is need for close surveillance of patients with Barrett's oesophagus and particularly with dysplasia, and some workers have advocated prophylactic resection in these circumstances, (Skinner et al., 1983). Whilst there remains doubt concerning regression of Barrett's epithelium after anti-reflux surgery (vide supra), there is evidence that effective anti-reflux surgery may both reduce the risk of neoplastic transformation and promote regrowth of squamous epithelium over the Barrett's mucosa (Skinner et al., 1983) suggesting the alternative of anti-reflux surgery and careful surveillance in cases with less florid dysplasia.

Rare variants of adenocarcinoma are adenosquamous carcinoma, adeno-acanthoma, and choriocarcinoma. Adenosquamous lesions comprise coexisting adeno and squamous carcinomas and are felt to represent areas of squamous metaplasia within adenocarcinoma arising from oesophageal mucous glands. In adeno-acanthoma, the squamous component comprises mature squamous epithelium and the likely origin is from areas of ectopic gastric mucosa. These tumours spread extensively via the blood stream, the submucosa and within the perimural spaces and are consequently associated with a poor prognosis. Choriocarcinoma of the oesophagus is extremely rare, representing trophoblastic-like differentiation in adenocarcinomas, resulting in atypical giant cells which have been found to contain human chorionic gonadotrophin.

Spread of oesophageal tumours

Spread of oesophageal carcinoma can occur by local extension, lymphatic spread or by blood-borne metastases. Local extension can be both through the oesophageal wall, ultimately to invade contiguous structures, or longitudinally. In our series (Watson, 1990) only 30% were confined to the oesophageal wall, and of these, the majority were squamous lesions. The peri-oesophageal tissues are firstly involved by extra-oesophageal spread, but subsequently, depending on the level of the lesion, invasion of the aorta, bronchi, pericardium or vertebrae may occur. Complications of such extra-oesophageal extension may be recurrent laryngeal nerve paresis, tracheo-oesophageal fistula or rarely, in advanced cases, extensive transmediastinal spread involving most contiguous organs. As might be expected, extra-oesophageal spread adversely affects the prognosis. The incidence of nodal metastases rises progressively from 14% in T1a lesions to 72% in T3 lesions (Giuli, 1984) and where contiguous structures are involved, 5-year survival rarely exceeds 5% (Mannell, 1982).

   In addition to the macroscopic longitudinal invasion previously alluded to, it is well recognized that both squamous and adenocarcinoma can extend submucosally for considerable distances from the apparent macroscopic tumour limits (Miller, 1962; McKeown, 1979). This is more likely to occur proximally rather than distally, and can be for a distance of up to 9 cm. For this reason, clearance of 10 cm from the apparent macroscopic limits is recommended in radical resection, as even frozen section can be inaccurate as normal epithelium may overlie submucosal deposits, which may be present as skip lesions (Mannell, 1982).

   Lymphatic spread can occur both by embolization of tumour cells into submucosal lymphatics, producing skip or satellite nodules, and into contiguous and subsequently more distant lymph nodes. The para-oesophageal nodes are first involved, but because of the distance which submucosal lymphatics can run before connecting with para-oesophageal lymphatics, the nodal deposits may be at considerable distances from the primary tumour. Subsequently tracheobronchial, hilar, posterior mediastinal, cervical and coeliac nodes may be involved, depending on the level of the tumour. Akiyama et al. (1981) showed that coeliac nodes may be involved in over 30% of patients with upper and middle third tumours, and in patients with lower third tumours, nodal metastases occur in about 10% in the superior mediastinal group of nodes. Nodal metastases occur more frequently in advanced lesions, and are most commonly present at the time of surgery in adenocarcinomas. Lesions less than 3 cm in length and T1 lesions rarely have lymph node metastases. Conversely T3 lesions and those longer than 5 cm almost invariably have nodal metastases (Yamada, 1979; Giuli, 1984). In our series, lymph node metastases were present in 85% of adenocarcinomas at the time of surgery, compared with 54% for squamous lesions (Watson, 1990). The effect of nodal metastases on long-term survival is pronounced, 5-year survival varying from 7 to

15% in node-positive cases compared to 12–54% for node-negative cases (Akiyama *et al.*, 1981; Huang, 1981; Lam *et al.*, 1981). In our own series, 5-year survival for node-positive cases was 6% compared to 50% for node-negative cases. Distant lymph node involvement is invariably associated with incurable disease, both Postlethwait (1979) and Lam *et al.* (1981) reporting no 5-year survivors where supraclavicular or scalene nodes were involved.

Blood-borne metastases can occur to most organs, particularly liver, lungs, brain and bone and clearly signify incurable disease.

Clinical features

The classical presenting symptom of oesophageal carcinoma is dysphagia. Despite the rather dramatic nature of this symptom, patients rarely present early, usually modifying the consistency of their diet in order to preserve nutrition. In the historical review of Earlam and Cunha-Melo (1980a) the mean duration of symptoms prior to diagnosis was 7.5 months. However, currently there is some improvement, the mean duration of symptoms in our series being 4.1 months.

Despite this, however, 72% of resected growths had not only penetrated the entire oesophagus but had also metastasized to lymph nodes, whilst only 10% had not breached the muscularis propria (Watson, 1982). Clearly, education is needed both amongst the general public and general practitioners that dysphagia is a potentially sinister symptom which merits urgent investigation. Dysphagia usually begins as an awareness of the passage of particularly solid foods such as bread and meat, progressively followed by an inability to swallow these foods, other solids and even semi-solids. However, some patients do not present until they are only able to tolerate liquids. The site of the dysphagia as experienced by the patient is not a reliable guide to the level of the lesion, Edwards and Lobello (1982) having shown a lack of correlation in up to 30% of people between the respective levels.

An inevitable consequence of reduced dietary intake consequent on progressive oesophageal narrowing is impaired nutrition and weight loss, most patients having lost some 10% of their body weight at the time of presentation. This may be exacerbated by the metabolic effects of the tumour itself and hypoalbuminaemia is common at presentation, which is an unwelcome prelude to the prospect of major surgical intervention.

Pain is an uncommon form of presentation of oesophageal cancer. It may reflect very advanced disease with local infiltration into the spine or intercostal nerves. However, the presence of pain does not invariably mean such extensive disease. In some patients with dysphagia, the act of swallowing and particularly the impaction of a food bolus may produce excruciating oesophageal pain or odynophagia, felt retrosternally and radiating into the back and occasionally the jaws and arms.

Rarely, oesophageal tumours may present with bleeding. This may be in the form of occult bleeding producing anaemia, but exceptionally, oesophageal carcinoma may present with an acute gastrointestinal bleed due to ulceration of a neoplasm, in the absence of any dysphagia. In some instances, oesophageal tumours may be detected relatively early in these circumstances. Massive bleeding due to erosion into a major vessel is an unusual circumstance, except as a terminal event.

Very occasionally, oesophageal tumours may present by virtue of extension into contiguous organs or by the development of metastases. Hoarseness or respiratory problems may indicate recurrent laryngeal nerve paresis or tracheo-oesophageal fistula. More rarely, metastatic nodes in the neck or hepatic metastases may have their primary origin in an oesophageal tumour, but the vast majority have local manifestations before this stage is reached.

Physical signs are usually few. An epigastric mass may be present where tumours arise from the cardia and are extensive, but otherwise physical signs relate to the presence of nodal or hepatic metastases.

Diagnosis

The cornerstones of diagnosis are barium studies and endoscopy. The two are complimentary, since barium studies may give more accurate information concerning length of the tumour and gastric involvement, if present. In early cases, barium studies may be inconclusive unless a careful double-contrast technique is used which may identify mucosal lesions. However, in the more usual advanced lesions, the length, tortuosity and shouldering help differentiate from benign stricture or achalasia, although in some cases the diagnosis is not resolved until endoscopy.

Endoscopy, which nowadays principally means fibreoptic endoscopy, allows the diagnosis of early lesions or the confirmation or exclusion of neoplastic lesions highlighted on barium swallow. Typically, the haemorrhagic, exophytic nature of oesophageal cancer aids differentiation from benign stricture, but occasionally, the differentiation may be difficult. Even in macroscopically obvious cases, it is vital to have a tissue diagnosis and both punch biopsies and brush cytology are recommended. If the stricture is tight, punch biopsy allows only a limited portion of the lesion to be sampled and this may only be an inflammatory response at the edge of the tumour, leading to a false negative result. It has been shown that the combination of brush cytology with punch biopsy leads to an accurate diagnosis in over 90% of cases (Tytgat, 1984). Whilst a diagnostic endoscopy is being performed, the opportunity may be taken to dilate the stricture, which not only allows examination of the length and distal limits of the tumour, but also may facilitate improvement of nutritional status during consideration for surgery. In particularly stenotic lesions, it is sometimes advisable to pass a fine-bore feeding tube at endoscopy if enteral nutrition is considered preferable to intravenous feeding.

Staging

Staging of oesophageal tumours is rather more difficult than many tumours elsewhere because of their relative inaccessibility. Whilst staging may be academic in patients presenting with widely disseminated disease and those whose general health precludes consideration of aggressive therapy, it is necessary in the majority of patients in order to plan a therapeutic strategy. One of the worst tragedies which may befall patients suffering from this distressing disease is inappropriate surgical intervention. In the historical review of Earlam and Cunha-Melo (1980a), 33% of patients in whom resection was intended were operated on and their lesions found to be irresectable.

Basic information relevant to staging can be obtained from physical examination, barium studies and endoscopy, from the standpoint of tumour length and obvious disseminated spread. Further information can be obtained relatively simply by chest X-ray, looking for the presence of pulmonary metastases, mediastinal nodes, transmediastinal spread and respiratory tract involvement. Real-time ultrasound gives accurate information regarding hepatic metastases and frequently the presence of coeliac axis nodes. However, whole body imaging is being used increasingly to obtain more detailed staging data.

Computerized tomography has been used extensively with a view to not only increasing the accuracy of detection of pulmonary and hepatic metastases, but to obtain data on tumour extent, adherence to contiguous structures and presence of lymph node metastases. The tumour itself is seen as a thickening of the oesophageal wall producing an eccentric lumen or circumferential thickening, and extension beyond the oesophageal wall results in obliteration of the peri-oesophageal fat planes. Whilst specificity for these parameters is high, its overall sensitivity for detection of invasion of contiguous structures is low at approximately 40% and even lower at 25% for the presence of lymph node metastases (Laas et al., 1986). Overall accuracy in this latter series was around 80% for invasion of contiguous structures and 60% for the presence of enlarged lymph nodes. Furthermore, the presence of enlarged lymph nodes does not necessarily mean involved lymph nodes, and inflammatory adherence to contiguous structures cannot be distinguished from neoplastic infiltration. Clearly, however, broncho-scopy is indicated where any infiltration into the bronchial tree is suspected. CT scanning is more accurate in the hopelessly inoperable situation of extensive transmediastinal spread, where accuracy is over 90% (Moss et al., 1981).

Other staging modalities have been used in an attempt to increase accuracy. Magnetic resonance imaging has been used by some workers, but in comparison with CT scanning, it appears even less reliable (Lehr et al., 1986). On the other hand, endoscopic ultrasound has been more recently applied to preoperative staging and in a preliminary study, had an overall accuracy of 85% (Tio and Tytgat, 1986). This technique appears promising and needs further evaluation, but is presently available in only a few specialized centres. More invasive techniques such as azygos venography, pneumomediastinography and mediastinoscopy have been used to try to increase accuracy, and whilst specificity is relatively high, low sensitivity of less than 50% in some series does not appear to justify the invasiveness of these procedures (DuBrow, 1985).

Our own practice is to stage patients by conventional radiography, endoscopy, liver ultrasound and CT scanning, using bronchoscopy only where indicated. The first 72 of our resected patients were staged without CT scanning, and in this group the resectability rate of those undergoing surgery was 97% (Watson, 1987).

Treatment

The objectives of treatment in oesophageal carcinoma are firstly to restore euphagia and hopefully avoid an unpleasant death due to starvation, secondly to prolong useful survival, the ultimate ambition being cure of the disease and thirdly the therapeutic modality employed to achieve these objectives should have an acceptably low mortality. Whilst many forms of therapy have had their vogue, only surgical resection has stood the test of time in producing the best quality and durability of palliation, with the bonus of cure in a proportion of patients. Whilst historical, retrospective reviews have painted a dismal picture of the results of resection (Earlam and Cunha-Melo, 1980a) with operative mortality of 33% and 5-year survival of 4%, more recent reports from specialist centres treating large numbers of patients are considerably more optimistic, with operative mortality around 10% or less and 5-year survival between 10% and 20% (Ellis and Gibb, 1979; McKeown, 1979; Dark, Moussali and Vaughan, 1981; Skinner et al., 1986; Watson, 1990). The considerably more favourable reports from Japan and China, where earlier diagnosis is achieved, reinforce the strength of surgical resection, particularly in more favourable cases. In the Western world, however, where tumours are frequently advanced at the time of presentation, and patients often old, infirm and malnourished, careful selection must be employed to identify those patients in whom resection is appropriate, in order to maximize the return on therapeutic investment. In general terms, surgery remains the preferred option, provided that the tumour is not too far advanced to preclude this and the patient is considered fit enough to withstand a major surgical procedure which frequently includes thoracotomy.

The staging modalities discussed previously give useful guidance as to the likely operability of oesophageal tumours. Obvious contraindications to resection include distant metastases, gross involvement of contiguous organs, particularly the respiratory tract and thoracic aorta, and extensive transmediastinal spread as determined by CT scanning. The demonstration of enlarged para-oesophageal or left gastric nodes is not a contraindication to surgery, as enlarged lymph nodes may not necessarily be metastatic, and if so, there is not a linear correlation between the presence of lymph node metastases and survival. Postlethwait (1979) has shown evidence of poor survival in node-negative cases and prolonged survival in some node-positive cases, which accords with our own experience, particularly with squamous lesions. In patients with tumours considered operable, Wong (1981) has clearly demonstrated the significant influence of age and intercurrent disease on mortality associated with resection. Whilst biological age is clearly more relevant than chronological age, it is our policy to offer resection to few patients over the age of 75 because of the escalation in mortality above this age, and to exclude patients with significant degrees of cardiac disease or pulmonary insufficiency. Wong (1981) has shown also that severe degrees of diabetes and impairment of renal and hepatocellular function also increase mortality following resection.

On the basis of these assessments of tumour staging and patient fitness, the majority of clinical situations will resolve themselves into two principal categories, namely, where a radical or a palliative approach is appropriate. In Lancaster, where all referred cases from a catchment population of 200 000, with one of the highest incidences of oesophageal cancer in the UK are treated in one unit, we find, using the criteria outlined above that approximately 40% of patients are considered suitable for radical treatment. Whilst the decision to operate is somewhat subjective, there is usually a high price to be paid for over-zealousness in this context. Although 58% of the patients in the review of Earlam and Cunha-Melo (1980a) underwent surgery, only 39% had a resection. In a large series from the Mayo Clinic, 67% were subjected to surgery but only 45% underwent resection (Gunnlaugsson et al., 1970). Ong et al. (1978) showed that as resection rate increased from 45% to 58%, mortality increased from 18% to 44%.

Radical treatment usually means resection, though in squamous lesions with an enthusiastic radiotherapist, radical radiotherapy may be considered to be an alternative. Combination treatment using radiotherapy and/or chemotherapy as an adjunct to surgery has been employed in an attempt to improve survival. Where radical treatment is considered inappropriate, palliation aimed at relieving dysphagia is the objective, and may be achieved by intubation, laser therapy, surgical bypass or merely dilatation. Each of these treatment modalities will be discussed in turn.

Resection

As the only treatment modality which has been repeatedly associated with prolonged survival in the literature, albeit in a relatively small proportion of cases treated, resection must be strongly considered as the treatment of choice in a relatively fit patient with a relatively favourable tumour, at least until the results of controlled clinical trials are known. The only exception to this is in cervical or hypopharyngeal growths which, fortunately on account of the magnitude of surgery involved, are extremely radiosensitive. There are many reasons for the improvement in results following resection for oesophageal carcinoma which have been reported in recent years. Paramount amongst these has been the tendency towards management of these patients in specialized units dealing with a sufficient number of cases to enable a multidisciplinary approach between surgeons, physicians and anaesthetists, backed up by skilled nursing teams, where management policies can be defined based on a continuing review of results. Earlam (1984) reporting experience in the North-east Thames region in 1981 has shown how bad results can be when resection is undertaken by the occasional oesophagectomist. In contrast, Matthews, Powell and McConkey (1986), have shown how improvement in results parallels experience in the management of this condition. Other reasons for improved success have been careful selection as outlined above, and attention to preoperative preparation and postoperative management as well as to operative technique.

Preoperative preparation

As many patients with oesophageal carcinoma are malnourished, and some may be anaemic or dehydrated, it is often valuable to spend a few days correcting these deficiencies. The majority of patients are able to swallow liquids, and are able to tolerate a high calorie liquid diet of appropriate composition. In those with absolute dysphagia, the placement of a fine-bore feeding tube following gastroscopy and dilatation may facilitate this process, but where problems exist, parenteral nutrition may be used. Whilst nutritional support would appear rational from a general and immunological standpoint (Daly, Dudrick and Copeland, 1980), the measurable benefit to such patients undergoing resection remains controversial (Heatley, Williams and Lewis, 1979). In an attempt to reduce the incidence of respiratory, infective and thromboembolic complications, it is advisable to commence vigorous physiotherapy preoperatively, and to administer prophylactic antibiotics and low-dose subcutaneous heparin, unless obviously contraindicated.

Operative technique
A variety of operative approaches to the resection of oesophageal tumours have been described since the first successful resection and oesophagogastric anastomosis by Adams and Phemister in 1938. Common to these approaches has

been the desire to achieve as much clearance as possible and to minimize the risk of anastomotic dehiscence and consequent mediastinitis. Greater longitudinal clearance than normally practised in cancer surgery is necessary because of the well-documented propensity for both squamous and adenocarcinomas to extend submucosally for a considerable distance from the apparent macroscopic tumour limits (Morson, 1961; Miller, 1962), although there is recent evidence to suggest that this is primarily associated with distal oesophageal tumours (Wong, 1987). Intrathoracic oesophageal anastomoses are less likely to heal than other portions of the alimentary tract because of the relatively poor blood supply of the oesophagus, the absence of a serous coat and high intraluminal pressures associated with swallowing. As a result, anastomotic dehiscence is the greatest single cause of mortality in many series (Chassin, 1978) and this risk appears to be increased by the presence of residual microscopic tumour at the anastomosed ends (Inberg et al., 1971).

From the standpoint of addressing these two important principles governing resectional surgery of oesophageal cancer, the two-stage or three-stage procedures have been the most popular. The classical two-stage procedure was described both by Lewis (1946) and Tanner (1947). This approach remains the most popular, and involves mobilization of the stomach on a right gastric or gastro-epiploic arterial pedicle by a preliminary transabdominal approach, followed by a right thoracotomy through the fifth or sixth intercostal space, through which the proximal stomach and an appropriate length of intrathoracic oesophagus are excised and an oesophagogastric anastomosis constructed. A third cervical phase to this procedure was described by Ong and Kwong (1969) and McKeown (1972). The rationale of this additional phase was to construct the oesophagogastric anastomosis in the neck, where the oesophageal blood supply is better and anastomotic leakage is likely to be less serious, and it had the added advantage of achieving wider longitudinal clearance. However, the addition of a cervical phase prolongs what is already a major surgical procedure in a debilitated patient, and the benefits may not be as great as were initially envisaged. Firstly, clinically relevant anastomotic leakage is no longer a major problem with intrathoracic anastomoses, with recently reported rates of 1.5 and 2.3% (Watson, 1984b; Wong, 1987). Furthermore, a recent multicentre study has shown that leaks from cervical anastomoses frequently occur into the mediastinum (Giuli, 1984). As regards clearance, Wong's data have shown that for other than superior mediastinal tumours, proximal clearance of between 5 cm and 10 cm with an anastomosis at the apex of the mediastinum results in a very low rate of anastomotic recurrence. Our experience is in accord with that of Wong and it is our practice to perform a cervical phase only with proximally-placed tumours where resection of a portion of the cervical oesophagus is necessary to achieve the requisite clearance.

A further operative approach which has attracted considerable interest in recent years is that of transhiatal oesophagectomy without thoracotomy. Although first described by Turner in 1936, it is only since reports from Kirk (1974) and Orringer and Sloane (1978) that this technique has achieved greater popularity. The rationale behind this approach is to combine the presumed advantages of a cervical anastomosis and avoid the morbidity of thoracotomy. The stomach is initially mobilized by a transabdominal approach as with the Lewis–Tanner procedure, but, in addition, blunt dissection through the oesophageal hiatus enables much of the thoracic oesophagus to be mobilized, unless the tumour is particularly adherent. Mobilization of the upper oesophagus is carried out similarly through a cervical incision and the mobilized stomach brought through the posterior mediastinum to the neck for the oesophagogastric anastomosis. Orringer (1984a) has by far the greatest experience of the technique, and in his hands morbidity and mortality are low.

Comparative studies have been performed looking at morbidity and mortality comparing blunt transhiatal oesophagectomy with conventional 2- or 3-stage resection including thoracotomy. Giuli and Sancho-Garnier (1986) reporting the large multicentre OESO study reported perioperative mortality associated with transhiatal oesophagectomy of 19% compared with 13% using the Lewis–Tanner technique. The incidence of pulmonary complications was similar to that following thoracotomy, as was the requirement for temporary postoperative ventilatory support. Similar results were reported by Shahian et al. (1986) apparently emphasizing the fact that a well-conducted thoracotomy is not the hazardous procedure some would claim, and indeed both series showed that transhiatal oesophagectomy is associated with other complications not normally associated with a transthoracic approach such as tracheobronchial injuries, damage to the recurrent laryngeal nerve and to the thoracic duct. Occasionally, with locally advanced tumours in the middle third of the oesophagus, significant haemorrhage can ensue.

Certainly transhiatal oesophagectomy does not appear by any means to have replaced the conventional transthoracic approach to oesophageal tumours, because of its unproven advantages in the generality of its use and anxiety about its efficacy as a potentially curative procedure. However, Orringer has claimed equivalent long-term survival to that obtained by more radical operations, and the comparative study of Shahian et al. (1986) supports this view. It may well be that for early, curative lesions, either technique is appropriate and for advanced lesions, the poor prognosis is determined by the biology of the tumour rather than the extent of resection. In the multicentre study of Giuli and Sancho-Garnier (1986) 12% of the 790 resections were performed by the transhiatal technique, 12% by the 3-stage technique and 67% by the standard Lewis–Tanner technique. It would appear that the place of transhiatal oesophagectomy is in the treatment of proximal or distally placed tumours in circumstances where it is desirable to avoid thoracotomy, but the technique would appear to be contraindicated in locally advanced intrathoracic lesions.

Whilst the stomach is by far the commonest replacement organ used following oesophageal resection, other workers, notably Skinner (1983) and De Meester and Lafontaine (1985) have advocated the use of a colon interposition. This can be brought retrosternally, subcutaneously or via the posterior mediastinum, but has the disadvantage of a more prolonged procedure with multiple anastomoses, which depend on the accurate preservation of the colonic blood supply for their healing. The preference for colon over the stomach as the replacement organ usually coexists with the belief that ultraradical surgery is beneficial in appropriate tumours, and that this can be best achieved by employing a colonic conduit. Whilst many would espouse the recommendations of Akiyama et al. (1981) that lymph nodes at a considerable distance from the tumour may be involved and should preferably be removed, Skinner (1983) has advocated a radical en bloc mediastinectomy in patients with relatively localized tumours, which involves not only resection of 10 cm proximal and distal clearance and associated lymph nodes, but a block of tissue that includes both pleural surfaces, the posterior part of the pericardium, together with the azygos vein, thoracic duct and all adjacent lymphatic and fibro-areolar tissue. Orringer (1984b) takes an opposing view that survival is determined by the biological behaviour of the tumour, and claims similar results by transhiatal oesophagectomy, which removes the tumour, the oesophagus and a limited portion of its lymphatic drainage.

Other technical points which have aroused controversy are whether the oesophageal anastomosis should be sutured or stapled and whether pyloroplasty should be used when the stomach is employed as the replacement organ. As yet, no randomized controlled study has been performed of sutured against stapled anastomoses, but some data are available from comparative studies. Maillard, Goyer and Lortat-Jacob (1971) observed a reduction in anastomotic leakage from 41% with sutured anastomoses to 20.5% with stapled anastomoses. However, both Hopkins, Alexander and Postlethwait (1984) and Wong (1987), both of which series had leakage rates of approximately 3% with sutured anastomoses, found no significant difference when staples were used. However, both groups found a high incidence of anastomotic stricture following stapled anastomoses of 13.3 and 25% respectively. It is our practice to perform a hand-sewn anastomosis with a single layer of loosely tied horizontal mattress sutures with silk, our results showing a clinically relevant anastomotic leakage rate of 1.6% and a stricture rate of 8.8%.

With regard to the question of pyloroplasty, many workers feel it to be appropriate because a vagotomy is an inevitable part of oesophageal resection. However, there are certain differences between its use during oesophagogastrec-tomy and in ulcer surgery, as firstly the duodenum is unlikely to be diseased or deformed and secondly, as the pylorus comes to lie vertically at the oesophageal hiatus, gravity aids gastric emptying. Both Shapiro, Hamilton and Morgenstern (1972) and McKeown (1979) found pyloroplasty to be unnecessary. The only randomized controlled trial has been performed by Wong (1987). Whilst there was no statistically significant difference in complications associated with gastric outlet obstruction in patients with and without pyloroplasty, he concluded that there was an increased incidence of symptoms compatible with delayed gastric emptying in the latter group, and advocates pyloroplasty. It is our practice only to perform pyloroplasty if there is obvious pyloroduodenal disease, and otherwise merely to perform a blunt myotomy by finger invagination through the pylorus. Our experience is similar to that of Hennessy (1986), in that only approximately 5% of patients develop problems due to impaired gastric emptying and we prefer to deal with this small proportion of patients, which can often be managed by endoscopic balloon dilatation, than to subject the remaining 95% to duodeno-gastric alkaline reflux.

Postoperative management
It is advisable to manage patients in the early stages after oesophageal resection in the Intensive Care Unit where careful monitoring of cardiorespiratory parameters can be undertaken and ventilatory support provided, when required. Some centres advocate routine elective ventilation for the first 24 hours, and this has been our experience in the past. We have recently found the use of thoracic epidural analgesia to be a great advance in the prevention of postoperative pulmonary complications, by enabling patients to cooperate with physiotherapy with the minimum of systemic analgesia, and since employing this technique we rarely ventilate electively (Watson, 1988). Intensive physiotherapy is administered, and in patients with particularly excessive secretions, usually complicating longstanding pulmonary disease, tracheobronchial suction via a minitracheotomy device has

proved useful (Matthews and Hopkinson, 1984). Serial blood gas estimation and chest radiography are useful in monitoring respiratory status.

We routinely delay oral alimentation until a contrast swallow on the fifth postoperative day has demonstrated anastomotic integrity. Until this time, nutritional support is administered, the options being enterally, either via a jejunostomy tube or a fine-bore nasojejunal tube placed at the time of surgery, or parenteral nutrition.

Results following resection

The parameters which have attracted most attention in the literature are the perioperative mortality associated with resection and 5-year survival rate. Operative mortality varies greatly as shown in the historical review of Earlam and Cunha-Melo (1980a) in which operative mortality ranges from 1 to 83%. There are clearly many reasons for this gross variation in addition to operative technique and quality of management, important amongst these being the degree of selection employed, the aggressiveness of the surgeon and the experience of the centre in managing such patients. These factors have been alluded to previously, and in general terms, the major British and American units with a specialist interest in oesophageal disease are currently publishing operative mortality of around 10% or less. Both Ong *et al.* (1978) and Belsey and Hiebert (1974) have demonstrated that operative mortality can exceed 40% when the majority of tumours are resected, emphasizing the importance of careful selection if an acceptable mortality is to be achieved. The series from China (Huang, 1981) and Japan (Akiyama *et al.*, 1981), both with operative mortality around 2%, highlight the advantage of early detection of tumours before they are complicated by metabolic and nutritional problems.

Long-term survival also varies considerably in published reports, and appears to vary more with the characteristics and staging of the tumour than the extent of surgery undertaken. Overall, the recent major British and American series report 5-year survival rates between 10% and 20%, depending to some extent on whether long-term survivors are reported as a proportion of all patients treated, or those surviving the operation. However, such figures are considerably less optimistic than Eastern series, in which a 5-year survival rate up to 96% is reported in superficial lesions detected by screening (Huang, 1981).

The major determinants of prognosis appear to be depth of invasion, involvement of contiguous organs and the presence of nodal metastases, rather than tumour length, degree of differentiation and histological cell type *per se*. In general, adenocarcinomas fare less well than squamous lesions, but this probably reflects the fact that they are associated with greater degrees of local invasion and nodal metastases at the time of presentation (Watson, 1990). In the multi-centre study of Giuli (1984), the incidence of nodal metastases rose progressively from 14% in T1 lesions to 72% in T3 lesions. When lymph node metastases are present, the 5-year survival ranges from 7% to 15% as compared to 12% to 54% for node-negative cases (Akiyama *et al.*, 1981; Huang, 1981; Lam *et al.*, 1981).

Whilst no controlled studies have been done on the benefit of a radical surgical approach in the presence of nodal involvement, Skinner *et al.* (1986) have shown improved survival when relatively localized tumours with localized node involvement were submitted to radical *en bloc* oesophagectomy. However, it is unclear whether these relatively favourable results relate to the radical nature of the operation or the selection of patients likely to have a better prognosis by virtue of their more favourable tumours. Orringer (1984b) has claimed similar 2-year survival to that reported in more radical operations using blunt oesophagectomy without nodal dissection. In this rather controversial situation, where 5-year survivors with nodal involvement occur, but in the absence of easy determinants of which patients will follow this course, it is our practice to dissect involved and contiguous lymph node groups, including para-oesophageal and left gastric nodes, in all cases.

In Lancaster, 123 resections for oesophageal carcinoma have been performed between 1975 and 1988, with a standardized procedure-related mortality (mortality in hospital or within 30 days, whichever is the longer) of 8.3% overall. During the period 1985–88 when thoracic epidural analgesia was used routinely, 42 patients underwent resection with a standarized procedure-related mortality of 4.8%. Five-year survival (expressed as a percentage of all patients undergoing surgery) is 14.3%. Stratification of the survival data according to cell type and tumour staging showed that this 14.3% comprised 23.8% for squamous lesions and 7.1% for adenocarcinoma. The 1-year survival rates were 62% and 53.5% respectively. Nodal involvement occurred in 58.8% of squamous and 80.7% of adenocarcinoma, in which circumstances 5-year survival rate was 10% and 0% respectively. In node-negative cases, 5-year survival rate was 57.1% for squamous lesions and 40% for adenocarcinomas. Only 10.2% of lesions were confined to the oesophageal wall, all these being squamous lesions, and the 5-year survival rate in this group was 75%. Clearly, therefore, the small proportion of lesions which do present early are associated with prolonged survival equivalent to that of Eastern series and equivalent to other, e.g. colorectal tumours, or equivalent staging.

Radiotherapy

Whilst radiotherapy is the modality of choice in cervical and hypopharyngeal lesions, its role in other squamous lesions of the oesophagus remains controversial. Although there are many individual reports of tumours shrinking following radiotherapy, most cumulative series report unfavourable results from the standpoint of long-term survival. In a cumulative review of 49 series by Earlam and Cunha-Melo (1980b), the mean 5-year survival rate was only 6%. Only the series of Pearson (1977) has reported encouraging results using megavoltage radiotherapy with a tumour dose of 5000 cg, with 5-year survival of 16% in those patients able to complete the course of radiotherapy. Such results have never been repeated, and Cederquist et al. (1978), using a similar tumour dose, reported 5-year survival figures of 4%.

The principal theoretical advantage of radiotherapy is the avoidance of operative mortality. However, many would consider that a radical course of radiotherapy in a debilitated patient is not without its risks. In Cederquist's series, there was a 9% mortality during radical radiotherapy, and most series report patients unable to complete their course of radiotherapy because of side-effects. Continuing dysphagia is a major problem, necessitating continued treatment in 50% of patients in Pearson's series, intermittent dilatation or intubation being the treatment of choice.

The limitations of radiotherapy as a primary curative procedure would appear to relate to the inability to irradiate more than 5 cm beyond the tumour margin, which would result in an unacceptable reduction in tumour dose. For this reason, the concept of 'palliative radiotherapy' is difficult to define, as the dose delivered to long and extensive tumours is relatively low, and there is no evidence that patients receiving palliative radiotherapy fare better than those receiving no radiation at all (Miller, 1962). However, the recent development of intracavitary irradiation (Rowland and Pagliero, 1985) may overcome these objections.

There is, therefore, little evidence to support the use of radiotherapy as a primary treatment modality in patients who are otherwise candidates for resection. The principle value of radiotherapy would appear to be as part of a combination treatment programme.

Combination therapy

The disappointing overall results of surgery and radiotherapy in terms of prolonged survival have led to several studies of adjuvant radiotherapy and/or chemotherapy in combination with surgical resection. The theoretical advantages include the down-staging of tumours to render an increasing proportion of tumours resectable, the sterilization of micrometastases and the ablation of residual tumour following resection for locally advanced lesions. Most of the studies of radiotherapy combined with surgery recommend the use of radiotherapy 2–4 weeks prior to surgery (Akakura et al., 1970; Parker and Gregorie, 1976; Fraser et al., 1978). Whilst tumour shrinkage and increased resectability are reported, this appears to be at the expense of increased mortality and morbidity associated with resection, with no convincing evidence that long-term survival is superior to other series where preoperative irradiation is not used (Gignoux et al., 1987).

Several chemotherapeutic agents have been applied to the management of oesophageal carcinoma, principally bleomycin (Ravry et al., 1973) and more recently cisplatinum in combination with bleomycin alone or in combination regimes including methotrexate, Adriamycin, 5-fluorouracil or vincristine (Gissel-brecht et al., 1983; Kelsen, 1984). The results have been conflicting with objective response varying from 0 to 80%, but most responses, when occurring, were of short duration lasting only a few months. The lack of convincing evidence of the efficacy of radiotherapy or chemotherapy as an adjunct to surgery has led to studies using both modalities prior to resection. Werner (1979) reported that in 27% of patients receiving preoperative radiotherapy and methotrexate, no residual tumour was found in resected specimens. However, the operative mortality following surgery was 14.5%, and long-term survival was no better than other series using surgery alone. More recently, Wolfe et al. (1987) have reported the use of combination chemotherapy and high-dose radiotherapy with surgery 4 months later. Whilst many patients had no residual tumour at the time of surgery and operative mortality was low, over half the patients initially deemed operable were no longer operable by virtue of tumour staging or general condition after the 4 months' adjunctive treatment, and no overall survival advantage could be claimed. Similarly encouraging short-term results were reported by Hilgenberg et al. (1988) using preoperative chemotherapy, resection and selective postoperative radiotherapy but in the absence of control data, no survival advantage could be demonstrated.

In the current state of knowledge, therefore, any benefit claimed in terms of downstaging tumours must be weighed against the delay in submitting patients to resection and increased morbidity and mortality associated with surgery and indeed the adjunctive treatment itself. There is currently no convincing evidence of improved long-term survival using these regimens, but the situation will be clarified by the emergence of results from randomized prospective controlled trials.

Intubation

In a significant proportion of patients, varying with the selection criteria employed, the aggressiveness of the surgeon and the operative mortality he is prepared to accept, a palliative procedure to restore the ability to swallow is all that is appropriate. A variety of intubation techniques have been used, ranging from the placement of a Souttar's tube via the rigid endoscope, the placement of a Celestin or Mousseau–Barbin tube at laparotomy and, more recently, the less invasive technique of fibreoptic endoscopic intubation. The former method is rarely used nowadays, on account of the small calibre of the tubes employed via the rigid endoscope and their capacity to erode through the tumour into the mediastinum. Surgical intubation, with the passage of a Celestin or Mousseau–Barbin tube at laparotomy, was a popular method of palliation until the advent of fibreoptic endoscopic intubation. Whilst surgical intubation is a relatively minor surgical procedure, it is associated with a perioperative mortality of around 40% (Lishman, Dellipiani and Devlin, 1980; Watson, 1982). This probably reflects the immunodepressive effect of surgery on an already debilitated patient, but it is likely also that perforation, due to splitting of the tumour, occurs more frequently than is realized. Probably the only place nowadays for surgical intubation is in the small number of patients where fibreoptic endoscopic intubation is not feasible because of extreme tortuosity of the neoplastic stricture, or where tumour is discovered to be unresectable at operation (Watson, 1985).

Fibreoptic endoscopic intubation has been the most popular palliative technique used during the last decade. The ability to pass either an Atkinson or Celestin tube placed over a guide wire after dilatation of the neoplastic stricture at fibreoptic endoscopy means that the procedure can be performed under sedation rather than general anaesthesia (Atkinson and Ferguson, 1977; Celestin, 1978). Consequently, the procedure is less invasive and better tolerated than surgical intubation, which is an important consideration in the management of debilitated patients whose life expectancy is short. Procedure-related mortality ranges from 6% to 11% (Ogilvie *et al.*, 1982; Watson, 1984b), and in our series mean hospital stay was 7.6 days compared to 13.0 days for surgical intubation in a similar group of patients. The principal complications of fibreoptic endoscopic intubation are perforation, tube migration and blockage of the tube. Early perforation occurred in 11% of patients in the Nottingham series, and is frequently, but not invariably, fatal. Late perforation occasionally occurs in patients who have subsequently received radiotherapy. Tube migration is less common since the design of tubes was modified to include a distal flange. Tube blockage may be caused by bolus obstruction, or by tumour overgrowth above or below the tube. *In vivo* destruction of tubes rarely occurs, as few patients survive longer than 1 year, with a mean survival of approximately 9 months following intubation.

The quality of palliation following intubation varies with the technique used. In our study of the quality of swallowing after various procedures, we found that 33% of people following fibreoptic intubation had normal swallowing compared to 15% after surgical intubation (Watson, 1982). Approximately 60% in each group had dysphagia for solids but were able to take a semi-solid or puréed diet. This is in sharp contrast to those patients who had undergone resection, of whom over 90% were restored to normal swallowing. Fibreoptic endoscopic intubation is, therefore, the most attractive of the intubation techniques in those patients for whom resection is inappropriate. It provides useful palliation also in those patients with tracheo-oesophageal fistula, with persistent dysphagia after radiotherapy and where local recurrence is a late complication of surgical resection.

Laser therapy

The increasing use of the neodymium -YAG laser has led to its application to the palliation of inoperable obstructing oesophageal tumours (Fleischer, 1981). Several reports have alluded to the quality of palliation achieved by this form of therapy (Krasner and Beard, 1984; Swain and Bown, 1984), although multiple treatments are necessary and there is a risk of perforation. Carter and Smith (1986) compared quality of palliation between 10 patients undergoing laser therapy and 10 undergoing intubation and concluded that the quality of palliation was better with laser therapy. The patients were not randomized and it was acknowledged that several courses of laser therapy were necessary in their patients in whom the mean survival was only 6 months.

On the available evidence, it would appear that the possibility of superior palliation needs to be weighed against the necessity of patients with a limited life span returning regularly to hospital, and the capital cost of the equipment. Until the results of randomized prospective controlled trials are known, laser therapy would appear to have most attraction to those patients in whom intubation is not feasible or has failed due to tumour overgrowth and in the case of proximally-sited tumours, where pharyngeal irritation may preclude patient tolerance of an endoscopic tube.

Surgical bypass procedures

Surgical bypass has declined in popularity in Britain as a palliative modality since the development of intubation and laser techniques. However, it is more commonly employed in the USA and the Far East, where these latter modalities are less commonly used. Surgical techniques include oesophagogastrostomy, where the stomach is brought into the chest and anastomosed to the oesophagus proximal to the tumour, the use of a reversed gastric tube and the insertion of a jejunal or colonic conduit between the stomach and the oesophagus proximal to the tumour. The advantage of surgical bypass is that it results in a degree of palliation comparable to that following resection. However the principal disadvantage is the morbidity and mortality resulting from major surgery in a debilitated group of patients with a limited life expectancy. Operative mortality is reported between 21 and 41%, with mean survival of around 5 months (Postlethwait, 1979; Wong et al., 1981).

With availability of endoscopic intubation and laser therapy, probably the only indication for palliative surgical bypass is if the tumour is only found to be inoperable at thoracotomy during a 2-stage procedure. With modern methods of staging, this should be a relatively infrequent occurrence.

Dilatation

Intermittent endoscopic dilatation has been recommended as a palliative procedure for inoperable oesophageal tumours (Graham, Dodds and Zubler, 1983). As one might expect, recurrent dysphagia usually occurs so rapidly that it has little application beyond that of a temporary measure or prior to endoscopic intubation.

Conclusion

Carcinoma of the oesophagus remains a formidable disease because of its late presentation in the West, by which time over 70% have metastasized to lymph nodes. Improved staging techniques have facilitated the selection process of the 40% of patients in whom an active surgical approach is justified, and minimized the frequency of inappropriate surgical intervention in the remainder. Advances in preoperative preparation, operative technique and postoperative management have enabled resection to be performed in specialized centres with an operative mortality of around 10% or less, with a prospect of cure in between 10 and 20% of patients and with restoration of normal swallowing in the majority. There is as yet, inconclusive evidence that these results can be improved by performing ultraradical resectional procedures or by using radiotherapy or chemotherapy as adjuncts to surgery.

In the current situation, a palliative procedure to improve swallowing and prevent an unpleasant demise from starvation will be the objective in approximately 60% of patients. Of the available palliative modalities, fibreoptic endoscopic intubation is the least invasive procedure which offers reasonable palliation to the majority of patients with the minimum of hospitalization. The role of laser therapy in palliation is being clarified and will be helped by the results of prospective controlled trials.

The favourable results obtained from the Far East in the management of early lesions, together with similar results obtained in the West in the small proportion of patients who present early, emphasize the need to direct our attention towards earlier diagnosis, to which careful surveillance of high-risk groups, notably those with dysplasia in Barrett's oesophagus, may contribute.

References

Adams, W. E. and Phemister, D. B. (1938) Carcinoma of the lower thoracic esophagus: Report of a successful resection and esophagogastrostomy. *Journal of Thoracic Surgery*, **7**, 621–632

Akakura, I., Nakamura, Y., Kakegawa, T. *et al.* (1970) Surgery of carcinoma of the esophagus with pre-operative radiation. *Chest*, **57**, 47–57

Akiyama, H., Tsurumaru, M., Kawamura, T. and Ono, Y. (1981) Principles of surgical treatment for carcinoma of the esophagus. Analysis of lymph node involvement. *Annals of Surgery*, **194**, 438–446

Atkinson, A. (1989) Barrett's oesophagus – to screen or not to screen? *Gut*, **30**, 2–5

Atkinson, M. and Ferguson, R. (1977) Fibreoptic endoscopic palliative intubation of inoperable oesophagogastric neoplasms. *British Medical Journal*, **1**, 266–267

Barrett, N. R. (1950) Chronic peptic ulcer of the oesophagus and oesophagitis. *British Journal of Surgery*, **38**, 175–182

Baruah, D. (1979) Cancer of the oesophagus in South Western Maharashtra and in adjacent parts of Karnataka. *Indian Journal of Radiology*, **33**, 254–258

Belsey, R. (1966) Functional disease of the esophagus. *Journal of Thoracic and Cardiovascular Surgery*, **52**, 164–188

Belsey, R. and Hiebert, C. A. (1974) An exclusive right thoracic approach for cancer of the middle third of the esophagus. *Annals of Thoracic Surgery*, **18**, 1–15

Bigelow, N. H. (1953) Carcinoma of the esophagus developing at the site of lye stricture. *Cancer*, **6**, 1159–1164

Brand, D. L., Ylvisaker, J. T., Gelford, M. and Pope, C. E. (1980) Regression of columnar esophageal (Barrett's) epithelium after antireflux surgery. *New England Journal of Medicine*, **302**, 844–848

Bremner, C. G. (1984) Barrett's oesophagus. In *Disorders of the Oesophagus* (ed. A. Watson and L. R. Celestin), Pitman, London, pp. 94–104

Cameron, A. J. and Payne, W. S. (1983) Barrett's oesophagus: Incidence of adenocarcinoma during long-term follow-up. *Gut*, **24**, 1007

Cameron, J. L. (1987) Discussant in: Early results with combined modality therapy for carcinoma of the esophagus (Wolfe, W. G., Burton, G. V., Seigler, H. F. *et al*.). *Annals of Surgery*, **205**, 563–571

Carter, R. and Smith, J. (1986) Oesophageal carcinoma: A comparative study of laser recanalisation versus intubation in the palliation of gastro-oesophageal carcinoma. *Lasers in Medical Science*, **1**, 245–252

Cederquist, C., Nielsen, J., Berthelsen, A. and Hansen, H. S. (1978) Cancer of the oesophagus. II. Theory and Outcome. *Acta Chirurgica Scandinavica*, **144**, 233–240

Celestin, L. R. (1978) New techniques of intubation. *Proceedings of the World Congress of Digestive Endoscopy*, 97

Chassin, J. L. (1978) Esophagogastrectomy: Data favouring end to side anastomosis. *Annals of Surgery*, **188**, 22–26

Cook-Mozaffari, P. J., Azordegan, F., Day, N. E. *et al*. (1979) Oesophageal cancer studies in the Caspian Littoral of Iran. Results of case control study. *British Journal of Cancer*, **39**, 293–309

Cooper, D. T., Holmes, G. K. T., Ferguson, R. and Cooke, W. T. (1980) Coeliac disease and malignancy. *Medicine (Baltimore)*, **59**, 249–261

Daly, J. M., Dudrick, S. J. and Copeland, E. M. (1980) The intravenous hyperalimentation: effect on delayed cutaneous hypersensitivity in cancer patients. *Annals of Surgery*, **192**, 587–592

Dark, J. F., Moussali, H. and Vaughan, R. (1981) Surgical treatment of carcinoma of the oesophagus. *Thorax*, **36**, 891–895

Day, M. E., Munoz, N. and Ghadirian, P. (1982) Epidemiology of esophageal cancer: A review. In *Epidemiology of Cancer of the Digestive Tract* (ed. W. H. Enszel and P. Correa), Nijhoff, The Hague, pp. 21–55

Dejong, U. W., Breslow, N., Goh Ewe Hong, J. *et al*. (1974) Aetiological factors in oesophageal cancer in Singapore Chinese. *International Journal of Cancer*, **13**, 291–303

De Meester, T. R. and Lafontaine, E. R. (1985) Surgical therapy of carcinoma of the esophagus and cardia. In *Cancer of the Esophagus* (ed. T. R. De Meester and B. Levin), Grune and Stratton, Orlando, pp. 141–198

Dooner, J. and Cleator, I. G. M. (1982) Selective management of benign esophageal strictures. *American Journal of Gastroenterology*, **77**, 172–177

Druckrey, H. (1972) Organospecific carcinogenesis in the digestive tract. In *Topics in Chemical Carcinogenesis* (ed. W. Nakahara, S., Takayama, T., Sugimura, T. *et al*.), University Park Press, Tokyo, pp. 73–103

DuBrow, R. A. (1985) Imaging of cancer of the esophagus. In *Cancer of the Esophagus* (ed. T. R. De Meester and B. Levin), Grune and Stratton, Orlando, pp. 75–88

Earlam, R. (1984) Oesophageal cancer treatment in North-east Thames Region, 1981: Medical Audit Using Hospital Activity Analysis Data. *British Medical Journal*, **288**, 1892–1894

Earlam, R. and Cunha-Melo, J. R. (1980a) Oesophageal squamous cell carcinoma. I: A critical review of surgery. *British Journal of Surgery*, **67**, 381–390

Earlam, R. and Cunha-Melo, J. R. (1980b) Oesophageal squamous cell carcinoma. II: A critical review of radiotherapy. *British Journal of Surgery*, **67**, 457–461

Edwards, D. A. W. (1974) Carcinoma of the oesophagus and fundus. *Postgraduate Medical Journal*, **50**, 223–227

Edwards, D. A. W. and Lobello, R. (1982) Site of referral of the sense of obstruction to swallowing. *Gut*, **23**, 435

Ellis, F. G. (1960) The natural history of achalasia of the cardia. *Proceedings of the Royal Society of Medicine*, **53**, 663–666

Ellis, F. H. and Gibb, S. P. (1979) Esophagogastrectomy for carcinoma. *Annals of Surgery*, **190**, 699–705

Fleischer, D. (1981) Palliative therapy for oesophageal carcinoma by endoscopic Nd-YAG Laser. *Laser Endoscopy*, **2**, 17–20

Fraser, R. W., Wara, W. M., Thomas, A. N. *et al*. (1978) Combined treatment methods for carcinoma of the esophagus. *Radiology*, **128**, 461–465

Gignoux, M., Roussel, A., Paillot, B. *et al*. (1987) The value of pre-operative radiotherapy in oesophageal cancer; results of a study of the EORTC. *World Journal of Surgery*, **11**, 426–432

Gisselbrecht, C., Calvo, F., Mignot, L. *et al.* (1983) Fluorouracil, Adriamycin and Cisplatin: Combination chemotherapy of advanced esophageal carcinoma. *Cancer*, **52**, 974–977

Giuli, R. (ed.) (1984) *Cancer of the Esophagus* (Proceedings of First Polydisciplinary International Congress of OESO), Maloine S. F. Editeur, Paris

Giuli, R. and Sancho-Garnier, H. (1986) Diagnostic, therapeutic and prognostic features of cancers of the esophagus: results of the international prospective study conducted by the OESO group (790 patients). *Surgery*, **99**, 614–622

Graham, D. Y., Dodds, S. M. and Zubler, M. (1983) What is the role of prosthesis insertion in oesophageal carcinoma? *Gastrointestinal Endoscopy*, **29**, 1–5

Gunnlaugsson, G. H., Wychulis, A. R., Roland, C. and Ellis, F. H. (1970) Analysis of the records of 1657 patients with carcinoma of the esophagus and cardia of the stomach. *Surgery, Gynecology and Obstetrics*, **130**, 997–1005

Haggitt, R. C., Reid, B. J., Rabinovitch, P. S. (1988) Barrett's esophagus: correlation between mucin histochemistry, flow cytometry and histologic diagnosis for predicting increased cancer risk. *American Journal of Pathology*, **131**, 53–61

Haggitt, R. C., Tryzelaar, J., Ellis, F. H. (1978) Adenocarcinoma complicating columnar epithelium-lined (Barrett's) esophagus. *American Journal of Clinical Pathology*, **70**, 1–5

Hamilton, S. R., Hutcheon, D. F., Ravich, W. J. *et al.* (1984) Adenocarcinoma in Barrett's esophagus after elimination of gastroesophageal reflux. *Gastroenterology*, **86**, 356–360

Harper, P. S., Harper, R. M. J. and Howel-Evans, A. W. (1970) Carcinoma of the esophagus with tylosis. *Quarterly Journal of Medicine*, **39**, 317–333

Heatley, R. V., Williams, R. H. P. and Lewis, M. H. (1979) Pre-operative intravenous feeding – a controlled trial. *Postgraduate Medical Journal*, **55**, 541–545

Hennessy, T. P. J. (1986) Tumours of the oesophagus. In *Surgery of the Oesophagus* (ed. T. P. J. Hennessy and A. Cuschieri), Baillière-Tindall, London, pp. 307–351

Hilgenberg, A. D., Carey, R. W., Wilkins, E. W. *et al.* (1988) Pre-operative chemotherapy, surgical resection and selective post-operative therapy for squamous cell carcinoma of the esophagus. *Annals of Thoracic Surgery*, **45**, 357–363

Hill, L. D., Gelfand, M. and Bauermeister, D. (1970) Simplified management of reflux esophagitis with stricture. *Annals of Surgery*, **172**, 638–646

Hirayama, T. (1979) Epidemiological evaluation of the role of naturally occurring carcinogens and modulators of carcinogens. In *Proceedings of the Ninth International Symposium of the Princess Takamatasu Cancer Research Fund*, Tokyo, pp. 359–380

Holmes, G. K. T., Stokes, P. L., McWalter, R. *et al.* (1974) Coeliac disease, malignancy and gluten-free diet. *Gut*, **15**, 339

Hopkins, R. A., Alexander, J. C. and Postlethwait, R. W. (1984) Stapled esophagogastric anastomosis. *American Journal of Surgery*, **147**, 283–287

Huang, K. C. (1981) Diagnosis and surgical treatment of early esophageal carcinoma. In *Medical and Surgical Problems of the Esophagus* (ed. S. Stipa, R. H. R. Belsey and A. Moraldi), Academic Press, New York, pp. 296–299.

Inberg, M. V., Linna, M. I., Scheinin, T. M. and Vänttinen, E. (1971) Anastomotic leakage after excision of esophageal and high gastric carcinoma. *American Journal of Surgery*, **122**, 540–544

Joint Iran-International Agency for Research on Cancer Study Group (1977) Esophageal cancer studies in the Caspian Littoral of Iran: Results of Population Studies – A prodrome. *Journal of the National Cancer Institute*, **59**, 1127–1138

Kelsen, D. (1984) Chemotherapy of esophageal cancer. *Seminars in Oncology*, **11**, 159–168

Kirk, R. M. (1974) Palliative resection of oesophageal carcinoma without formal thoracotomy. *British Journal of Surgery*, **61**, 689–690

Kirk, R. M. (1987) Oesophageal carcinoma: features and assessment. In *Diseases of the Gut and Pancreas* (ed. J. J. Misiewicz, R. E. Pounder and C. W. Venables), Blackwell Scientific Publications, Oxford, pp. 169–178

Kiviranta, U. K. (1952) Corrosion carcinoma of the esophagus. *Acta Oto-laryngologica*, **42**, 89–95

Krasner, N. and Beard, J. (1984) Laser irradiation of tumours of the oesophagus and gastric cardia. *British Medical Journal*, **288**, 829

Laas, J., Scheller, E., Haverich, A. *et al.* (1986) How accurate is the pre-operative staging with computed tomography in esophageal cancer? In *Proceedings of the Third World Congress of the International Society for Diseases of the Esophagus*, p. 40

Lam, K. H., Wong, J., Lim, S. T. K. (1981) Results of esophagectomy. In *Medical and Surgical Problems of the Esophagus* (ed. S. Stipa, R. H. R. Belsey and A. Moraldi), Academic Press, New York, pp. 353–359

Lambert, R., Audigier, J. C. and Tuyns, A. J. (1978) Epidemiology of oesophageal cancer in France. In *Carcinoma of the Oesophagus* (ed. W. Silber), A. A. Blakema, Cape Town, pp. 23–28

Lansing, P. B., Ferrante, W. A. and Oschner, J. L. (1969) Carcinoma of the esophagus at the site of lye stricture. *American Journal of Surgery*, **118**, 108–111

Lehr, L., Rupp, N., Reiser, M. *et al.* (1986) Pre-operative evaluation of resectability of esophageal cancer by CT and MR imaging. In *Proceedings of the Third World Congress of the International Society for Diseases of the Esophagus*, p. 36

Lewis, I. (1946) The surgical treatment of carcinoma of the oesophagus with special reference to a new operation for growths of the middle third. *British Journal of Surgery*, **34**, 18–20

Lishman, A. H., Dellipiani, A. W. and Devlin, H. B. (1980) The insertion of oesophagogastric tubes in malignant oesophageal strictures: Endoscopy or surgery? *British Journal of Surgery*, **80**, 257–259

Lortat-Jacob J. L., Richard, C. A., Fekete, F. and Testart, J. (1969) Cardiospasm and esophageal carcinoma. Report of 24 Cases. *Surgery*, **66**, 969–975

McKeown, K. C. (1972) Trends in oesophageal resection for carcinoma. *Annals of the Royal College of Surgeons of England*, **51**, 213–238

McKeown, K. C. (1979) Carcinoma of the oesophagus, *Journal of the Royal College of Surgeons of Edinburgh*, **24**, 253–274

Maillard, J. N., Goyer, B. and Lortat-Jacob, J. L. (1971) Comparison chez l'homme des anastomoses oesophagogastriques à la pince PKS 25 et à la suture. *Annals de Chirurgie*, **33**, 374–378

Mannell, A. (1982) Carcinoma of the esophagus. *Current Problems in Surgery*, **19**, 557–647

Marasas, W. F., Van Rensburg, S. J. and Mirocha, C. J. (1979) Incidence of fusarium species and the mycotoxins deoxynivalenol and zeatalone in corn produced in esophageal cancer areas in Transkei. *Journal of Agriculture and Food Chemistry*, **27**, 1108–1112

Matthews, H. R. and Hopkinson, R. B. (1984) Treatment of sputum retention by minitracheotomy. *British Journal of Surgery*, **71**, 147–150

Matthews, H. R., Powell, D. J. and McConkey, C. C. (1986) Effect of surgical experience on the results of resection for oesophageal carcinoma. *British Journal of Surgery*, **72**, 621–623

Miller, C. (1962) Carcinoma of the thoracic oesophagus and cardia. A review of 405 cases. *British Journal of Surgery*, **49**, 507–522

Moghissi, K. (1979) Conservative surgery in reflux stricture of the oesophagus associated with hiatal hernia. *British Journal of Surgery*, **76**, 221–225

Morson, B. C. (1961) The spread of carcinoma of the oesophagus. In *Tumours of the Oesophagus* (ed. N. C. Tanner and D. W. Smithers), Livingstone, Edinburgh, pp. 136–145

Moss, A. A., Schnyder, P., Thoeni, R. F. and Margulis, A. R. (1981) Esophageal carcinoma: Pre-therapy staging by computed tomography. *American Journal of Roentgenology*, **136**, 1051–1056

Munoz, N. and Crespi, M. (1984) Studies in the aetiology of oesophageal carcinoma. In *Disorders of the Oesophagus* (ed. A. Watson and L. R. Celestin), Pitman, London, pp. 147–154

Naef, A. P., Savary, M. and Ozello, L. (1975) The columnar lined lower oesophagus: An acquired lesion with malignant predisposition. Report on 140 cases of Barrett's oesophagus with 12 adenocarcinomas. *Journal of Thoracic and Cardiovascular Surgery*, **70**, 826–835

Napalkov, N. P. and Pozharisski, K. M. (1969) Morphogenesis of experimental tumours of the esophagus. *Journal of the National Cancer Institute*, **42**, 922–940

Norell, S., Ahlbom, A., Lipping, H. and Österblom, L. (1983) Oesophageal cancer and vulcanisation work. *Lancet*, **1**, 462–463

Ogilivie, A. L., Dronfield, M. W., Ferguson, R. and Atkinson, M. (1982) Palliative intubation of oesophagogastric neoplasms at fibreoptic endoscopy. *Gut*, **23**, 1060–1067

Ogilvie, A. L., Ferguson, R. and Atkinson, M. (1980) Outlook with conservative treatment of peptic oesophageal stricture. *Gut*, **21**, 23–25

Ong, G. B. and Kwong, K. H. (1969) The Lewis–Tanner operation for cancer of the oesophagus. *Journal of the Royal College of Surgeons of Edinburgh*, **14**, 3–19

Ong, G. B., Lam, K. H., Wong, J. (1978) Factors influencing morbidity and mortality in esophageal carcinoma. *Journal of Thoracic and Cardiovascular Surgery*, **76**, 745–749

Orringer, M. B. (1984a) Transhiatal esophagectomy with thoracotomy for carcinoma of the thoracic esophagus *Annals of Surgery*, **200**, 282–288

Orringer, M. B. (1984b) Is it illusory to envisage extended lymph node dissection? In Cancer of the Esophagus (*Proceedings of the First Multi-disciplinary International Congress of OESO*) (ed. R. Giuli), Maloine S. A. Editeur, Paris, pp. 138–140

Orringer M. B. and Sloane, H. E. (1978) Esophagectomy with thoracotomy. *Journal of Thoracic and Cardiovascular Surgery*, **76**, 643–654

Parker, E. F. and Gregorie, H. B. (1976) Carcinoma of the esophagus: long-term results. *Journal of the American Medical Association*, **235**, 1018–1020

Paull, A., Trier, J. S., Dalton, M. D. *et al.* (1976) The histologic spectrum of Barrett's oesophagus. *New England Journal of Medicine*, **295**, 476–480

Pearson, J. G. (1977) The present status and future potential of radiotherapy in the management of esophageal cancer. *Cancer*, **39**, 882–890

Postlethwait, R. W. (ed.) (1979) *Surgery of the Esophagus*. Appleton Century-Crofts, New York.

Ravry, M., Moertel, C. G., Schutt, A. J. *et al.* (1973) Treatment of advanced squamous cell carcinoma of the gastro-intestinal tract with bleomycin. *Cancer Chemotherapy Reports*, **57**, 493–496

Reid, B. J., Weinstein, W. M., Lewin, K. J. *et al.* (1988) Endoscopic biopsy can detect high-grade dysplasia or early adenocarcinoma in Barrett's esophagus without grossly recognizable neoplastic lesions. *Gastroenterology*, **94**, 81–90

Reuber, M. D. (1977) Histopathology of pre-neoplastic and neoplastic lesions of the esophagus in BUF rats ingesting diethylnitrosamine. *Journal of the National Cancer Institute*, **58**, 313–321

Robertson, C. S., Mayberry, J. F., Nicholson, D. A. *et al.* (1988) Value of endoscopic surveillance in the detection of neoplastic change in Barrett's oesophagus. *British Journal of Surgery*, **75**, 760–763

Rosenberg, J. C., Franklin, R. and Steiger, Z. (1981) Squamous cell carcinoma of the thoracic esophagus: An interdisciplinary approach. *Current Problems in Cancer*, **5**, 1–52

Rowland, C. G. and Pagliero, K. M. (1985) Intracavitary irradiation in palliation of carcinoma of oesophagus and cardia. *Lancet*, **2**, 981–982

Rubiro, C. A. (1985) Experimental models. In *Cancer of the Esophagus* (ed. T. R. De Meester and B. Levin), Grune and Stratton, Orlando, pp. 21–42

Shafer, R. B. (1971) Adenocarcinoma in Barrett's columnar-lined esophagus. *Annals of Surgery*, **103**, 411–413

Shahian, E. M., Neptune, W. B., Ellis, F. H. and Watkins, E. (1986) Transthoracic versus extra-thoracic esophagectomy: mortality, morbidity and long-term survival. *Annals of Thoracic Surgery*, **40**, 321–322

Shapiro, S., Hamilton, D. and Morgenstern, I. (1972) The fate of the pylorus in esophagogastrostomy. *Surgery, Gynecology and Obstetrics*, **135**, 216–218

Sjogren, R. W. and Johnson, L. F. (1983) Barrett's oesophagus: A Review. *American Journal of Medicine*, **74**, 313–321

Skinner, D. B. (1983) En bloc resection for neoplasms of the esophagus and cardia. *Journal of Thoracic and Cardiovascular Surgery*, **85**, 59–69

Skinner, D. B. (1985) The columnar-lined esophagus and adenocarcinoma. *Annals of Thoracic Surgery*, **40**, 321–322

Skinner, D. B., Little, A. G., Ferguson, M. K. *et al.* (1986) Selection of operation for esophageal cancer based on staging. *Annals of Surgery*, **204**, 391–401

Skinner, D. B., Walther, B. C., Riddell, R. H. *et al.* (1983) Barrett's esophagus: Comparison of benign and malignant cases. *Annals of Surgery*, **198**, 554–565

Smith, R. L., Hamilton, S. R., Boitnott, J. K. and Rogers, E. L. (1984) The spectrum of carcinoma arising in Barrett's esophagus. *American Journal of Surgical Pathology*, **8**, 563–573

Spechler, S. J., Robbins, A. H., Rubins, H. B. *et al.* (1984) Adenocarcinoma and Barrett's esophagus. An over-rated risk? *Gastroenterology*, **87**, 927–933

Stephen, S. J. and Uragoda, C. G. (1970) Some observations on esophageal carcinoma in Ceylon including its relationship to betel chewing. *British Journal of Cancer*, **24**, 11–15

Swain, C. P. and Bown, S. G. (1984) Laser recanalization of obstructing foregut cancer. *British Journal of Surgery*, **71**, 112–115

Tanner, N. C. (1947) The present position of carcinoma of the oesophagus. *Postgraduate Medical Journal*, **23**, 109–139

Tio, T. L. and Tytgat, G. N. J. (1986) The role of endoscopic ultrasonography in pre-operative staging of oesophagus malignancy. In *Proceedings of the Third World Congress of the International Society for Diseases of the Oesophagus*, p. 38

Troncoso, P. and Riddell, R. H. (1985) Pathology of cancer of the esophagus. In *Cancer of the Esophagus* (ed. T. R. De Meester and B. Levin), Grune and Stratton, Orlando, pp. 89–118

Turner, G. G. (1936) Carcinoma of the oesophagus. The question of its treatment by surgery. *Lancet*, **1**, 67–72, 130–134

Tuyns, A. J., Pequiqnot, G. and Abbatucci, J. S. (1979) Oesophageal cancer and alcohol consumption: Importance of type of beverage. *International Journal of Cancer*, **23**, 443–447

Tytgat, G. N. J. (1984) Non-radiological investigation of the oesophagus. In *Disorders of the Oesophagus* (ed. A. Watson and L. R. Celestin), Pitman, London, pp. 24–36

Van Der Veen, A. H., Dees, J., Blankensteijn, J. D. and Blankenstein, M. V. (1989) Adenocarcinoma in Barrett's oesophagus: an over-rated risk. *Gut*, **30**, 14–18

Watson, A. (1982) A study of the quality and duration of survival following resection, endoscopic intubation and surgical intubation in oesophageal carcinoma. *British Journal of Surgery*, **69**, 585–588

Watson, A. (1984a) The role of anti-reflux surgery combined with fibreoptic endoscopic dilatation in peptic esophageal stricture. *American Journal of Surgery*, **148**, 346–349

Watson, A. (1984b) Therapeutic options and patient selection in the management of oesophageal carcinoma. In *Disorders of the Oesophagus* (eds. A. Watson and L. R. Celestin), Pitman, London, pp. 167–186

Watson, A. (1985) Palliative intubation in inoperable esophageal neoplasms. *Annals of Thoracic Surgery*, **39**, 501–502

Watson, A. (1986) Survival following resection, endoscopic intubation and surgical intubation in oesophageal carcinoma. In *Proceedings of the Second International Congress of the International Society for Diseases of the Esophagus* (eds. G. Castrini, P. Trentino and G. Pappalardo), Publisher Assisi: S. Maria Degli Angeli, pp. 377–386

Watson, A. (1987) Management of carcinoma of the oesophagus. In *Diseases of the Gut and Pancreas* (ed. J. J. Misiewicz, R. E. Pounder and C. W. Venables), Blackwell Scientific Publications, Oxford, pp. 179–192

Watson, A. (1988) Surgery for carcinoma of the oesophagus. *Postgraduate Medical Journal*, **64**, 860–864

Watson, A. (1990) Pathologic changes affecting survival in esophageal cancer. In *International Trends in General Thoracic Surgery* (ed. N. C. Delarue and H. Eschapasse), Mosby, St Louis, pp. 90–97

Werner, I. D. (1979) The multi-disciplinary approach in the management of squamous carcinoma of the esophagus. *Frontiers of Gastrointestinal Research*, **5**, 130–135

Wesdorp, I. C., Bartelsman, J., Schipper, M. E. and Tytgat, G. N. J. (1981) Effect of long-term treatment with Cimetidine and antacids in Barrett's oesophagus. *Gut*, **22**, 724–727

Wolfe, W. G., Burton, G. V., Seigler, H. F. *et al.* (1987) Early results with combined modality therapy for carcinoma of the esophagus. *Annals of Surgery*, **205**, 563–571

Wong, J. (1981) Management of carcinoma of the oesophagus: Art or Science? *Journal of the Royal College of Surgeons of Edinburgh*, **26**, 138–148

Wong, J. (1987) Esophageal resection for cancer: The Rationale of Current Practice. *American Journal of Surgery*, **153**, 18–24

Wong, J., Lam, K. H., Wei, W. I. and Ong, G. B. (1981) Results of the Kirschner operation. *World Journal of Surgery*, **5**, 547–552

Yamada, A. (1979) Radiologic assessment of resectability and prognosis in oesophageal carcinoma. *Gastrointestinal Radiology*, **4**, 213–218

Yang, C. S. (1980) Research of esophageal cancer in China: A Review. *Cancer Research*, **40**, 2633–2644

Young, M. and Russell, W. T. (1926) An investigation into the statistics of cancer in different trades and professions. *Medical Research Council Special Report 1926*. Series No. 99, HMSO, London

Chapter 2

The management of gastric cancer

D. Cunningham

Incidence and aetiology

The most recent statistics from England and Wales show that 11 553 cases of stomach cancer were registered in 1983 (Table 2.1) (Office of Population Censuses and Surveys, 1986). It is the third most common cause of cancer deaths in males and the fourth most common cause of cancer deaths in females (Office of Population Censuses and Surveys, 1985). There is a marked male preponderance with a male to female ratio of 2:1 and it is more common among lower

Table 2.1 Site of primary tumours (Source OPCS)

Site description	Number	%
Males		
All sites (ECD 140–208)	100 645	100
Trachea, bronchus and lung	26 403	26
Skin, other than melanoma	11 317	11
Prostate	9 127	9
Stomach	7 060	7
Bladder	6 683	7
Colon	6 488	6
Rectum, rectosigmoid junction and anus	5 171	5
Pancreas	2 881	3
Oesophagus	2 294	2
Kidney and other unspecified urinary organs	1 894	2
Others	21 327	21
Females		
All sites (ICD 140–208)	97 604	100
Breast	21 297	22
Skin, other than melanoma	10 419	11
Trachea, bronchus and lung	9 475	10
Colon	8 124	8
Ovary and other uterine adnexa	4 521	5
Stomach	4 493	5
Rectum, rectosigmoid junction and anus	4 329	4
Cervix uteri	3 875	4
Body of uterus	3 346	3
Pancreas	2 752	3
Other	24 973	26

socio-economic groups. During the past 50 years there has been a steady, unexplained decline in the number of cases affecting both sexes (Sandler and Holland, 1987) but the crude 5-year survival has remained between 7% and 11%. On a worldwide scale, the incidence of gastric cancer varies considerably (Table 2.2) (Hattori, Asai and Segi, 1984). The incidence in Japan exceeds any other country and is more than 2.5 times that of the UK and nine times that of the USA. Japanese migrants to the USA have a lower incidence of stomach cancer but it remains five times that of the indigenous population (Waterhouse *et al.*, 1983). The marked inter-county variation in the incidence of gastric cancer, and the studies of migrant populations have implicated environmental factors in its aetiology. The most important of these is thought to be diet but other factors such as exposure to coal dust or asbestos are also relevant (Mewhouse, 1981).

Table 2.2 Age-adjusted death rates for cancer of the stomach in the world

Country	Males	Females
Japan	50.4	25.4
Chile	46.0	23.4
Hungary	33.4	15.8
Austria	26.1	13.6
Italy	23.4	11.2
Spain	21.4	11.1
Scotland	18.8	9.2
England and Wales	18.1	8.1
Mauritius	16.3	7.4
Sweden	13.4	7.0
France	13.1	6.0
Canada	10.5	4.8
USA	6.4	3.13
Nicaragua	0.1	0.4

There have been a number of studies which have attempted to identify the dietary constituents which lead to an increased risk of gastric cancer. The results have been conflicting. For Japanese migrants to Hawaii the ingestion of salted and dried fish was found to be a strong risk factor (Haenszel *et al.*, 1972) but this was not confirmed in a further study from Japan (Haenszel *et al.*, 1976). Similarly in south Louisiana, smoked foods and home cured meat were associated with an increased risk of gastric cancer in the black population but not in the white (Correa *et al.*, 1985). One recent study from Greece identified pasta, beans and nuts (Trichopoulos *et al.*, 1985) and another from Canada identified chocolate and carbohydrate as risk factors (Risch *et al.*, 1985). In Columbia, which has one of the highest incidences of gastric cancer outside Japan, people from areas with a high incidence of gastric cancer were found to eat fava beans in far larger amounts than equivalent groups from low incidence areas (Correa *et al.*, 1983). However, the only consistent finding from all of these studies was the protective effect of the ingestion of vegetables, particularly lettuce and citrus fruits and that alcohol and cigarettes have no proven link with the development of gastric cancer.

Nitrites have been implicated in the aetiology of gastric cancer. They are used as a preservative and a colouring agent in a variety of fish and meat products especially home-cured meats, dried fish and sausages. Also, nitrates in the diet can be converted to nitrites by bacterial action in the food or in the stomach (Hall *et al.*, 1986). Dietary nitrates are mainly derived from crop fertilizer. They are taken up by the crops, and may also contaminate fresh water supplies. These factors have led to a general increase in the amount of dietary nitrate in the past 20 years (Reid, 1977). Nitrites can also interact with Japanese soy sauce (Wakabayashi *et al.*, 1983) and with fava beans to make them mutagenic (Yang *et al.*, 1984). One possible mechanism for the development of gastric cancer which incorporates these nitrite/nitrates data was suggested by Correa *et al.* (1975). In this hypothesis gastric atrophy played a key role by leading to a reduction in gastric acid secretion and permitting bacterial colonization of the stomach; this would not be possible in an acid environment. These bacteria, it was postulated, could reduce dietary nitrate to nitrite and form N-nitroso compounds through the nitrosation of dietary amines. N-nitroso compounds are known to be carcinogenic in animals (Ogiu, Nakadate and Odashima, 1975) and could therefore act on the atrophic gastric mucosa causing intestinal metaplasia, dysplasia and ultimately cancer. It has been suggested that the decline of gastric cancer in the USA and the UK is linked to more widespread refrigeration of foodstuffs with a resultant reduction in the use of nitrites. In the USA during the last 50 years there has been a 75% reduction in the nitrite content of meat, used to prevent botulism (Binkerd and Kolari, 1975). However, two studies from the UK failed to show a positive association between nitrate in the drinking water (Beresford, 1985) or in the saliva and gastric cancer. Levels of salivary nitrate, which are taken to be a good marker of the dietary intake of nitrate, showed an inverse correlation with the risk of developing gastric cancer (Forman, Al-Dabbagh and Doll, 1985). These findings cast doubt on the importance of nitrates as a factor in the development of gastric cancer. Nevertheless, it should be emphasized that in the UK the largest proportion of dietary nitrate is derived from vegetables which are abundant in vitamin C and may therefore prevent the formation of carcinogenic N-nitroso compounds by blocking the chemical reaction between nitrites and dietary amines in the stomach (Mirvish *et al.*, 1972).

A high intake of salt may also be relevant to the development of gastric cancer. Salt has been shown to increase the uptake by the stomach of carcinogens in an animal model (Capoferro and Torgersen, 1974). Thus, in man, the salt in dried fish and other cured meats may be an important prerequisite to the carcinogenic effects of nitrites in the diet. The balance between dietary nitrite, ascorbic acid and nitrate is clearly of major importance and its complex inter-relationship could account for the difficulties which still exist in this area of epidemiology. However, there is other evidence favouring the Correa hypothesis. Conditions such as pernicious anaemia (Borch, 1986; Svendsen *et al.*, 1986), hypogammaglobulinaemia (Hermans, Diax-buxo and Stobo, 1976) and gastric surgery for peptic ulcer (Caygill *et al.*, 1986, Viste *et al.*, 1986) are associated with hypochlorhydria and predispose to gastric cancer. In a Scandinavian study 10 (8%) of 123 patients with pernicious anaemia screened endoscopically were found to have gastric neoplasms; 5 were carcinoid, 4 adenocarcinoma and 1 adenomatous polyp (Borch, 1986). It has also been shown that the gastric juice of these patients contains bacteria capable of reducing nitrate to nitrite (Ruddell *et al.*, 1976). Nevertheless, a recent study of the gastric aspirate from three groups of patients – one with pernicious anaemia, one following polya gastrectomy and a control group, whilst confirming these findings, failed to show a direct correlation between an alkaline pH and an increase in the production of nitrosamines. Indeed the reverse applied – there was a definite trend in favour of increased nitrosamine production at an acid pH (Hall *et al.*, 1986). These results suggest the formation of N-nitroso compounds in the stomach is more likely to occur at an acid pH which favours the chemical reaction between nitrites and amines (Douglass *et al.*, 1978), rather than at an alkaline pH which favours bacterial colonization but not necessarily nitrosation.

These results also imply that the Correa model for carcinogens in the stomach is not totally accurate. Bacterial colonization in an alkaline pH may not be an essential step. It could well be that the achlorhydria is a marker for abnormal gastric mucosa, such as the atrophic gastritis associated with ageing or pernicious anaemia, and it is this alteration in the mucosal barrier rather than the bacterial colonization which is important. Similarly, after gastric surgery patients develop dysplastic changes in the residual gastric mucosa as a result of bile reflux (Thomas *et al.*, 1984) which may predispose to gastric cancer.

Pathology

Adenocarcinoma of the stomach accounts for 97% of gastric malignancies. There are several histological classifications of this tumour in current use. The classification devised by the World Health Organisation (WHO) recognizes tubular, papillary, mucinous and signet ring forms of gastric cancer (Oota and Sobin, 1977). It has not gained wide acceptance partly because many tumours have a mixture of more than one type, especially the tubular and papillary forms, but also because the four histological groups do not correlate well with known epidemiological data.

Table 2.3 Histology of gastric cancer according to the Lauren classification

	Intestinal	*Diffuse*
Histology	Cells similar to intestinal epithelium and tend to grow in clumps. Little fibrous reaction. Usually there is an inflammatory infiltrate	Cells often single or arranged in 'indian file'. Gives rise to the signet ring cell tumours. Stromal reaction marked
Epidemiology	More common in areas with a high incidence of gastric cancer. Male:Female 2:1	Hereditary form of gastric cancer. More common in young age groups. Male:Female 1:1 Associated with blood group A
Progress	Outlook better than the diffuse type	Submucosal spread frequent. Therefore resection margin involvement more common than with the intestinal type

The most widely used classification was proposed by Lauren in 1965 (Table 2.3). Lauren described two basic types of gastric cancer – intestinal and diffuse. The intestinal type is characterized by cells which grow in a tubular arrangement similar to small intestinal epithelium. They commonly have a striated border and are very cohesive, expanding into surrounding normal tissue in a well-circumscribed fashion. There is usually little fibrous tissue reaction but often an inflammatory cell infiltrate. In the diffuse type the cells are usually single or arranged in indian file and infiltrate diffusely into surrounding tissue. These cells may be devoid of cytoplasm or contain much cytoplasm leading to the so-called signet ring cell, in which the nucleus is pushed to the side of the cell by the cytoplasm. There is usually a marked stromal reaction. However, in a considerable proportion of cases, approximately 15% (Correa *et al.*, 1973), there is a mixture of intestinal and diffuse forms and in some reviews it has not been possible to classify a further 25% of cases (Caygill, Day and Hill, 1986).

It has been shown that the two histological types of gastric cancer, intestinal and diffuse, appear to have a distinctive aetiology. The diffuse type is considered to be the 'endemic' form of gastric cancer. It affects both sexes equally and is associated with blood group A (Correa *et al.*, 1973) and younger age groups (Grabiec and Owen, 1985; Tso *et al.*, 1987). It appears to have to have a strong hereditary basis and has a similar incidence in high and low incidence areas. On the other hand the intestinal type is the 'epidemic' form of gastric cancer (Correa *et al.*, 1973; Munoz and Connelly, 1971). It is more common in males with a 2:1 male female ratio and is the most usual form of gastric cancer in the elderly (Esaki, Hirokawa and Yamashiro, 1987). In countries with a high incidence of gastric cancer such as Japan, the increased number of cases are mainly of the intestinal type (Correa *et al.*, 1973; Munoz and Connelly, 1971). These features point towards a strong environmental component in the development of intestinal type of gastric cancer. However, it has not always been possible to demonstrate such a close correlation between the two different histological subtypes and these features. A recent report from the UK showed the reverse; there was a higher incidence of diffuse gastric cancer in the high risk areas for gastric cancer (Caygill, Day and Hill, 1986). One possible reason for this inconsistency is the heterogeneous nature of the histology. In reality, the architecture of these tumours often has a mixture of intestinal and diffuse forms and morphologically, commonly consist of both well- and poorly-differentiated cells, which must make histological assessment extremely difficult.

Kubo (1974) suggested that well-differentiated tumours tended to be intestinal and poorly-differentiated diffuse and that these morphological characteristics are of more importance than the pattern of growth. Using this simple classification in Japan and New Zealand, he was unable to show any of the usual demographical and epidemiological correlations of the Lauren classification (Kubo, 1971; 1973). Ming (1977) has proposed a classification for gastric cancer with two histological categories; an expanding type and an infiltrating type. In his series, the expanding type of gastric cancer constituted 67% of all cases. Of the expanding tumours 63% were fungating, 20% ulcerated, 10% polypoid, 4% superficial and 3% diffuse. The infiltrative carcinoma was diffuse in 68%, ulcerated in 27% and fungating in 5% of cases. Therefore, the histological type has a significant influence on the macroscopic appearance of the tumour. The infiltrative carcinoma with a diffuse macroscopic appearance gives rise to 'linitis plastica' or leather bottle stomach. The Ming classification does appear to have some merit although it offers relatively little advantage over the Lauren classification.

It is most important that a histological classification should be clinically and biologically relevant. Despite the obvious difficulties in classifying a proportion of cases, the Lauren classification is the closest to satisfying these criteria. Patients with the intestinal type of gastric cancer have a better prognosis than those with the diffuse type, independent of the type of surgical treatment (Cady *et al.*, 1977).

Also, with the diffuse type microscopic infiltration occurs beyond the macroscopic boundary of the tumour therefore it is recommended that the surgical resection margins for diffuse tumours should be 5 cm compared to the 2 cm margin for intestinal tumours. Taking these factors and the epidemiological data into account I would suggest, where possible, the Lauren classification of gastric cancer should be used.

The most common sites for gastric cancer are the pylorus and pyloric antrum which account for 70% of cases. Carcinoma of the proximal third of the stomach and lower oesophagus now constitute up to 30% of cases compared to 15–20% 30 years ago (Antonioli and Goldman, 1982). This change in the pattern of distribution may be related to the unique association between carcinoma of the cardia and lower oesophagus with Barrett's oesophagus (Barrett, 1950). Thus the apparent increase of carcinoma at these sites is due to a relative decline of carcinoma of the pylorus and pyloric antrum. Barrett's oesophagus is characterized by a shifting of the squamocolumnar junction to at least 3 cm above the lowermost part of the oesophagus. Within the columnar epithelium there is usually gastric parietal and chief cells, junctional epithelium and epithelium which resembles intestinal mucosa with an abundance of mucus-secreting glands (Hawe et al., 1973; Paull et al., 1976). Epithelial dysplasia and carcinoma-in-situ are well described in Barrett's oesophagus and are premalignant conditions. Up to 86% of oesophageal adenocarcinomas are thought to arise in Barrett's oesophagus and carcinoma is found in 7–46% of Barrett's oesophagus at diagnosis (Berenson et al., 1978; Haggitt et al., 1978). The precise aetiology of Barrett's oesophagus is not established although it is likely to be related to reflux of the gastric contents. Between 2 and 11% of patients with reflux oesophagitis develop Barrett's oesophagus (Berenson et al., 1978) and a proportion of these will ultimately develop malignant change. Efforts to ameliorate the risks of malignancy have produced the proponents of radical anti-reflux surgery because this is known to reverse the epithelial change whereas medical treatment does not (Brand et al., 1980). However, since the risk of developing cancer in Barrett's oesophagus may be as low as 1 in 175 patient years (Spechler et al., 1984), and the average age of patients with Barrett's oesophagus is 60 years, the decision regarding surgery is not clear-cut.

Molecular biology

During the past ten years there have been enormous advances in our understanding of the molecular biology of cancer. The learning curve seems to be exponential as we unravel the complex interrelationship between cellular oncogenes, viral oncogenes, polypeptide growth factors and cancer. The proto-oncogenes are genes present in normal mammalian cells which are homologous with the viral genes responsible for the tumorigenic properties of RNA tumour viruses. They are also known as cellular oncogenes. In normal cells they are responsible for growth and maturation but when transferred to non-malignant cell lines (transfection) they can promote the development of tumours. Oncogenes are over-expressed in a variety of solid tumours and it is now clear that they are an integral part of the mechanism of carcinogenesis.

A number of oncogenes have been identified in gastric cancer and gastric cancer cell lines. These include the genes H-ras, myc and erb B-2 (Kota et al., 1985;

Fukshige *et al.*, 1986; Yokota *et al.*, 1986). Using *in situ* hybridization the H-ras gene was found to be over-expressed relative to normal tissues in a small series of primary stomach cancers and was also found in intermediate amounts in areas of dysplastic gastric mucosa (Ohuchi *et al.*, 1987). In a more extensive study of formalin-fixed, paraffin-embedded tissue the presence of the ras protein was demonstrated using monoclonal antibodies to the oncogene product. There was no correlation between tumour differentiation or depth of invasion and expression of H-ras although there was a tendency for more advanced tumours to express comparatively larger amounts of H-ras (Ohuchi *et al.*, 1987). These findings may have diagnostic and prognostic implications for the future. The ras oncogene is normally activated through point mutations at the 12, 13 or 61 codons. In a gastric cancer cell line a point mutation of the 12th codon (guanine to thymine) was found in cells which over-express H-ras (Deng *et al.*, 1987).

The erb B-2 oncogene is also amplified in gastric cancer. This oncogene codes for a protein which is a truncated form of the epidermal growth factor (EGF) receptor (Yokota *et al.*, 1986). The erb B-1 oncogene codes for EGF receptor and the possession of EGF receptor is known to be a poor prognostic factor in breast cancer (Sainsbury *et al.*, 1985). It is therefore of particular interest that EGF has also been found in primary gastric cancer and that the prognosis was worse for patients whose tumours elaborated EGF (Tahara *et al.*, 1986). The promoter regions for erb B-1 (Ishii *et al.*, 1985) and erb B-2 have recently been characterized. These areas regulate the production of receptors by the gene and are potential targets for therapy. Chromosomal abnormalities are also found in gastric cancer and recently deletions of the long arms of chromosomes 1 and 5 have been demonstrated (Fey *et al.*, 1989). Loss of the chromosomal material may deprive the cell of an anti-oncogene allele or tumour-associated antigen allele.

Natural history

In Europe and the USA gastric cancer presents late in its natural history. By the time of diagnosis the majority of patients have locally advanced disease or have evidence of metastases. Presenting symptoms related to gastric cancer are non-specific and include upper abdominal pain (78%), weight loss (67%), vomiting (48%), anorexia (45%) and weakness (42%) (Lundh *et al.*, 1974). These symptoms may predate the diagnosis by 12–24 months but patients usually present within 12 months of their onset. Once suspected the diagnosis can normally be confirmed using either barium studies or endoscopy (Kurtz and Sherlock, 1985).

Gastric cancer in general, is an intra-abdominal disease. The tumour typically spreads by local invasion of the stomach and surrounding structures. It metastasizes to local and then regional lymph nodes and often spreads by the transcoelomic route to the peritoneum and omentum or occasionally to the ovaries giving rise to a Kruckenberg tumour. Haematogenous spread to the liver is via the portal vien. At laparotomy up to 70% of patients will have evidence of tumour in the regional lymph nodes, 25% will have liver metastases and a similar proportion will have peritoneal metastases (Lundh *et al.*, 1974). There is direct infiltration of the pancreas in 23% and of the colon in 5%. The net effect of these findings is that relatively few patients have tumours which can be surgically cured despite the absence of metastases outside the abdomen. Only 5–10% of patients will be alive 5 years after diagnosis and the majority of patients will die within the first two years

(Swynnerton and Truelove, 1952; Gilbertson, 1969; Cassell and Robinson, 1976; Dupont *et al.*, 1978).

The pattern of recurrence at post-mortem reflects the original mode of dissemination of the tumour, except that liver metastases are more frequent (54%) and that lung metastases can be detected in almost 25% of cases (Dupont *et al.*, 1978). The pattern of failure after successful surgical removal of the primary tumour was studied by Gunderson and Sosin (1982). In this series, 107 patients were subjected to periodic re-operation. Eighty-six developed recurrent disease and of these 87% had local–regional recurrence which was defined as tumour in the gastric bed, lymph node recurrence or a localized peritoneal recurrence. Distant metastases were present in 30% of patients but were the sole site of recurrence in only 5%.

In Japan, due to earlier diagnosis the natural history is more favourable; the 5-year survival for patients with gastric cancer having a curative resection is 50% (78). However, Kato (1989) highlighted that the annual death rate from gastric cancer in Japan has remained stable between 1975 and 1984 at 50 000 from an estimated annual incidence of 70 000 cases. The latter figure is derived from cancer registries, which in Japan do not allow for dual counting which occurs when a patient is seen in more that one hospital. Therefore at best, the overall 5-year survival rate in Japan is 29%.

Early gastric cancer and screening for gastric cancer

Early gastric cancer is defined as tumour which has not penetrated the submucosa. Lesions may be protuberant, elevated, flat, depressed or excavated (Murakami, 1979). Their average diameter is between 2 and 3 cm (Esaki, Hirokawa and Yamashiro, 1987) but lesions as large as 12.5 cm may occur (Sato, Kamata and Goto, 1985). This has led some to suggest that because these tumours can be slow growing (Fujita, 1978), almost regardless of when the diagnosis is established, their natural history is such that they remain confined to the submucosa and are therefore easily cured by surgery. However, this seems unlikely because the Japanese have increased the proportion of cases with early gastric cancer from 1% before 1951 (Muto *et al.*, 1968) to over 40% in a population exposed to a screening programme with a concomitant improvement in overall survival (Oshima *et al.*, 1986).

In Japan over 4 million people are screened each year, with the detection of around 4000 new cases of gastric cancer. Indeed, it has become Japanese public health policy to make one screening investigation available to all adults over the age of 40 years once every 3 years. The screening method involves the use of a double-contrast barium meal in conjunction with photofluorographic apparatus that takes 5–7 exposures per examination. The examination usually takes place in a mobile unit staffed by skilled technicians. Suspicious cases are referred for endoscopy. Although it seems likely that screening improves survival (Oshima *et al.*, 1986), in the absence of any randomized trial of screening versus no screening, it is not possible to unequivocally prove this assertion. At the present time, case-control studies are used as an alternative to the randomized trial. In a recent case-control study from Nosetown in Osaka, the odds ratio of dying from gastric cancer in screened compared with unscreened individuals was 0.595 for males and 0.382 for females, thus supporting the notion that screening improves mortality rates (Oshima *et al.*, 1986).

In the UK it is now accepted that early gastric cancer is identical to the Japanese variety (Evans *et al.*, 1978). In the 1960s the detection rate for early gastric cancer was as low as 0.7% (Fielding *et al.*, 1980) although more recent data puts it at 10% (Houghton *et al.*, 1985). In Bristol the number of early gastric cancers doubled during the two 10-year periods of 1965–1975 and 1975–1985. The survival rate of the patients with early gastric cancer was extremely good; 71% were alive at least five years (adjusted mortality 92%) (Houghton *et al.*, 1985). However, although the screening programme has been successful in Japan the detection rate is low (1 in 1000 screened) and in the context of the lower rates of gastric cancer in the USA and Europe screening of all the population would be difficult to justify (Chamberlain *et al.*, 1986). An alternative is to screen high-risk groups. In Birmingham, England, all patients, from six general practices, who were over the age of 40 years and complained of dyspepsia were referred to a dyspepsia clinic for endoscopy. Over a 2-year period 15 gastric cancers were diagnosed and 2 (15%) had early gastric cancer (Allum *et al.*, 1986). Sixty-seven per cent of patients had a radical resection which is higher than the 18% reported previously from the same group.

Surgical treatment and staging

During the past 50 years there have been many reviews of the surgical treatment of gastric cancer which have produced remarkably similar findings. A summary of 7 studies (Swynnerton and Truelove, 1952; Gilbertson, 1969; Cassell and Robinson, 1976; Cady *et al.*, 1977; Dupont *et al.*, 1978; Bizer, 1983; Ziliotto *et al.*, 1987) is shown in Table 2.4. Almost 80% of patients will have an operation. The remaining

Table 2.4 Results of surgery taken from 7 studies (1952–1987)

No. of patients	Operation rate (%)	Resection rate (%)	5-year survival (%)
7044	79	62	12

patients will be deemed unsuitable for surgery because of metastatic disease or because they are considered a poor operative risk. Approximately 60% of patients will have the tumour resected. In some of the reviews it is not stated what proportion of these resections are considered curative, but usually this applies to 50% of cases. In any event the assessment of curative resection is very subjective and may not accurately reflect the adequacy of the surgery. Laparotomy and biopsy or a palliative bypass procedure is performed in 20%. The results of surgery have remained remarkably static during the past 30 years. The only real area of improvement has been the reduction in the operative mortality rates. These have declined in one group's experience from 22.5% in the period 1969–1977 to 11.76% in the period 1978–1982 (Gall and Hermanek, 1985). Gilbertson (1969) reviewed the surgical experience in gastric cancer of the University of Minnesota between 1936 and 1963 and concluded that more extensive surgery excisions did not lead to an improvement in survival. Indeed, he argued that patients fared worse under an aggressive surgical policy; the 5-year survival of patients having a curative resection between 1950 and 1958 was 28% compared to a 17% survival for 1958–1963 when more radical surgery was performed. This finding was explained by an increase in operative mortality for partial gastrectomy (25.6%) and total gastrectomy (33.3%) during the second period. With the recent improvements in postoperative care this argument may now be spurious.

We recently reviewed 328 patients with histologically proven gastric adenocarcinoma diagnosed between 1974 and 1984 (Cunningham *et al.*, 1987b). The types of operation and survival of patients for each subgroup are shown in Table 2.5 and Figure 2.1. Almost all of the long-term survivors came from the 128 patients in the curative resection group, a group which survived significantly longer ($P<0.001$) than any other. However, despite curative resection, only 24% of these patients were alive 5 years after diagnosis. For these patients, serosal involvement was the main determinant of survival (Table 2.6). The group with serosal involvement had

Table 2.5 Survival of patients with gastric cancer according to surgical procedure

Primary treatment	No. of patients (%)	Percentage surviving at years					Median survival (months)
		1	2	3	4	5	
Curative resection	128 (39.0)	63	47	36	30	24	21
Palliative resection	32 (9.8)	27	14	3	3	0	6
Gastroenterostomy	33 (10.1)	8	0	0	0	0	4
Celestin tube	26 (7.9)	8	4	4	4	0	2
Laparotomy alone	58 (17.7)	9	0	0	0	0	2
No surgery	51 (15.5)	12	6	3	3	3	1

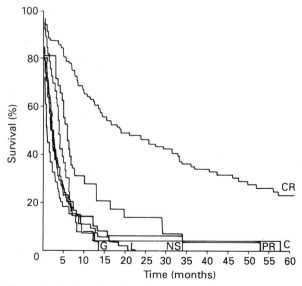

Figure 2.1 Survival by surgical procedure in 328 patients with gastric cancer. (CR, curative resection: n=128; PR, palliative resection: n=32; G, gastro-enterostomy: n=33; C, Celestin tube: n=26; L, laparotomy: n=58; NS, no surgery: n=51.) Survival of CR v. PR: $P < 0.001$. Survival of PR versus G+L+NS: $P < 0.01$

Table 2.6 Survival by serosal involvement, resection margin involvement and lymph node involvement in 128 patients and undergoing curative resection for gastric cancer

	No. of patients	Percentage surviving at years					p value
		1	2	3	4	5	
Serosa							
Positive	90	54	35	26	18	13	0.0004
Negative	38	85	78	59	59	47	
Margins							
Positive	33	41	7	7	0	0	0.0005
Negative	95	69	58	43	36	28	
Nodes							
Positive	65	55	37	27	22	17	0.04
Negative	63	71	57	45	37	31	

a 5-year survival rate of 13% compared to 47% for the group without serosal involvement. One explanation for the strong correlation between serosal involvement and survival, is that these patients have malignant cells in the peritoneal cavity (Nakajima *et al.*, 1978). Therefore it is likely that they have intraperitoneal micrometastases at presentation. Although lymph node involvement is generally regarded as a major prognostic factor in gastric cancer (Miwa, 1979), in our experience this only applied to patients without serosal involvement.

Resection margin involvement is also associated with a poor prognosis. Approximately 20–24% of patients having an apparently curative resection will have resection margin involvement (Papachristou *et al.*, 1980; British Stomach Cancer Group, 1984; Cunningham *et al.*, 1987b). This is a more common finding in patients with tumours of the diffuse type because these tumours infiltrate submucosally, thus the tumour margins are difficult to define macroscopically. Examination of the resection margins by frozen section may overcome this problem. In our series 31 of the 128 patients who had a curative resection had resection margin involvement and of these 31 patients 84% also had serosal involvement; therefore, by inference, their progress would have been poor regardless of resection margin involvement. In this regard it is of interest that in one study only 23% of the 73 patients with resection margin involvement developed anastomotic recurrence, the majority died of metastatic disease. Therefore, similar to serosal involvement, resection margin involvement may be indicative of a particularly aggressive gastric tumour. Tumours which involve the cardia have a poorer prognosis than those arising in the body or antrum of the stomach. This is due to the higher operative mortality for proximal tumours and the more frequent occurrence of resection margin involvement with tumours of the cardia (Gall and Hermanek, 1985). Patients with a long history of presenting symptoms fare significantly better than those with a short history. This finding was first reported by Swynnerton and Truelove in 1952 and may reflect differences in tumour biology.

The two basic types of operation for gastric cancer are subtotal resection and total resection of the stomach. Subtotal resection can be curative for antral tumours but for proximal tumours total resection is likely to be necessary. Both may be combined with an R1 lymph node resection (left and right cardiac nodes, nodes along the greater and lesser curvature) or an R2 resection (R1 plus gastric artery nodes, coeliac artery nodes, common hepatic artery nodes, lymph nodes of the splenic hilum, supra and infra pyloric nodes, splenic artery nodes) or R3 resection (R2 plus lymph nodes in the hepatoduodenal ligament, retropancreatic nodes, lymph nodes at the root of the mesentery, diaphragmatic and para-oesophageal nodes, splenectomy and for all except antral lesions the removal of the distal half of the pancreas). The value of radical surgery in the treatment of gastric cancer is unknown (Cuschieri, 1986). In particular, there is still controversy over the type of surgical procedure which should be performed for tumours of the body and antrum. There are proponents of both subtotal gastrectomy and total gastrectomy (McNeer et al., 1951; Gennari et al., 1986) but as yet no randomized trial has addressed this issue. From retrospective studies it is clear that the major problem in making the comparison of survival following either surgical procedure is that although one would expect total gastrectomy to produce more long-term survivors, this advantage is offset by the higher operative mortality for total gastrectomy (11.5–37.2%) compared to subtotal gastrectomy 3.2–23.7%) (Gennari et al., 1986).

Although the main aim of surgery in gastric cancer is to effect a cure, the palliative role of surgery should not be underestimated. Even in the presence of solitary or multiple liver metastases palliative resection may contribute to improved survival (Koga et al., 1980; Boddie et al., 1983) and may alleviate symptoms of upper gastrointestinal obstruction. Palliative bypass on the other hand did not appear to improve survival in our group of patients (Table 2.5) when compared to those patients who had laparotomy alone, hence it could be argued that this procedure should be reserved for those patients with tumours deemed likely to give rise to obstructive symptoms.

The Japanese experience with gastric cancer is considerable and the results which they have obtained with surgery are better than has been achieved in the USA or Europe. In a review of 4946 patients treated surgically in the National Cancer Centre, Tokyo between 1962 and 1984 Maruyama (1986) reported that 4734 patients (95.4%) underwent tumour resection and that the 5-year survival for these patients was 51%. The postoperative mortality rate was only 1.6%. Admittedly over 50% of patients had tumours which had not penetrated the serosa but even so the results are impressive. What can be learned from the Japanese experience? The emphasis must be on early diagnosis and low postoperative mortality. The Japanese perform, by US and European standards, radical surgery (Japanese Research Society for Gastric Cancer, 1981) but their results cannot be taken to indicate that a radical approach is necessarily best because there are no randomized trials in the Japanese literature which have addressed this issue.

The staging of gastric cancer is extremely important because it allows valid comparisons of the results from different centres and different surgical approaches to this tumour. In 1984 a new staging system was devised to replace the three other systems in current use (UICC, Japanese Research Society for Stomach Cancer (JRSSC) and the American Joint Committee on Cancer) and thus unify the description of gastric cancer in the USA, Europe and Japan. Essentially, it is a TNM system which recognizes four stages of gastric cancer. Its application depends upon the surgeon following the guidelines of the JRSGC (1981) coupled with a careful histological analysis of the resected tumour and regional lymph nodes. It is summarized in Table 2.7 and the corresponding survival figures from Maruyama (1986) show that the new staging effectively separates survival by stage.

Table 2.7 The new TNM classification with survival according to Maruyama (1986)

Stage		% Survival at 5 years
I	Ia T1 N0	
	Ib T1 N1	88
	T2 N0	
II	T1 N2	
	T2 N1	65
	T3 N0	
III	IIIa T2 N2	
	T3 N1	38
	T4 N0	
IV	ANY M1	5

T = Primary tumour
    T1 – Tumour limited to the mucosa and submucosa
    T2 – Tumour involves the subserosa
    T3 – Tumour penetrates the serosa

N = Regional lymph nodes
    N0 – No metastases to regional lymph nodes
    N1 – Involvement of perigastric lymph nodes within 3 cm from
        the primary tumour
    N2 – Involvement of regional lymph nodes more than 3 cm from
        the primary tumour

M = Distant metastases
    M0 – No evidence of distant metastases
    M1 – Evidence of distant metastases

Single agent chemotherapy

5-Fluorouracil (5-FU) has been extensively studied in gastric cancer and has an overall response rate of 22% with a response duration of 4–5 months (Comis and Carter, 1974). 5-FU has been given using a relatively intensive schedule of 15 mg/kg/24 hr × 5 i.v., then 7.5 mg/kg on alternate days to toxicity (Moertel, 1973a), or by administration as a continuous infusion (30 mg/kg/24 hr) for 72 hours every 2 weeks (Shah and McDonald, 1983). However, these different methods have not been associated with improved response rates and the conventional way of giving 5-FU as an intravenous bolus of 750–1000 mg/m^2 every week remains the mainstay of single agent treatment. The most common side-effects associated with 5-FU are stomatitis, diarrhoea, leucopenia and alopecia. Alopecia is dose-related and does not occur with low-dose regimens. Whereas giving 5-FU by continuous intravenous infusion has not been conclusively shown to be associated with higher response rates it is associated with less toxicity.

As a single agent, mitomycin-C has similar activity to 5-FU, with a response rate of 24% (Schein et al., 1978). Its use is associated with cumulative myelosuppression, mainly thrombocytopenia. In view of this the drug should be given as an intravenous bolus at no shorter than 6-weekly intervals. Mitomycin-C has also been linked to the development of the haemolytic-uraemic syndrome; it was reported in 8.5% of 251 patients receiving adjuvant mitomycin-C and 5-FU. Doxorubicin (Adriamycin) is relatively active in gastric cancer and produces tumour regression in 15–24% of patients (Moertel and Levin, 1979; Gastrointestinal Tumor Study

Group, 1979). Its use leads to alopecia, and at doses above $550\,mg/m^2$, it may cause a congestive cardiomyopathy. Epirubicin (Pharmarubicin) a derivative of doxorubicin is less cardiotoxic and produces less stomatitis than the parent compound and may offer some therapeutic advantages. Mitoxantrone a bis-substituted anthraquinone that binds to DNA, showed no activity in a group of 32 patients with advanced gastric cancer (De Simone, Gams and Birch, 1986). In one study, etoposide was shown to have modest activity in gastric cancer (Kelsen *et al.*, 1982).

The nitrosourea, methyl-CCNU has been used in combination with other cytotoxic drugs in a number of studies (Gastrointestinal Tumor Study Group, 1979; 1982), despite showing little efficacy as a single agent; Moertel reported only 8% of 37 patients responded (Moertel *et al.*, 1976). BCNU in limited testing had moderate activity (18%) in gastric cancer (Moertel, 1973b). Other cytotoxic drugs including methotrexate have received remarkably little attention. A report from the Gastrointestinal Tumor Study Group (GITSG) suggests little activity for methotrexate in patients who had been treated with previous chemotherapy but did show promising results for another folate antagonist triazinate (Bruckner, Likich and Stablein, 1982).

Cisplatin has significant activity in gastric cancer, with response rates of 25% in studies where some of the patients were pretreated with chemotherapy (Beer *et al.*, 1983; Leichman *et al.*, 1984; Lacave *et al.*, 1985). Cisplatin is highly emetogenic and nephrotoxic. Carboplatin, an analogue of cisplatin with less gastrointestinal renal toxicity, has been tested in a small number of patients with gastric cancer but so far the results show no significant activity (Einzig *et al.*, 1985) and the same applies to the cisplatin analogue TNO-6 (Cunningham *et al.*, 1986).

Combination chemotherapy

The Mayo Clinic were among the first to investigate combination chemotherapy. In one study patients were randomly allocated to 5-FU and methyl-CCNU alone. Response to the combination was 40% and the patients survived significantly longer following treatment with 5-FU but a subsequent study failed to confirm these results (Baker *et al.*, 1976; Moertel *et al.*, 1976). Doxorubicin has been added to the combination of 5-FU and methyl-CCNU (Gatrointestinal Tumor Study Group, 1979; 1982; 1984). When the results of these studies are combined the response rate is only 35% (14 of 40 patients with measurable disease). Levi, Dalley and Aroney (1979) treated 35 evaluable patients with the combination of 5-FU, Adriamycin and BCNU (FAB) and found 18 (51%) of patients responded with a median duration of response of 10 months. However, a subsequent randomized study showed no difference in the survival of patients treated with single agent Adriamycin compared with FAB (Levi *et al.*, 1986). Also Schnitzler *et al.* (1986) randomized 77 patients to either FAB or 5-FU and BCNU in combination (FB) and reported that only 24% of patients responded to FAB and 11% responded to FB with no difference in survival between the 2 groups. Triazinate the antifolate has been combined with mitomycin-C to treat advanced gastric cancer. Using this combination O'Connell *et al.* (1987) have treated 33 patients, 29 of whom had failed previous chemotherapy. Nine (27%) patients had a partial response.

The FAM regimen has been extensively investigated. Preliminary results indicated that over 50% of patients would respond to the combination but subsequent Phase II data have shown the figure to be lower (Table 2.8).

Table 2.8 Details of FAM regimen and response to treatment

Drug/dose/days/reference		No. of patients	Complete response (CR)	Partial response (PR)	CR + PR (%)
5-FU 600 mg/m^2 days 1, 8, 29, 36 Adriamycin i.v. 30 mg/m^2 days 1, 29 Mitomycin C i.v. 10 mg/m^2 days 1 MacDonald *et al.* (1980)	} Every 8 weeks	62	–	26	42
5-FU 600 mg/m^2 days 1, 8, 29, 36 Adriamycin i.v. 30 mg/m^2 days 1, 29 Mitomycin C i.v. 10 mg/m^2 days 1 Cunningham *et al.* (1984)	} Every 8 weeks	81	4	24	35
5-FU 600 mg/m^2 days 1, 8, 29, 36 Adriamycin i.v. 30 mg/m^2 days 1, 29 Mitomycin C i.v. 10 mg/m^2 days 1 Fraschini *et al.* (1983)	} Every 8 weeks	47	1	20	45

Furthermore, two randomized studies have failed to show a benefit of FAM over 5-FU in terms of overall survival (Cullinan *et al.*, 1985; Beretta *et al.*, 1989). Bertino *et al.* (1977) were the first to demonstrate a synergism between 5-FU and methotrexate. Klein *et al.* (1983) utilized this effect in the treatment of gastric cancer and reported a very high response rate to the combination of 5-FU, methotrexate and Adriamycin (FAMTX) and emphasized the lack of toxicity. These data and the results from two other studies are shown in Table 2.9. The combination has significant activity in gastric cancer but it can be myelosuppressive. In the EORTC phase II study (Wils *et al.*, 1986) its use was associated with 4 toxic deaths although 3 of them occurred in patients where the treatment protocol had not been closely adhered to. Analysis of a subsequent randomized EORTC study of FAM versus FAMTX shows no difference in toxicity between the two arms and a significantly ($P = 0.004$) higher response rate to FAMTX (44%) compared to FAM (14%) but it is too early to assess survival (Wils *et al.*, 1989).

Because cisplatin has shown such promising activity as a single agent (Beer *et al.*, 1983; Leichman *et al.*, 1984; Lacave *et al.*, 1985) it has been incorporated into a

Table 2.9 Details of FAMTX regimen

Drug/dose/days/reference	No. of patients	Complete response (CR)	Partial response (PR)	CR + PR (%)
Wils *et al.* (1986)	67	9	13	33
Cunningham *et al.* (1985)	11	–	2	18
Klein *et al.* (1983)	30	2	17	63
Total	(108)	(11)	32	40

FAMTX regimen
Methotrexate 1.5 g/m^2 day 1 followed by 5-fluorouracil (1 hour later) 1.5 g/m^2 day 1 }
Folinic acid 15 mg/m^2 every 6 hours for 48 hours beginning after chemotherapy   } Every 28 weeks
Adriamycin i.v. 30 mg/m^2 day 15 }

number of phase II studies of combination chemotherapy (Table 2.10). The addition of cisplatin to other agents such as 5-FU and doxorubicin results in relatively high response rates. Moreover, the three-drug combination, cisplatin, etoposide and doxorubicin (EAP), has been investigated in a large phase II study with extremely encouraging results (Table 2.10). EAP has also been used to treat patients with inoperable primary tumours where there was no evidence of metastatic disease. In a group of 35 patients the overall response to EAP was 69% including a 23% complete response rate. Twenty of the responders had a resection after chemotherapy and 6 were confirmed as complete pathological remissions (Preusser *et al.*, 1989). The GITSG have compared 5-FU, doxorubicin and semustine (FAMe) with 5-FU, doxorubicin and triazinate (FAT) with 5-FU, doxorubicin and cisplatin (FAP) in a randomized trial of 249 patients with gastric cancer. The survival of patients in the FAT and FAP arms was significantly better than FAMe arm; the 1-year survival in the FAT arm was 30%, in the FAP arm 32% and in the FAMe arm 15% (Gastrointestinal Tumor Study Group, 1988).

Further trials of chemotherapy are required to determine new, active cytotoxic drugs and to optimize the best presently available cytotoxic drugs for clinical use. Promising addition to the list of active single agents include cisplatin and triazinate

Table 2.10 Phase II studies of cisplatin combinations in gastric cancer

Drug/dose/days/reference		No. of evaluable patients	Complete response (CR)	Partial response (PR)	CR + PR (%)
Cisplatin infusion 100 mg/m^2 24 hr i.v. 5-FU 1000 mg/m^2 infusion over 5 days beginning on day 2 Lacave *et al.* (1989)	Repeat every 3 weeks	56	2	20	41
Cisplatin 20 mg/m^2 i.v. days 1–5 5-FU 300 mg/m^2 i.v. days 1–5 Doxorubicin 50 mg/m^2 i.v. day 1 Wagener *et al.* (1985)	Repeat every 3 weeks	18	–	9	50
Cisplatin 75 mg/m^2 i.v. day 1 5-FU 600 mg/m^2 i.v. days 1–5 Doxorubicin 40 mg/m^2 i.v. day 1 Cazap *et al.* (1986)	Repeat every 4 weeks	35	–	10	29
Cisplatin 100 mg/m^2 day 2 5-FU 1 g/m^2 per day i.v. infusion over 5 days Rougier *et al.* (1989)	Repeat every 4 weeks	50	4	19	52
Total		159	6	58	172
Cisplatin 40 mg/m^2 i.v. days 2 and 8 Etoposide 120 mg/m^2 i.v. days 4, 5 and 6 Doxorubicin 20 mg/m^2 i.v. days 1 and 7 Wilke *et al.* (1989)	Repeat every 4 weeks	145	22	61	57
Etoposide 100 mg i.v. days 1–3 Adriamycin 20 mg/m^2 i.v. days 1 and 8 Cisplatin 40 mg/m^2 i.v. days 1 and 8	Repeat every 4 weeks	25	3	15	72
Total		170	25	76	129

and survival benefit from combination chemotherapy regimens containing these drugs are now evident. For some of these patients successful treatment may result in sufficient tumour regression to allow the resection of a primary tumour initially deemed to be inoperable. Therefore, the potential benefits from chemotherapy of this subgroup of patients are considerable, particularly if side-effects of treatment such as nausea and vomiting can be abolished, and with the new 5-HT$_3$ antagonists (Cunningham *et al.*, 1987b) this may become possible.

Adjuvant chemotherapy

As yet there is no convincing evidence that chemotherapy can improve the survival of patients after surgical resection of the primary tumour. In a large randomized series (1616 patients), in the mid sixties, the Veterans Administration failed to show any benefit from intra-operative and adjuvant thiotepa – indeed the treatment group fared slightly worse (Longmire, Kirzma and Dixon, 1968; Dixon, Longmire and Holden, 1971). They also studied adjuvant floxuridine in 400 patients but again showed no difference in survival between control and treatment groups (Serlin *et al.*, 1969). 5-FU in combination with methyl-CCNU has been reported in three large series (Douglas and Stanlein, 1982; Higgins *et al.*, 1983; Engestrom *et al.*, 1985). The first of these from the GITSG showed significant benefit (40 deaths in 71 control patients; 29 deaths in 71 treated patients) at a median follow-up time of 48 months (Douglas and Stanlein, 1982). However, in a similar study where 200 patients were randomized to intravenous 5-FU and oral methyl-CCNU for a period of 2 years, or no treatment after surgical resection, there was no significant difference in disease-free survival or overall survival between the 2 groups (Engestrom *et al.*, 1985). The third study of 5-FU and methyl-CCNU whilst showing an early survival advantage for the treatment group, showed no difference in survival between treatment and control groups at a median follow-up of 42 months (Higgins *et al.*, 1983). The British Stomach Group has conducted a randomized trial of 5-FU and mitomycin-C, with or without an induction course of 5-FU, vincristine, cyclophosphamide and vincristine against no treatment after surgery. They were unable to show any overall survival benefit from chemotherapy in this large well-designed study which accrued over 400 patients (Allum, Hallissey and Kelley, 1989). Adjuvant FAM has also been studied with a negative result as an adjuvant to surgery in a multicentre study (Wils *et al.*, 1986).

There have been a number of adjuvant studies from Japan. However, because adjuvant chemotherapy is now accepted as a standard treatment following surgery in many centres in Japan, the most recent studies do not possess non-treatment control arms (Inokuchi *et al.*, 1984; Hattori *et al.*, 1986). This is disappointing because many of the earlier studies in the Japanese literature, taken to indicate definitive evidence of the value of adjuvant chemotherapy show only marginal benefits. Imanaga and Nakazota (1977) reported benefit from adjuvant mitomycin-C (0.08 mg/kg × 2 weekly for 5 weeks after surgery) in a randomized study of 520 patients, with a 5-year survival of 68% in the treatment group compared to 54% in the control group. However, these results could not be reproduced in a subsequent phase of the study where the same treatment formed one of 3 arms. The other 2 arms were mitomycin-C, 5-FU and cytosine arabinoside and a control arm. Survival was not significantly improved with either chemotherapy (Imanaga and Nakazato, 1977). In a recent study from Japan the survival of 2873 patients was analysed after random allocation to one of 3 treatments (Hattori *et al.*, 1986). Group A were given bolus mitomycin-C with no further therapy. Group B were given bolus mitomycin-C and oral futraful for 1 year and group C were given oral futraful alone for 1 year. There was no difference in the 5-year survival of the 3 groups.

Radiotherapy

There is relatively little information on the efficacy of radiation therapy in the treatment of gastric cancer. Many reviews cite the experience of Wieland and Hymmen (1970) who reported an 11% 3-year survival and a 7% 5-year survival in 82 patients treated with radiation (60 Gy) alone. These results published in 1970 are taken to show that radiation therapy is effective in gastric cancer. They are further supported by the findings of Hoshi (1968) who gave radiation preoperatively and reported histological evidence of radiation damage to the resected tumour in 25–88% of cases depending on the dose of radiation administered. However, Falkeson and Falkeson (1969) found no responders in a group of patients with measurable lesions treated with radiation alone, compared to a 17% response rate for patients treated with 5-FU and a 55% response for patients treated with a combination of 5-FU and radiation.

The promising results from the combination of radiation and 5-FU were also shown by a study from the Mayo Clinic in which patients with unresectable gastric cancer were randomly allocated to radiation therapy (35–40 Gy) and placebo or the same dose of radiation plus 5-FU given at a dose of 15 mg/kg daily over 3 days prior to radiation (Moertel *et al.*, 1969). Forty-eight patients entered the trial; the mean survival for the combined treatment arm was 13 months and 3 patients were alive at 5 years compared to a mean survival of 5.9 months for the radiation and placebo arm and all patients in this group were dead at 5 years. More intensive chemotherapy regimens have subsequently been used in combination with radiation therapy. One study randomized 90 patients with locally unresectable gastric cancer to receive chemotherapy consisting of 5-FU and methyl-CCNU or radiation (50 Gy) given concurrently with 5-FU and then later the same combination of 5-FU and methyl-CCNU (Schein and Novak, 1982). Although there was a median survival advantage for the chemotherapy alone group (70 weeks versus 36 weeks for the combined modality group) the analysis at 5 years favoured the combined modality treatment; 16% of the combined treatment arm were alive compared to 7% in the chemotherapy arm. The reason for this was the early, higher mortality related to the combined modality therapy. A randomized study from the Eastern Cooperative Oncology Group (Klaassen *et al.*, 1985) failed to confirm the Mayo Clinic data (Moertel *et al.*, 1969). Fifty-seven patients with histologically confirmed, unresectable gastric cancer were allocated to 5-FU 600 mg/m^2 once weekly or radiation therapy (40 Gy) combined with 5-FU 600 mg/m^2 i.v. for the first 3 days of radiotherapy and then 5-FU 600 mg/m^2 i.v. weekly. The survival of both treatment groups was almost identical; for 5-FU alone the median survival was 9.3 months, 5-FU plus radiation 8.2 months. Toxicity was more marked with combined modality treatment.

The toxicity related to combined modality therapy was also highlighted in a study from O'Connell *et al.* (1985). In this pilot study patients with locally advanced gastric cancer were treated with 5-FU and Adriamycin followed by concurrent radiation and 5-FU, Adriamycin and methyl-CCNU. Patients experienced severe and prolonged nausea, weight loss and sepsis, and despite the achievement of local control of tumour all but 2 patients had progression of distant metastases.

Intra-operative radiation treatment has been pioneered by Abe *et al.* (1975). The radiation is delivered as a single fraction (30–40 Gy) to the tumour bed and surrounding lymph glands. In a non-randomized trial (patients received intra-operative radiation therapy depending on the day of surgery) there were survival advantages for the group treated with intra-operative radiation therapy. This advantage was particularly marked in those patients where the tumour had penetrated the serosa and invaded surrounding structures such as the pancreas. For this group the 5-year survival was 27% when treated with intra-operative radiation therapy compared to 0% when treated by surgery alone (Abe and Takahashi, 1981). These results have yet to be confirmed in a randomized trial.

References

Abe, M. and Takahashi, M. (1981) Intraoperative radiotherapy: the Japanese experience. *International Journal of Radiation, Oncology, Biology and Physics*, **7**, 863–868

Abe, M., Takahashi, M., Yabumoto, E. *et al.* (1975) Techniques, indications and results of intraoperative radiotherapy of advanced cancers. *Radiology*, **116**, 693–702

Allum, W. H., Hallissey, M. T., Dorrell, A. *et al.* (1986) Programme for early detection of gastric cancer. *British Medical Journal*, **293**, 541

Allum, W. H., Hallissey, M. T. and Kelley, K. A. (1989) Adjuvant chemotherapy in operable gastric cancer. *Lancet*, **1**, 571–574

Antonioli, D. A. and Goldman, H. (1982) Changes in the location and type of gastric adenocarcinoma. *Cancer*, **50**, 775–781

Baker, L.H., Talley, R. W., Matter, R. *et al.* (1976). Phase III comparison of the treatment of advanced gastrointestinal cancer with bolus weekly 5-FU vs methyl-CCNU plus bolus weekly 5-FU. *Cancer*, **38**, 1–8

Barrett, N. F. (1950) Chronic peptic ulcer of the oesophagus and oesophagitis. *British Journal of Surgery*, **38**, 175–182

Beer, M., Cocconi, G., Ceci, G. *et al.* (1983) A phase II study of cisplatin in advanced gastric cancer. *European Journal of Cancer and Clinical Onocology*, **19**, 717–720

Berenson, M. M., Riddell, R. H., Skinner, D. B. and Freston, J. W. (1978) Malignant transformation of esophageal columnar epithelium. *Cancer*, **41**, 554–561

Beresford, S. A. A. (1985) Is nitrate in the drinking water associated with the risk of cancer in the urban UK? *International Journal of Epidemiology*, **14**, 57–63

Beretta, G., Arnoldi, E., Beretta, G. D. *et al.* (1989) A randomized study of fluorouracil versus FAM polychemotherapy in gastric carcinoma. *Proceedings of the EORTC Symposium on Advances in Gastrointestinal Tract Cancer Research and Treatment*, p. 48

Bertino, J. R., Sawicki, W. L., Lindquist, C. A. and Gupta, V. S. (1977) Schedule-dependent antitumour effects of methotrexate and 5-fluorouracil. *Cancer Research*, **37**, 327–334

Binkerd, E. F. and Kolari, O. E. (1975) The history and use of nitrate and nitrite in the curing of meat. *Food and Cosmetic Toxicology*, **13**, 655–661

Bizer, L. D. (1983) Adenocarcinoma of the stomach: current results of treatment. *Cancer*, **51**, 743–745

Boddie, A. W., McMurtrey, M. J., Giacco, C. G. and McBride, C. M. (1983) Palliative total gastrectomy and oesophagogastrectomy: a re-evaluation. *Cancer*, **51**, 1195–1200

Borch, K. (1986) Epidemiologic, clinicopathologic and economic aspects of gastroscopic screening of patients with pernicious anaemia. *Scandinavian Journal of Gastroenterology*, **21**, 21–30

Brand, D. L., Ylvisaker, J. T., Gelfand, M. and Pope, C. E. (1980) Regression of columnar oesophageal (Barrett's epithelium after anti-reflux surgery. *New England Journal of Medicine*, **302**, 844–848

British Stomach Cancer Group (1984) Resection line disease in stomach cancer. *British Medical Journal*, **289**, 601–603

Bruckner, H. W., Likich, J. J. and Stablein, D. M. (1982) Studies of Baker's Antifol methotrexate and razosxone in advanced gastric cancer: A Gastrointestinal Tumour Study Group Report. *Cancer Treatment Reports*, **66**, 1713–1717

Cady, B., Ramsden, D. A., Stein, A. and Haggitt, R. C. (1977) Gastric cancer. Contemporary aspects. *American Journal of Surgery*, **133**, 423–429

Capoferro, R. and Torgersen, O. (1974) The effect of hypertonic saline on the uptake of tritiated 7,12-dimethylbenz(a) antrancene by the gastric mucosa. *Scandinavian Journal of Gastroenterology*, **9**, 343–349

Cassell, P. and Robinson, J. O. (1976) Cancer of the stomach: a review of 854 patients. *British Journal of Surgery*, **63**, 603–607

Caygill, C., Day, D. W. and Hill, M. J. (1986) Gastric cancer in Norfolk. *British Journal of Cancer*, **52**, 145–147

Caygill, C. P. J., Hill, M. J., Kirkham, J. S. and Northfield, T. C. (1986) Mortality from gastric cancer following gastric surgery for peptic ulcer. *Lancet*, **i**, 929–931

Cazap, E. L., Gisselbrecht, C., Smith, F. P. *et al.* (1986) Phase II trials of 5-FU, doxorubicin and cisplatin in advanced, measurable adenocarcinoma of the lung and stomach. *Cancer Treatment Reports*, **70**, 781–783

Chamberlain, J., Day, N. E., Hakama, M. *et al.* (1986) UICC workshop of the project on evaluation of screening programmes for gastrointestinal cancer. *International Journal of Cancer*, **37**, 329–334

Comis, R. L. and Carter, S. K. (1974) A review of chemotherapy in gastric cancer. *Cancer*, **34**, 1576–1586

Correa, P., Cuello, C., Fajardo, L. F. *et al.* (1983) Diet and gastric cancer: nutrition survey in a high risk area. *Journal of the National Cancer Institute*, **70**, 673–678

Correa, P., Fontham, E., Pickle, L. W. *et al.* (1985) Dietary determinants of gastric cancer in South Louisiana inhabitants. *Journal of the National Cancer Institute*, **75**, 645–654

Correa, P., Haenszell, W., Cuello, C. *et al.* (1975) A model for gastric cancer epidemiology. *Lancet*, **ii**, 58–60

Correa, P., Sasano, N., Stemmermann, G. N. *et al.* (1973) Pathology of gastric carcinoma in Japanese populations: comparisons between Miyagi Prefecture, Japan and Hawaii. *Journal of the National Cancer Institute*, **51**, 1449–1459

Cullinan, S. A., Moertel, C. G., Fleming, T. R. *et al.* (1985) A comparison of three chemotherapeutic regimens in the treatment of advanced pancreatic and gastric carcinoma. *Journal of the American Medical Association*, **253**, 2061–2067

Cunningham, D., Gilchrist, N. L., Forrest, G. J. *et al.* (1985) Chemotherapy in advanced gastric cancer. *Cancer Treatment Reports*, **69**, 927–928

Cunningham, D., Hawthorn, J., Pople, A. *et al.* (1987a) Prevention of emesis in patients receiving cytotoxic drugs by GR38032F, a selective 5-HT3 receptor antagonist. *Lancet*, **i**, 1461–1462

Cunningham, D., Hole, D., Carter, D. C. *et al.* (1987b) An evaluation of the prognostic factors in gastric cancer: the effect of chemotherapy on survival. *British Journal of Surgery*, **74**, 715–720

Cunningham, D., Soukop, M., McArdle, C. S. *et al.* (1984) Advanced gastric cancer: experience in Scotland using 5-fluorouracil, adriamycin and mitomycin-C. *British Journal of Surgery*, **71**, 673–676

Cunningham, D., Soukop, M., Gilchrist, N. L. *et al.* (1986) TNO-6 has no effect in gastrointestinal cancer: N-acetyl-glucosaminidase shows renal damage. *Medical Oncology and Tumour Pharmacotherapy*, **3**, 25–28

Cuschieri, A. (1986) Gastrectomy for gastric cancer: definitions and objectives. *British Journal of Surgery*, **73**, 513–514

De Simone, P. A., Gams, R. and Birch, R. (1986). Phase II evaluation of mitoxantrone in advanced carcinoma of the stomach: a South-eastern Cancer Study Group Trial. *Cancer Treatment Reports*, **70**, 1043–1044

Deng, G., Ju, Y., Chen, S. *et al.* (1987) Activated c-Ha-ras oncogene with a guanine to thymine transversion at the twelfth codon in a human stomach cancer cell line. *Cancer Research*, **47**, 3195–3198

Dixon, W. J., Longmire, W. P. and Holden, W. D. (1971) Use of triethylenethiophosphoramide as an adjuvant to the surgical treatment of gastric and colorectal carcinoma: ten year follow up. *Annals of Surgery*, **173**, 16–23

Douglas, H. O. and Stanlein, D. M. (1982) Controlled trial of adjuvant chemotherapy following curative resection for gastric cancer. *Cancer*, **49**, 1116–1122

Douglass, M. L. Kabacoff, B. L., Anderson, G. A. and Cheng, M. C. (1978) The chemistry of nitrosamine formation, inhibition and destruction. *Journal of the Society of Cosmetic Chemistry*, **29**, 581–606

Dupont, J. B., Lee, J. R., Burton, G. R. and Cohn, I. (1978) Adenocarcinoma of the stomach: review of 1497 cases. *Cancer*, **41**, 941–947

Einzig, A., Kelsen, D. P., Cheng, E. *et al.* (1985) Phase II trial of carboplatin in patients with adenocarcinomas of the upper gastrointestinal tract. *Cancer Treatment Reports*, **69**, 1453–1454

Engestrom, P. F., Lavin, P. T., Douglass, H. O. and Brunner, K. W. (1985) Postoperative adjuvant 5-fluorouracil plus methyl-CCNU therapy for gastric cancer patients. *Cancer*, **55**, 1868–1873

Esaki, Y., Hirokawa, K. and Yamashiro, M. (1987) Multiple gastric cancers in the aged with special reference to intramucosal cancer. *Cancer*, **59**, 560–565

Evans, D. M. D., Craven, J. L., Murphy, F. and Cleary, L. (1978) Comparison of 'early gastric cancer' in Britain and Japan. *Gut*, **19**, 1–19

Falkeson, G. and Falkeson, H. C. (1969) Fluorouracil and radiotherapy in gastrointestinal cancer. *Lancet*, **ii**, 1252–1253

Fey, M. F., Hesketh, C., Wainscoat, J. S. *et al.* (1989) Clonal allele loss in gastrointestinal cancers. *British Journal of Cancer*, **59**, 750–754

Fielding, J. L. W., Ellis, D. J., Jones, B. G. *et al.* (1980) Natural history of 'early gastric' cancer: results of a 10-year regional survey. *British Medical Journal*, **281**, 965–967

Forman, D., Al-Dabbagh, S. and Doll, R. (1985) Nitrates, nitrites and gastric cancer in Great Britain. *Nature*, **313**, 620–625

Fraschini, P., Beretta, G., Arnoldi, E. *et al.* (1983) Confirmed activity of FAM polychemotherapy in advanced gastric carcinoma. *Tumori*, **69**, 59–64

Fujita, S. (1978) Biology of early gastric carcinoma. *Pathology Research and Practice*, **163**, 297–309

Fukshige, S. I., Matsubara, K. I., Yoshida, M. *et al.* (1986) Localization of a novel v-erbB-related gene, C erbB-2 on human chromosome 17 and its amplification in a gastric cancer cell line. *Molecular and Cellular Biology*, **63**, 955–958

Gall, F. P. and Hermanek, P. (1985) New aspects in the surgical treatment of gastric carcinoma – a comparative study of 1936 patients operated on between 1969 and 1982. *European Journal of Surgical Oncology*, **11**, 219–225

Gastrointestinal Tumor Study Group (GITSG) (1979) Phase II-III chemotherapy studies in advanced gastric cancer. *Cancer Treatment Reports*, 1871–1876

Gastrointestinal Tumor Study Group (GITSG) (1982) A comparative clinical assessment of the combination chemotherapy in the management of advanced gastric cancer. *Cancer*, **49**, 1362–1366

Gastrointestinal Tumor Study Group (GITSG) (1984) Randomized study of combination chemotherapy in unresectable gastric cancer. *Cancer*, **53**, 13–17

Gastrointestinal Tumor Study Group (GITSG) (1988) Triazinate and platinum efficacy in combination with 5-fluorouracil and doxorubicin: results of a three-arm randomized trial in metastatic gastric cancer. *Journal of the National Cancer Institute*, **80**, 1011–1015

Gennari, L., Bozzetti, F., Bonfanti, G. *et al.* (1986) Subtotal versus total gastrectomy for cancer of the lower two-thirds of the stomach: a new approach to an old problem. *British Journal of Surgery*, **73**, 534–538

Gilbertston, V. A. (1969) Results of treatment of stomach cancer. *Cancer*, **23**, 1305–1308

Grabiec, J. and Owen, D. A. (1985) Carcinoma of the stomach in young persons. *Cancer,* **56**, 380–396

Gunderson, L. L. and Sosin, H. (1982) Adenocarcinoma of the stomach: areas of failure in a reoperation series (second of symptomatic looks): clinicopathologic correlation and implications for adjuvant therapy. *International Journal of Radiation Oncology Biology and Physics*, **8**, 1–11

Haenszel, W., Kurihara, M., Locke, F. B. *et al.* (1976) Stomach cancer in Japan. *Journal of the National Cancer Institute*, **56**, 265–274

Haenszel, W., Kurihara, M., Segi, M and Lee, R. C. K. (1972) Stomach cancer among Japanese in Hawaii. *Journal of the National Cancer Institute*, **49**, 969–988

Haggitt, R. C., Tryzellar, J., Ellis, F. H. and Colcher, H. (1978) Adenocarcinomá complicating columnar epithelium-lined (Barrett's) oesophagus. *American Journal of Clinical Pathology*, **70**, 1–5

Hall, C. N., Darkin, D., Briblecombe, R. *et al.* (1986) Evaluation of the nitrosamine hypothesis of gastric carcinogenesis in precancerous conditions. *Gut*, **27**, 491–498

Hattori, T., Inokuchi, K., Taguchi, T. and Abe, O. (1986) Postoperative adjuvant chemotherapy for gastric cancer, the second report. *Japanese Journal of Surgery*, **16**, 175–180

Hattori, H., Asai, C. and Segi, R. (eds) (1984) Age adjusted death rates for cancer for selected sites (A-classification) in 46 countries in 1978. Nagoya, Japan: *Segi Institute of Cancer Epidemiology*.

Hawe, A., Payne, S. W., Weiland, L. H. and Fontana, R. A. (1973) Adenocarcinoma in the columnar epithelium lined lower (Barrett) esophagus. *American Journal of Clinical Pathology*, **70**, 1–5

Hermans, P. E., Diax-buxo, J. A. and Stobo, J. D. (1976) Idiopathic late-onset immunoglobulin deficiency. Clinical observation in 50 patients. *American Journal of Medicine*, **61**, 221–237

Higgins, G. A., Amadeo, J. H., Smith, D. E. *et al.* (1983) Efficacy of prolonged intermittent therapy with combined 5-FU and methyl-CCNU following resection for gastric carcinoma. *Cancer*, **52**, 1105–1112

Hoshi, H. (1968) Histologic studies on the effect of preoperative irradiation on gastric cancer. *Tokohu Journal of Experimental Medicine*, **6**, 293

Houghton, P. W. J., Mortenson, N. J. McC., Allan, A. *et al.* (1985) Early gastric cancer: the case for long term surveillance. *British Medical Journal*, **291**, 305–308

Imanaga, H. and Nakazato, H. (1977) Results of surgery for gastric cancer and effect of mitomycin-C on cancer recurrence. *World Journal of Surgery*, **1**, 213–221

Inokuchi, K., Hattori, T., Taguchi, T. *et al.* (1984) Postoperative adjuvant chemotherapy for adjuvant therapy. *Cancer*, **52**, 2393–2397

Ishii, S., Xu, H. Y., Stratton, R. H. *et al.* (1985) Characterization and sequence of the promotor region of the human epidermal growth factor receptor gene. *Proceedings of the National Academy of Science USA*, **82**, 4920–4924

Japanese Research Society for Gastric Cancer (1981) The general rules for the gastric cancer study in surgery and pathology. *Japanese Journal of Surgery*, **11**, 127–139

Kato, D. (1989) Surgery for gastric cancer. *Lancet*, **i**, 622

Katz, A., Gansl, R., Simon, S. *et al.* (1989) Phase II trial of VP-16, adriamycin and cisplatinum in patients with advanced gastric cancer. *Proceedings of the American Society of Clinical Oncology*, **8**, 98

Kelsen, D. P., Magill, G., Cheng, E. *et al.* (1982) Phase II trial of etoposide (VP-16) in the treatment of upper gastrointestinal malignancies. *Proceedings of the American Society of Clinical Oncology*, 96

Klaassen, D. J., MacIntyre, J. M., Catton, G. E. *et al.* (1985) Treatment of locally unresectable cancer of the stomach and pancreas: a randomized comparison of 5-fluorouracil alone with radiation plus concurrent and maintenance 5-fluorouracil – an Eastern Cooperative Oncology Study Group study. *Journal of Clinical Oncology*, **3**, 373–378

Klein, H. O., Dias Wickramanayake, P., Dieterle, F. *et al.* (1983) High-dose MTX/5-FU and adriamycin for gastric cancer. *Seminars in Oncology*, **10**, 29–31

Koga, S., Kawaguchi, H., Kishimote, H. *et al.* (1980) Therapeutic significance of noncurative gastrectomy for gastric cancer with liver metastases. *American Journal of Surgery*, **136**, 356–359

Kota, T., Matsushima, S., Saski, A. *et al.* (1985) C-myc gene amplification in primary stomach cancer. *Japanese Journal of Cancer Research*, **76**, 551–554

Kubo, T. (1971) Histologic appearance of gastric carcinoma in high and low mortality countries: comparison between Kyushu, Japan and Minnesota, USA. *Cancer*, **31**, 1498–1507

Kubo, T. (1973) Gastric carcinoma in New Zealand: some epidemiologic-pathologic aspects. *Cancer*, **31**, 1498–1507

Kubo, T. (1974) Geographic pathology of gastric carcinoma. *Acta Pathologica Japonica*, **24**, 465–479

Kurtz, R. C. and Sherlock, P. (1985) The diagnosis of gastric cancer. *Seminars in Oncology*, **12**, 11–18

Lacave, A. J., Buesa, J. M., Gracia, J. M. *et al.* (1989) Cisplatin and 5-fluorouracil in the treatment of advanced gastric cancer. *Proceedings of EORTC Symposium on Advances in Gastrointestinal Tract Cancer Research and Treatment*, 44

Lacave, A. J., Wils, J., Diaz-Rubio, E. *et al.* (1985) Cisplatin as second-line chemotherapy in advanced gastric adenocarcinoma. A phase II study of the EORTC Gastrointestinal Tract Cancer Cooperative Group. *European Journal of Cancer and Clinical Oncology*, **21**, 1321–1324

Lauren, P. (1965) The two histological main types of gastric carcinoma: Diffuse and so-called intestinal type carcinoma. *Acta Pathologica Microbiologica Scandinavia*, **64**, 31–49

Leichman, L., McDonald, B., Dindogru, A. *et al.* (1984) Cisplatin: an active drug in the treatment of disseminated cancer. *Cancer*, **53**, 18–22

Levi, J. A., Dalley, D. N. and Aroney, R. S. (1979) Improved combination chemotherapy in advanced gastric cancer. *British Medical Journal*, **2**, 1471–1473

Levi, J. A., Fox, R. M., Tattersall, M. H. *et al.* (1986) Analysis of a prospectively randomized comparison of doxorubicin versus 5-fluorouracil, doxorubicin and BCNU in advanced gastric cancer: implications for future studies. *Journal of Clinical Oncology*, **4**, 1348–1355

Longmire, W. P., Kirzma, J. W. and Dixon, W. J. (1968) The use of triethylenethiophosphoramide as an adjuvant to the surgical treatment of gastric carcinoma. *Annals of Surgery*, **167**, 293–312

Lundh, G., Burn, J. I., Kolig, G. *et al.* (1974) A cooperative international study of gastric cancer. *Annals of the Royal College of Surgeons of England*, **54**, 219–228

MacDonald, J. S., Schein, P. S., Wolley, M. D. *et al.* (1980) 5-fluorouracil, doxorubicin and mitomycin (FAM) combination chemotherapy for advanced gastric cancer. *Annals of Internal Medicine*, **93**, 533–536

McNeer, G., Vandenberg, H., Donn, F. Y. and Bowden, A. L. (1951) A critical evaluation of subtotal gastrectomy for the cure of cancer of the stomach. *Annals of Surgery*, **134**, 2–7

Maruyama, K. (1986) Results of surgery correlated with staging. In *Cancer of the Stomach* (eds P. E. Preece, A. Cuschieri and J. M. Wellwood) Grune and Stratton, London, pp. 145–163

Mewhouse, M. (1981) Epidemiology of asbestos related tumours. *Seminars in Oncology*, **8**, 250–257

Ming, S-C. (1977) Gastric carcinoma: a pathobiological classification. *Cancer*, **39**, 2475–2485

Mirvish, S. S., Wallcave, L., Eagen, M. and Shubik, P. (1972) Ascorbate-nitrate reaction: possible means of blocking the formation of carcinogenic N-nitroso compounds. *Science*, **177**, 65–68

Miwa, K. (1979) Cancer of the stomach in Japan. In *Recent Results of Cancer Treatment in Japan* (eds T. Kajitani, Y. Koyana, and Y. Umepaki), Japan Scientific Societies Press, Tokyo, pp. 61–75 (Gann monograph No. 22)

Moertel, C. G. (1973a) Clinical management of advanced gastrointestinal cancer. *Seminars in Drug Treatment*, **3**, 55–68

Moertel, C. G. (1973b) Therapy of advanced gastro-intestinal cancer with nitrosoureas. *Cancer Chemotherapy Reports*, **63**, 1863–1869

Moertel, C. G. (1986) The natural history of advanced gastric cancer. *Surgery Gynecology and Obstetrics*, **126**, 1071–1074

Moertel, C. G., Childs, D. S., Reitemeier, R. T. *et al.* (1969) Combined 5-fluorouracil and supervoltage radiation therapy of locally unresectable gastrointestinal cancer. *Lancet*, **ii**, 865–867

Moertel, C. G. and Levin, P. T. (1979) Phase II-III chemotherapy studies in advanced gastric cancer. *Cancer Treatment Reports*, **63**, 1863–1872

Moertel, C. G., Mittleman, J. A., Bakemeir, R. F. *et al.* (1976) Sequential and combination chemotherapy of advanced gastric cancer. *Cancer*, **38**, 678–682

Munoz, N. and Connelly, R. (1971) Time trends of intestinal and diffuse types of gastric cancer in the United States. *International Journal of Cancer*, **8**, 158–164

Murakami, T. (1979) Early cancer of the stomach. *World Journal of Surgery*, **3**, 685–692

Muto, M., Maki, T., Jamima, S. and Yamaguchi, I. (1968) Improvement in the end-results of surgical treatment of gastric cancer. *Surgery*, **63**, 229–235

Nakajima, T., Harashima, S., Hirata, M. and Kajitani, T. (1978) Prognostic and therapeutic values of peritoneal cytology in gastric cancer. *Acta Cytologica*, **22**, 225–229

O'Connell, M. J., Gunderson, L. L., Moertel, C. G. and Kvols, L. K. (1985) A pilot study to determine clinical tolerability of intensive combined modality therapy for locally unresectable gastric cancer. *International Journal of Radiation Oncology Biology and Physics*, **2**, 1827–1831

O'Connell, M. J., Schutt, A. J., Moertel, C. G. and Hahn, R. G. (1987) Phase II clinical trial of triazinate in combination with mitomycin-c for patients with advanced gastric cancer. *Journal of Clinical Oncology*, **5**, 83–85

Office of Population Censuses and Surveys (1985) *Cancer Statistics by Cause in England and Wales: 1982*. HMSO, London

Office of Population Censuses and Surveys (1986) *Cancer Statistics: 1983*. HMSO, London

Ogiu, T., Nakadate, M. and Odashima, S. (1975) Induction of leukaemias and digestive tract tumours in Donryu rats by 1-propyl-1-nitrosourea. *Journal of the National Cancer Institute*, **54**, 887–893

Ohuchi, N., Hand, P. H., Merlo, G. *et al.* (1987) Enhanced expression of c-Ha-ras p21 in human stomach adenocarcinomas defined by immunoassays using monoclonal antibodies and in situ hybridization. *Cancer Research*, **47**, 1413–1420

Oota, K. and Sobin, L. H. (1977) Histological typing of gastric and oesophageal tumours. WHO, Geneva

Oshima, A., Hirata, N., Ubukata, T. *et al.* (1986) Evaluation of a mass screening program for stomach cancer with a case-control study design. *International Journal of Cancer*, **38**, 829–833

Papachristou, D. N., Agnati, N., D'Agostine, H. and Fortnet, J. (1980) Histologically positive oesophageal margin in the surgical treatment of gastric cancer. *American Journal of Surgery*, **139**, 711–713

Paull, A., Trier, J. S., Dalton, M. D. *et al.* (1976) The histological spectrum of Barrett's oesophagus. *New England Journal of Medicine*, **295**, 476–480

Preusser, P., Wilke, H., Achterrath, W. *et al.* (1989) Neoadjuvant chemotherapy with the combination EAP (etoposide/adriamycin/cisplatin) in locally advanced, non-resectable gastric cancer. *Proceedings of the EORTC Symposium on Advances in Gastrointestinal Tract Cancer Research and Treatment*, 42

Reid, J. R. (1977) Nitrates in drinking water. *Report of a Meeting of a Working Group*. WHO, Geneva

Risch, H. A., Jain, M., Won Choi, N. *et al.* (1985) Dietary factors and the incidence of cancer of the stomach. *American Journal of Epidemiology*, **122**, 947–959

Rougier, P. H., Mahjoubi, M., Olivereira, J. *et al.* (1989) Treatment of advanced gastric adenocarcinoma (AGC) with 5-FU/platinum combination. *Proceedings of the EORTC Symposium of Advances in Gastrointestinal Tract Cancer Research and Treatment*, 45

Ruddell, W. S. J., Bone, E. S., Hill, M. J. *et al.* (1976) Gastric juice nitrite. A risk factor for cancer of the hypochlorhydric stomach. *Lancet*, **ii**, 550–552

Sainsbury, J. R. C., Sherbet, G. V., Farndon, J. R. and Harris, A. L. (1985) Epidermal growth factor receptors and oestrogen receptors in human breast cancer. *Lancet*, **i**, 364–366

Sandler, R. S and Holland, K. L. (1987) Trends in gastric cancer sex ratio in United States. *Cancer*, **59**, 1032–1035

Sato, O., Kamata, M. and Goto, S. (1985) Superficial spreading I + IIa type gastric cancer with an associated IIb lesion, report of a case. *Stomach and Intestine*, **20**, 63–70

Schein, P. S., MacDonald, J. S., Hoth, D. and Wooley, P. V. (1978) Mitomycin-C: experience in the United States; with emphasis on gastric cancer. *Cancer Chemotherapy and Pharmacology*, **1**, 73–75

Schein, P. S. and Novak, J. (1982) Combined modality therapy versus chemotherapy alone for locally unresectable gastric cancer. *Cancer*, **49**, 1771–1777

Schnitzler, G., Queisser, W., Heim, M. E. *et al.* (1986) Phase III study of 5-FU and carmustine versus 5-FU, carmustine and doxorubicin in advanced gastric cancer. *Cancer Treatment Reports*, **70**, 477–479

Serlin, O., Wolkoff, J. S., Amadeo, J. M. and Keehn, R. J. (1969) Use of 5-fluorodeoxyuridine (FUDR) as an adjuvant to the surgical management of carcinoma of the stomach. *Cancer*, **24**, 223–228

Shah, A. and MacDonald, W. (1983) Chemotherapy of advanced gastric cancer with 72 hour continuous intravenous 5-fluorouracil infusion at 2 week intervals. *Medical Pediatric Oncology*, **11**, 358–360

Spechler, S. J., Robbins, A. H., Rubins, H. A. *et al.*, (1984) Adenocarcinoma and Barrett's oesophagus. An overrated risk? *Gastroenterology*, **87**, 927–933

Svendsen, J. H., Dahl, C., Svendsen, L. B. and Christiansen, P. M. (1986) Gastric cancer in achlorhydric patients. A long term follow up study. *Scandinavian Journal of Gastroenterology*, **21**, 16–20

Swynnerton, B. F. and Truelove, S. C. (1952) Carcinoma of the stomach. *British Medical Journal*, **1**, 287–292

Tahara, E., Symiyoshi, H., Hata, J. *et al.* (1986) Human epidermal growth factor in gastric carcinoma as a biologic marker of high malignancy. *Japanese Journal of Cancer Research*, **77**, 145–152

Thomas, W. E. G., Cooper, M. J., Mortensen, N. J. McC. *et al.* (1984) The clinical assessment of duodenogastric reflux by scintigraphy and its relation to histological changes in gastric mucosa. *Scandinavian Journal of Gastroenterology*, **92**, 195–199

Trichopoulos, D., Ouranos, G., Day, N. E. *et al.* (1985) Diet and cancer of the stomach: a case-control study in Greece. *International Journal of Cancer*, **36**, 291–297

Tso., P. L., Bringaze, W. L., Dauterive, A. H. *et al.* (1987) Gastric carcinoma in the young. *Cancer,* **59,** 1362–1365

Viste, A., Bjornstead, E., Opheim, P. *et al.* (1986) Risk of carcinoma following gastric operations for benign disease. *Lancet,* **ii,** 502–504

Wagener, D. J., Yap, S. H., Wobbes, T. *et al.* (1985) Phase II trial of 5-fluorouracil, adriamycin and cisplatin (FAP) in advanced gastric cancer. *Cancer Chemotherapy Pharmacology,* **15,** 86–87

Wakabayashi, K., Ochiai, M., Saito, H. *et al.* (1983) Presence of 1-methyl-1,2,3,4-tetrahydro-B-carboline-3-carboxylic acid, a precursor of a mutagenic nitroso compound, in soy sauce. *Proceedings of the National Academy of Science USA,* **80,** 2912–2916

Waterhouse, J., Shanmugaratnam, K., Muir, C. and Powell, J. (eds) (1983) *Cancer Incidence in Five Continents.* Volume 4. Lyon: WHO. (International Agency for Research on Cancer. Scientific Publications No. 42)

Wieland, C. and Hymmen, U. (1970) Megavolttherapie maligner neoplasien des magens. *Strahlentherapie,* **40,** 20–26 (English Abstract)

Wilke, H., Preusser, P., Fink, U. *et al.* (1989) Clinical outcome and prognostic factors in 145 patients with advanced gastric cancer treated with EAP. *Proceedings of the EORTC Symposium on Advances in Gastrointestinal Tract Cancer Research and Treatment,* 43

Wils, J., Bleiberg, H., Dalesio, O. *et al.* (1986) An EORTC Gastrointestinal Group Evaluation of the combination of sequential methotrexate and 5-fluorouracil combined with adriamycin in advanced measurable gastric cancer. *Journal of Clinical Oncology,* **4,** 1799–1803

Wils. J., Coombes, R. C. and Chilvers, C. (1988) Randomized trial of FAM (5-FU, doxorubicin and mitomycin-C) chemotherapy versus control as adjuvant treatment for resected gastric carcinoma. *Proceedings of the American Society of Clinical Oncology,* **7,** 97

Wils, J., Klein, H. O., Wagener, D. Th. *et al.* (1989) Phase III study of sequential high dose MTX and 5-FU combined with adriamycin (FAMTX) versus FAM in advanced gastric cancer. *Proceedings of the EORTC Symposium on Advances in Gastrointestinal Tract Cancer Research and Treatment,* 46

Yang, D., Tannenbaum, S. R., Buchi, G. and Lee, G. C. (1984) 4-Chloro-6-methoxyindole is the precursor of a potent mutagen (4-chloro-6-methoxy-2-hydroxy-1-nitroso-indolin-3-one oxime) that forms during nitrosation of the fava bean (*Vicia faba*). *Carcinogenesis,* **5,** 1219–1224

Yokota, J., Yamamoto, T., Toyoshima, K. *et al.* (1986) Amplification of c-erbB-2 oncogene in human adenocarcinomas *in vivo. Lancet,* **i,** 364–366

Ziliotto, A., Kunzle, J. E., Souza, A. and Colicchio-Filho, O. (1987) Evolutive and prognostic aspects in gastric cancer. *Cancer,* **59,** 811–817

Chapter 3

Carcinoma of the pancreas and biliary system

D. C. Carter

Introduction

The nature of the problem

This chapter will be concerned principally with the common problem of ductal adenocarcinoma of the pancreas and the less common problem of cholangiocarcinoma. However, the opportunity will be taken to review the diagnosis and management of periampullary cancer as this relatively rare neoplasm has a comparatively favourable prognosis and can easily be misdiagnosed as pancreatic cancer.

Pancreatic cancer

Ductal adenocarcinoma of the pancreas remains a major diagnostic and therapeutic challenge. Of the three malignacies referred to above, it is by far the commonest cause of biliary obstruction. In 1982, 5720 deaths were registered as due to pancreatic cancer in England and Wales (Allen-Mersh and Earlam, 1986) and as in other Western countries, there has been a progressive rise in mortality rate throughout the century. In the USA there has been a three-fold increase in incidence in the past fifty years and this cancer ranks fourth and sixth in men and women respectively as a cause of cancer death (Aoki and Ogawa, 1978). Registration rates now exceed 10 per 100 000 of the population in many countries and Scotland and England and Wales rank among the first five countries in this grim league table. It should be stressed, however, that registration rates are notoriously inaccurate, given that not all patients have histologically proven carcinoma and that many may not even have undergone surgery. In a recent review, Gudjonsson (1987) found that the rate of histological confirmation in various series ranged from 43% to 75% and the true frequency of pancreatic cancer may be lower than current estimates suggest. It is also important to appreciate that while this chapter is concerned with ductal adenocarcinoma, other rarer pancreatic neoplasms, notably acinar-cell carcinoma, cystadenoma and cystadenocarcinoma, and various APUDomas also arise in the pancreas and in some cases, may carry a much better prognosis.

These considerations apart, carcinoma of the pancreas carries an appalling prognosis. It is predominantly a disease of the elderly (half of all patients are older than 70 years of age at diagnosis), diagnosis is usually made late in the natural history of the disease, 90% of patients are dead within a year of diagnosis and survival beyond five years is exceptional. Although studies in experimental animals (notably those using carcinogenic nitrosamines in the Syrian golden hamster and the azaserine treated rat) have elucidated the relationship between diet, hormones such as cholecystokinin and secretin, the development of pancreatic cancer (Morgan and Wormsley, 1977; Pour *et al.*, 1977; Howatson and Carter, 1985), the cause of its development in man remains uncertain. Aetiological factors linked firmly to human pancreatic cancer include increasing age, cigarette smoking, high fat–high protein diet, urbanization, immigration to Western countries, occupational exposure to carcinogens and hereditary pancreatitis. Controversial factors include coffee drinking, alcohol, diabetes and chronic pancreatitis. Eradication of pancreatic cancer by identification of its cause and elucidation of its pathogenesis remains an elusive and very distant goal.

Cholangiocarcinoma

The lethality of cholangiocarcinoma rivals that of pancreatic cancer although its exact incidence is even more difficult to determine. Gallbladder cancer is an uncommon neoplasm and although gallstones are found in almost every case, the risk of cancer developing in a patient with untreated gallstones is probably less than 1%. Cholangiocarcinoma affecting the bile ducts is even less common than gallbladder cancer and does not appear to have any association with gallstones. Ductal cholangiocarcinoma is, however, associated with congenital cysts (e.g. choledochal cysts, Caroli's syndrome), liver fluke infestation, ulcerative colitis (with or without sclerosing cholangitis) and with biliary cirrhosis due to congenital biliary atresia, although in the majority of Western patients no aetiological factor can be identified. Bengmark, Blumgart and Launois (1986) estimate that one case of ductal cancer will be encountered in every 100 bile duct operations and in every 1000 autopsies, and bile duct cancer is thought to account for 4500 new patients a year in the United States (Tompkins *et al.*, 1981). In contrast to the female sex preponderance of gallbladder cancer, ductal cholangiocarcinoma is at least as common in men. Cholangiocarcinoma is classically a disease of the elderly and in the case of gallbladder cancer, late diagnosis means that virtually the only long-term survivors are those in whom cancer is discovered as an incidental and unsuspected finding after removal of the gallbladder for cholelithiasis. Ductal cholangiocarcinoma also increases in incidence with advancing age and while allowance must be made for the effect of improved diagnosis, bile duct cancer may be increasing in incidence (Tompkins, 1982). Resectability rates and prospects of cure depend in great measure on the location of the cancer, both being highest in the case of cancers affecting the lower reaches of the extrahepatic ductal system.

Periampullary cancer

Periampullary cancer is the term usually employed to describe malignancy arising at or within 1 cm of the papilla of Vater. The diagnosis probably embraces tumours of the papilla, duodenum, lower common bile duct and pancreas developing in this area, and it is clear that the wide spectrum of histological type and degree of differentiation is paralleled by a wide range of behaviour extending from benignity to frankly invasive cancer. As already mentioned, this form of cancer may be difficult to distinguish from cancer of the head of the pancreas at laparotomy and it is likely that its true incidence is underestimated. Allen-Mersh and Earlam (1986) found only 126 patients registered as having periampullary cancer in England and Wales in one year, as opposed to 5881 thought to have pancreatic cancer. The disease affects the sexes equally and has its peak incidence in the seventh decade (Robertson *et al.*, 1987).

Diagnosis of malignant obstructive jaundice

Clinical presentation

All three forms of cancer present most frequently with obstructive jaundice. The patient is often elderly and in addition to the symptoms of obstructive jaundice (icterus, dark urine, pale stool, pruritus) frequently complains of anorexia, nausea and vomiting, weight loss and abdominal discomfort or pain. The classical teaching that cancer of the head of the pancreas presents with painless obstructive jaundice is incorrect; most of these patients experience discomfort or frank pain in the abdomen and/or the back. Cancer of the body and tail of the pancreas tends to present late and without jaundice, and pain may be associated with the presence of a palpable mass. Anaemia can be particularly marked in the case of periampullary cancer and the hypochromic, microcytic pattern is often associated with a positive faecal occult blood test. In some patients, metastases may dominate the clinical presentation with findings such as hepatomegaly and the presence of palpable peritoneal deposits. The recent onset of diabetes mellitus is a strong pointer to pancreatic malignancy and the gallbladder is often palpable in patients who develop malignant obstruction of the lower common bile duct. In patients with ductal cholangiocarcinoma, the cystic duct may become obstructed leading to gallbladder enlargement because of mucocoele or empyema formation. Most patients with malignant obstruction do not have infected bile but those who develop cholangitis may manifest the classical triad of jaundice, pain and fever with rigors.

Biochemical and haematological evaluation

After obtaining a full history and conducting a thorough physical examination, blood is withdrawn for determination of haemoglobin concentration, full blood count and biochemical evaluation. Liver function tests will confirm the presence of icterus and obstructive jaundice is reflected in gross elevation of the serum alkaline phosphatase concentration in association with relatively little rise in serum transaminase levels. Hypoalbuminaemia may reflect malnutrition and the urea and creatinine concentrations are used to check renal function, particularly in those with longstanding jaundice. Clotting status (prothrombin time, thrombin time, kaolin cephalin coagulation time and platelet count) is assessed routinely in all jaundiced patients although in reality the prothrombin time alone is usually an adequate reflection of derangement in these patients. Hepatitis B antigen status should be recorded routinely to avoid confusing malignant obstruction with hepatitis.

A vast literature now exists regarding the use of circulating tumour markers in the diagnosis of pancreatic cancer. Serum concentration of tissue polypeptide antigen (TPA) is a more sensitive index than carcinoembryonic antigen (CEA), as are levels of gastrointestinal cancer antigens with carbohydrate immunodeterminants which can be defined by monoclonal antibodies such as CA 19–9. However, despite sensitivities of the order of 80–90%, none of these markers are 100%

specific. At present they add little to the results of radiological investigations in symptomatic patients and none has found application in the screening of asymptomatic populations.

Pancreatic function tests such as the Lundh test meal and secretin stimulation test have sensitivities and specificities which can approach 80% in skilled hands, but have been superseded by the newer radiological methods of diagnosis.

Imaging investigations

Ultrasonography is still the first specific imaging procedure used to delineate the liver, biliary tree and pancreas in patients thought to have malignant biliary obstruction. It is non-invasive, inexpensive and a valuable means of targetting suspicious lesions for biopsy or aspiration cytology. Liver size and homogeneity of texture can be assessed, the degree of biliary obstruction can be measured and the level of any such obstruction can be defined. Gallbladder size is readily determined and although ultrasonography is an accurate means of displaying gallbladder stones, it is not as reliable in detecting calculi in the lower common bile duct. In one recent Dutch report, ultrasonography showed the space-occupying lesion in 54% of patients with carcinoma of the head of the pancreas (Nix et al., 1984).

Percutaneous transhepatic cholangiography (PTC) using a thin flexible needle is an acceptably safe method of outlining the biliary tree and in skilled hands, it is almost always successful in patients with dilatation following obstruction (Figure 3.1). It used to be practised routinely in most centres once ultrasound had confirmed the presence of large duct obstruction. However, the procedure is uncomfortable and despite precautions, cholangitis and intraperitoneal bleeding may develop in jaundiced patients.

Endoscopic retrograde cholangiopancreatography (ERCP) is often less distressing for the patient and the use of benzodiazepines in sedation frequently leaves the patient with no recollection of the investigation. ERCP also has the advantages that it allows inspection of the stomach and duodenum (permitting biopsy of periampullary tumours), enables a pancreatogram to be obtained thus allowing the diagnosis of pancreatic lesions not defined by cholangiography, and allows endoscopic papillotomy to relieve jaundice and allow stenting of an obstructed biliary system. As will be discussed, insertion of an endoprosthesis from 'above' is of course possible at PTC, but endoscopic insertion is now generally preferred. PTC may still be indicated when ERCP fails or when a stricture cannot be stented from below, and a combined approach is indicated. Both techniques allow material to be aspirated for cytological assessment. The drawback of both procedures is that infection may be introduced into an obstructed but previously sterile biliary tree, and this may prove problematic in patients with high biliary obstruction in whom palliative surgical bypass may be indicated (vide infra). In the study by Nix et al. (1984), ERCP was the radiological method that most frequently led to the diagnosis of carcinoma of the head of the pancreas. In 76% of patients it was the first technique to give the diagnosis and its diagnostic accuracy was 93%. Endoscopic ultrasonography is a relatively new technique which may prove useful in detecting small pancreatic mass lesions (Yasuda et al., 1988).

Computerized tomography (CT) has approximately the same ability as ultrasound to detect mass lesions in the pancreas (Nix et al., 1984) and is not used routinely in the preoperative assessment of such patients. CT criteria for

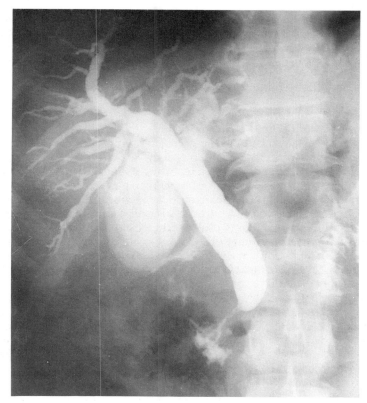

Figure 3.1 Percutaneous transhepatic cholangiogram showing dilatation of the biliary tree caused by a carcinoma in the head of the pancreas

unresectability of cancer of the head of the pancreas include evidence of hepatic and distant metastasis and/or evidence of locally advanced disease (extension to contiguous structures, vascular encasement/invasion and local lymphadenopathy). However, recent reports indicate that CT prediction of unresectability may be unreliable and are not a basis for electing to manage pancreatic cancer by non-operative means (Ross *et al.*, 1988). However, in patients with bile duct cancer, CT may be more valuable given its ability to relate bile duct anatomy to that of the liver. In patients with high bile duct cancer, a case can be made for reliance on CT (with targetted fine-needle aspiration cytology) and avoidance of unnecessary preoperative cholangiography with its risk of introducing sepsis.

Selective angiography adds little to the methods mentioned above as a means of diagnosis. It is true that vascular encasement will be detected in some two-thirds of patients with pancreatic cancer and portal vein invasion or displacement may be apparent in the venous phase. However, some surgeons no longer regard venous invasion/displacement as an indication of inoperability if wider dissemination is not found at operation (Fortner, 1984; Trede, 1985). It should be stressed that pancreatic cystadenocarcinoma may produce portal vein obstruction/displacement while remaining operable and indeed curable. If angiography no longer commands a routine place in diagnosis, a strong case can still be made for its use in defining vessel invasion and congenital anomalies when pancreatic resection is contemplated. An even stronger case can be made when contemplating resection of high bile duct cancer (Blumgart *et al.*, 1984) and bilateral vessel involvement is normally taken as an indication of irresectability. On the other hand, unilateral involvement of the hepatic artery and portal vein may not preclude curative partial hepatectomy, and some surgeons are willing to resect and repair the main trunk of the portal vein in patients with otherwise curable lesions.

Other radiological investigations such as barium meal, hypotonic duodenography and pancreatic scintiscanning are of historic interest only.

Laparoscopy has some advocates as a means of assessing patients with pancreatic cancer. Warshaw, Tepper and Shipley (1986) studied 40 patients with biopsy-proven adenocarcinoma, all of whom had been considered theoretically curable by surgery after conventional investigation. Fourteen patients showed evidence of spread (to liver, peritoneum or omentum) that precluded cure but laparoscopy failed to detect liver metastases in 3 patients who proved to have them at operation. The course of treatment was altered in 14 of the 40 patients by laparoscopy. Although not used widely, in this context, perhaps more consideration should be given to laparoscopy when resection is contemplated.

Cytological and histological diagnosis

We must not be lulled into a false sense of security by the apparent accuracy of modern imaging investigations. An impacted gallstone should no longer be misdiagnosed as 'operable pancreatic cancer' solely on the findings at operation, but a number of benign conditions (notably chronic pancreatitis, sclerosing cholangitis and compression of the common hepatic duct by an inflamed gallbladder can all masquerade radiologically and at operation as malignancy. Furthermore, a number of malignant conditions such as lymphoma and deposits from breast and bronchogenic carcinoma can simulate primary malignant obstruction of the biliary tree (Figure 3.2). It cannot be over-emphasized that histological or cytological confirmation remains the key to correct diagnosis and management of these conditions, many of which carry a far better prognosis than pancreatic cancer and cholangiocarcinoma following institution of appropriate therapy.

A preoperative diagnosis of pancreatic cancer can be obtained safely by percutaneous fine needle aspiration cytology or Trucut biopsy once a lesion has been targetted by radiology or ultrasonography. False positivity is extremely rare but sampling error can give rise to false negativity. While some recent reports suggest that diagnostic accuracy can be 100% (Yamamoto *et al.*, 1985), collected reviews indicate that a more representative figure may be around 80% (McLoughlin *et al.*, 1978). If a tissue diagnosis has not been made before operation, fine needle sampling can be employed at laparotomy although with less reliable results than radiologically targetted sampling. Trucut biopsy, performed trans-duodenally where possible may be 80–90% accurate although it carries a minimal risk of causing bleeding, pancreatitis, abscess and fistula formation. With all sampling techniques, multiple passes are best avoided as there is a small but real danger of causing track dissemination and serosal spread of tumour.

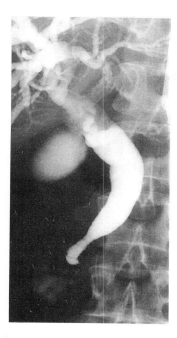

Figure 3.2 Malignant biliary obstruction thought originally to be due to pancreatic cancer but which proved to be due to the presence of lymphoma on histological examination

In the case of cholangiocarcinoma, preoperative diagnosis is frequently difficult given the small fibrotic nature of many of the lesions. While some prefer to rely on radiological diagnosis (Cameron, Broe and Zuidema, 1982) others advocate targetted fine-needle aspiration or cytological examination of bile recovered at PTC. Other methods include curettage, brush cytology and choledochoscopically directed punch biopsy at the time of surgery. In lesions which are diagnosed radiologically as cholangiocarcinoma it can be argued that resection is indicated wherever possible, regardless of whether the lesion proves to be benign or malignant. Failure to define the true nature of the diagnosis assumes much greater importance when resection is not performed and the patient is treated by intubation or palliative bypass. An added factor to be taken into account in diagnosis is the recognition that polypoid and papillary neoplasms carry a much better prognosis than nodular, scirrhous and diffusely infiltrating forms of cholangiocarcinoma (Todoroki *et al.*, 1980). Using a combination of preoperative and intraoperative methods, Blumgart *et al.* (1984) were able to obtain a positive tissue diagnosis in all but 3 of their 94 patients with hilar cholangiocarcinoma, and this approach must be encouraged.

Periampullary cancer is the most accessible cause of malignant obstruction and multiple biopsies can be obtained endoscopically (Figure 3.3). While the diagnosis of invasive carcinoma is secure, in many cases the pathologist is unable to give a confident diagnosis in a biopsy from a neoplastic lesion which shows only suggestive evidence of malignancy. Under these circumstances excision of the entire neoplasm is the only way to clarify the diagnosis, and provide information on such adverse factors as perineural invasion and lymph node metastases.

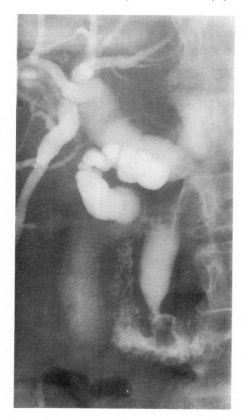

Figure 3.3 Periampullary cancer causing biliary obstruction. The tumour is obvious on percutaneous transhepatic cholangiography as a prominence bulging into the junction between the second and third part of the duodenum. The diagnosis was confirmed by endoscopic biopsy

Treatment

Treatment of pancreatic cancer

Resection
From the outset, it is clear that pancreatic cancer is rarely cured but that surgery holds out the only prospect of eradicating the disease. The study of registration data in England and Wales indicates that in 1979 only 200 resections were performed as opposed to 1700 bypass procedures to relieve jaundice (Allen-Mersh and Earlam, 1986). This suggests a resectability rate of 12% for all surgical patients and of less than 5% for all patients with the disease. As might be anticipated, specialist referral centres have higher resectability rates, ranging recently from 14% to 22% (Andren-Sandberg and Ihse, 1983; Morrow, Hilaris and Brennan, 1984; Nix *et al.*, 1984; Trede, 1985). Although modern methods of investigation do not appear to have influenced survival rates (Kairaluoma *et al.*, 1985), there is recent evidence that tumour size at operation has fallen while resectability rates have risen (Nix *et al.*, 1984; Trede, 1985). It must be emphasized that all considerations of resection apply only to cancer arising in the head of the pancreas; tumours arising in the body and tail are seldom, if ever, resectable.

The question of tumour size at the time of operation is important. A recent study from Japan showed that a resectability rate of 99% was achieved in 106 patients with tumours less than 2 cm in diameter (Tsuchiya *et al.*, 1986). Operative mortality was only 4% but no less than 44% of the patients proved to have disseminated disease, emphasizing that small cancer is not necessarily early or localized cancer. Nevertheless, the cumulative 5-year survival rate in these patients was 30%, supporting the need for improved screening and diagnostic methods. Of course, it can be argued that these patients with small cancers may be a group in which the natural history or the tumour is more favourable. The rarity of small cancer is underlined by the fact that these 106 patients were identified from a parent group of no less than 3315 patients with pancreatic cancer.

When resection is deemed feasible, the Whipple operation of pancreatico-duodenectomy is the standard procedure, although not without its shortcomings. The risks of major surgery in an elderly, ill group of jaundiced patients cannot be overemphasized (Blamey *et al.*, 1983). Attempts to reduce operative morbidity and mortality by a period of percutaneous transhepatic drainage have proved disappointing (McPherson *et al.*, 1984; Pitt *et al.*, 1985) but preliminary endoscopic papillotomy and stenting is advisable when resection is contemplated in ill patients who in addition to jaundice may have problems such as sepsis, malnutrition or impaired renal function. If a potentially resectable tumour is encountered at laparotomy in such ill patients, the prudent course of action is to institute temporary biliary drainage and not proceed immediately to resection. Temporary drainage may be achieved by cholecystojejunostomy but subsequent resection is simpler if tube drainage is instituted, either by cholecystostomy or by placing a T-tube in the common hepatic duct.

The Whipple operation is technically demanding and has a high potential for the development of intraoperative and postoperative problems. The operation entails *en bloc* resection of the gastric antrum, duodenum and first few inches of jejunum, the head and neck of pancreas, gallbladder and common bile duct. Detailed operative considerations are outwith the scope of this chapter but some points deserve stress:

1. It is often recommended that resectability should be assessed early in the operation by running the index fingers of both hands along the anterior surface of the portal vein, one from above and one from below, to check that it is not infiltrated by cancer from the neck of the pancreas. In my view this has been overvalued. Considerable dissection is required before this step can be achieved. More importantly, the tunnel between the portal vein and the back of the neck of the pancreas may be clear, yet tumour will still be found to have infiltrated the right posterior aspect of the portal vein in the final stages of resection and will have to be dealt with by inclusion of the involved part of the portal vein with the resection specimen.
2. Division of the extrahepatic biliary tree at the level of the common bile duct may compromise the radicality of resection. Furthermore, division at this level may devitalize the lowermost portion of the remaining bile duct, given that the blood supply for this area comes predominantly from below. For these reasons, the gallbladder should be removed with the resection specimen and biliary-enteric continuity restored using the common hepatic duct.
3. While preservation of the pylorus is now practised by some surgeons when resecting for chronic pancreatitis, this is used less widely when dealing with

pancreatic cancer. However, Grace, Pitt and Longmire (1986) advocate pylorus preservation on the grounds that the operation may be easier to perform than the Whipple operation, may cause less long-term nutritional upset, and may not adversely affect the prospects of long-term survival.

Marginal ulceration is a recognized problem after pancreaticoduodenectomy and probably reflects the relative lack of alkaline pancreatic exocrine secretion in the upper gastrointestinal tract. This means that it is advisable to combine antrectomy with vagotomy, or undertake more extensive gastric resection in the form of hemigastrectomy. It is our practice to prescribe an H_2-receptor antagonist routinely for at least two months following pancreaticoduodenectomy as a further safeguard against acute manifestations of the peptic ulcer diathesis.

4. The pancreaticojejunal anastomosis remains the Achilles heel of pancreatico-duodenectomy. Numerous techniques have been described to minimize the risk of leakage and include removal of the entire pancreas, ligation of the pancreatic duct (with or without occlusion by substances such as Ethibloc), use of separate jejunal loops for the biliary–enteric and pancreatico–jejunal anastomosis, and pancreaticogastrostomy rather than pancreaticojejunostomy (Kapur, 1986). In my view the body and tail of pancreas should be conserved whenever possible if only to minimize the risk of developing brittle diabetes. It is, however, good practice to trim back the pancreatic remnant so that uninflamed and non-friable tissue can be used for anastomosis. This manoeuvre has the added advantage that the pancreatic duct comes to occupy a more central rather than posterior position on the cut surface of the pancreatic remnant. If the pancreatic duct is grossly dilated then it is my practice to use mucosa-to-mucosa apposition in the pancreatico–jejunal anastomosis; if it is not dilated I prefer to use two layers of interrupted sutures to invaginate the entire cut surface of pancreas into the side of the jejunum. I prefer to place the pancreatico–jejunal anastomosis upstream of the gastro–jejunal and hepatico–jejunal anastomoses, and begin by constructing this, the most dangerous of the three anastomoses. Opinions vary as to whether the pancreatico–jejunal anastomosis should be splinted by a tube but this is no longer my practice.

5. Given the magnitude of the surgery and the complexity of the reconstruction, patients undergoing pancreaticoduodenectomy in my unit are commenced on tube enteral nutrition from the time of surgery. This allows nutritional status to be maintained and avoids pressure to commence oral feeding before one is convinced that anastomotic healing is complete. A proportion of these patients are diabetic before surgery and a number of patients may manifest hyperglycaemia and glycosuria postoperatively, albeit transiently. The importance of careful monitoring of blood glucose levels and meticulous insulin therapy cannot be overstressed.

Review of the Whipple operation by Shapiro (1975) indicated that mean operative mortality in 496 collected patients was 21%. This figure was clearly unacceptable, but improvements in operative technique and perioperative care, aided by concentration of experience in specialist centres has brought operative mortality rates down below 5% in recent years (Trede, 1985; Crist, Sitzmann and Cameron, 1987; Trede and Schwall, 1988). This has greatly weakened the case for total pancreatectomy as a means of reducing the unacceptable morbidity and mortality of the Whipple operation, and indeed the reported risks of total pancreatectomy indicate that it is at least as dangerous (Ihse *et al.*, 1977; Trede, 1985). It can be argued that total pancreatectomy is a more radical cancer operation which removes any anxiety about multifocality of cancer and which removes potentially involved nodes left behind by the less radical Whipple procedure (Cubilla, Fortner and Fitzgerald, 1978). However, the failure of total pancreatectomy or the more extended regional resections proposed by Fortner (1984) to affect long-term survival rates suggests that pancreatic cancer may be analogous to breast cancer in that regional lymph node spread denotes distant metastases.

It is clear that few patients with pancreatic cancer are candidates for resection and in turn that few of the resected patients will be cured of their disease. It must also be borne in mind that even 5-year survival does not always equate to cure and that independent review of histopathology is advisable in all long-term survivors thought to have had pancreatic cancer. It is our current practice to offer resection to good practice to offer resection to good risk patients in whom preoperative and intraoperative assessment shows no tumour dissemination outwith the head of pancreas. Gudjonsson (1987) reviewed reports incorporating 37 000 patients of whom 4100 had undergone resection; only 156 survived 5 years (of whom 12 had not undergone resection), an overall survival rate of 0.42%. Advocates of resection stress that it represents the only prospect of cure and that palliation may be superior to that achieved by bypass. The Japanese experience indicates that patients with small cancer can be cured (Tsuchiya *et al.*, 1986) and the recent Johns Hopkins study of 50 pancreatic cancer patients shows an *actuarial* 5-year survival rate of 18%, rising to 48% in those without lymph node involvement. It remains to be seen whether adjuvant therapy in the form of chemotherapy and/or radiotherapy (intraoperative and postoperative) will improve survival rates following potentially curative resections.

Palliative surgery

Following an extensive literature review Sarr and Cameron (1982) recommend cholecystojejunostomy as the safest and simplest means of relieving obstructive jaundice, reserving hepaticojejunostomy for those in whom the tumour encroaches on the junction of the cystic duct and the common hepatic duct. Concomitant gastroenterostomy is also usually recommended in that 10–15% of patients will otherwise develop duodenal obstruction. However, Doberneck and Berndt (1987) found that gastric emptying was delayed despite gastroenterostomy in 26% of their patients, while Weaver *et al.* (1987) found that patients with duodenal impingement of cancer more often had a poor outcome after gastroenterostomy (70%) than those without (40%). It is an unfortunate paradox that those who need gastroenterostomy most appear less likely to benefit from it.

It is not surprising that palliative surgical bypass carries a mean operative mortality of 19% in this patient population and mean duration of survival thereafter is only 5.4 months (Sarr and Cameron, 1982). We now reserve surgical bypass for good-risk patients in whom resection is contraindicated and consider insertion of an endoprosthesis in those who are ill and elderly (*vide infra*).

Non-surgical treatment

The indifferent results of palliative surgery has led to the assessment of alternative means of relieving jaundice in patients with unresectable pancreatic cancer. A prospective trial in Cape Town showed that 30-day mortality after percutaneous transhepatic placement of a biliary prosthesis was 8% as opposed to 20% in patients undergoing surgical bypass (Bornman *et al.*, 1986). In the Middlesex trial, stenting was assessed in patients with malignant obstructive jaundice deemed unfit for operation (Speer *et al.*, 1987); endoscopic stenting had a significantly higher success rate than percutaneous stenting (81% v. 61%) and a significantly lower 30-day mortality (15% v. 33%). There is no doubt that stenting has been a significant advance in management and that endoscopic stenting now obviates the need for hazardous surgery in ill elderly patients with malignant obstructive jaundice. However, it requires a skilled endoscopist, is not without the small but appreciable risks associated with papillotomy (bleeding, pancreatitis, perforation), and the stent frequently becomes blocked and requires replacement. Stent replacement may be performed on a day-patient basis and it seems clear that although long-term survival is not affected, stented patients spend less time in hospital than their surgically treated counterparts. The availability and success of stenting must not be allowed to obscure the need for histological or cytological confirmation of the diagnosis and patients with potentially curable causes of obstruction must not be denied surgical intervention.

Adjuvant therapy
Chemotherapy can increase the duration of survival in patients with inoperable pancreatic cancer and some 30–40% of patients show some response (Harvey and Schein, 1984). Combination chemotherapy (fluorouracil, methotrexate, vincristine and cyclophosphamide) extended median survival (44 v. 9 weeks) in the trial conducted by Mallinson *et al.* (1980), but other studies have questioned whether combination therapy confers any advantage to the effects of fluorouracil alone (Cullinan *et al.*, 1985). While some encouragement can be drawn from these studies the current results of chemotherapy are probably not good enough to justify its routine use in palliation. The regimes are not without side-effects and may erode the window of good quality life that remains to the patient once jaundice has been relieved.

The presence of oestrogen receptors and oestrogen-binding proteins in normal and neoplastic pancreas has given rise to hope that hormonal manipulation might be valuable (Greenway, 1987). Unfortunately, the results emerging to date have proved disappointing and the recent hopes that somatostatin and its analogues may be useful in management also appear ill-founded given the absence of somatostatin receptors in resected specimens of pancreatic cancer (Reubi *et al.*, 1988).

With regard to radiotherapy, controlled trials indicate that its effects can be enhanced by 5-fluorouracil in patients with locally unresectable pancreatic cancer (Moertel *et al.*, 1981). A report of 77 patients with locally advanced disease treated by high-energy neutrons showed symptomatic palliation in the majority, many patients died from metastatic disease rather than local recurrence, and at subsequent autopsy, extensive local reactive fibrosis was revealed (Cohen *et al.*, 1985). Further study is required to evaluate the effects of combining neutron irradiation with chemotherapy, to define the role of intraoperative radiotherapy (Mitsuyuki *et al.*, 1987; Roldnan *et al.*, 1988), and assess the value of local interstitial implantation (Morrow, Hilaris and Brennan, 1984). As with chemotherapy, more data are required before the routine use of radiotherapy can be advocated, alone or in combination with other treatments, in patients with pancreatic cancer.

Treatment of periampullary cancer

Review of 31 series indicates that the operative mortality in 2390 patients with periampullary cancer having pancreaticoduodenectomy was 19% while it was 25% in those having transduodenal excision (Wise, Pizzimbono and Dehner, 1976). A recent report from North-west England found that no less than 33 surgeons had been involved in the care of 61 patients (Knox and Kingston 1986). Radical surgery in 24 of these patients carried a mortality of no less than 30% while local excision was carried out in 25 without mortality. Our own experience in Glasgow Royal Infirmary in 41 patients collected over a 15-year period showed an operative mortality for pancreaticoduodenectomy of 8% compared to 25% for local excision and 17% for palliative bypass (Robertson *et al.*, 1987). The overall 5-year survival rate in our patients was 29%, emphasizing that this cancer carries a far better prognosis than pancreatic cancer. While Knox and Kingston (1986) report better survival rates following local excision, in our experience the 5-year survival rate after radical resection (34%) did not differ significantly from that following local excision (44%). In the review by Chiappetta *et al.* (1986) the 187 patients with negative lymph nodes had a 5-year survival rate of 39% after pancreaticoduodenectomy and these authors support the view that local excision should be reserved for high-risk patients. All are agreed that survival prospects after palliative bypass are poor and none of our own patients in this group survived five years.

While more data are required, I suggest that pancreaticoduodenectomy in experienced hands should still be the routine management of periampullary cancer. Transduodenal excision should be reserved for those deemed unfit for resection and endoscopic stenting or papillotomy alone should be considered as an option in patients who are considered unfit for any form of surgical intervention.

Treatment of cholangiocarcinoma

It is generally accepted that cholangiocarcinoma affecting the lower common bile duct should be dealt with by Whipple resection if the lesion appears potentially curable. Recent reports indicate resectability rates of 47–76% for lesions in the lower third of the extrahepatic biliary tree with operative mortality rates ranging from 0% to 8% (Langer *et al.*, 1985; Tsunoda *et al.*, 1985).

Resection rates for tumours in the middle third are usually lower than in the case of tumours in the lower one-third and are probably lowest of all for cancers in the upper third. However, Langer *et al.* (1985) report a resection rate of 22% in 54 patients with upper third lesions with only one death. Blumgart *et al.* (1984) undertook curative resection (with or without liver resection) in 18 of their 94 patients with cholangiocarcinoma at the confluence of the hepatic ducts and 2 patients died within 30 days of surgery, while none of the 18 patients with hilar cancer resected by Bismuth, Castaing and Traynor (1988) succumbed in the perioperative period. In Los Angeles, Tompkins *et al.* (1981) carried out resection in no less than 22 of their 47 patients with a mortality rate of 23%. Clearly resection should not be undertaken lightly and operation should be preceded by angiography and portography to assess vascular involvement. Major hepatic resection obviously increases the risk of surgery but an operative mortality of 17% has been reported when resection of high bile duct cancer also necessitates liver resection (Bengmark, Blumgart and Launois, 1986). Involvement of the caudate lobe by direct extension from hilar cancer has been emphasized recently (Mizumoto, Kawarada and Suzuki,

1986) and this lobe may have to be included in the resection in future. Pichlmayr and colleagues (1988) have recently practised liver transplantation in patients with unresectable tumours and no evidence of extrahepatic spread; the results of this policy are awaited with interest.

At the other end of the surgical spectrum, Terblanche (1979) has argued against resection for lesions in the area of the confluence, preferring to insert a U-tube and then treat with radiotherapy (Figure 3.4). While long-term survival has been described after such treatment, the reported results refer to small series of patients and in many patients treated by intubation, there has been no histological confirmation of the diagnosis. Cameron, Broe and Zuidema (1982) have elected to combine resection of proximal bile duct tumours with insertion of thick-walled silastic tubes into both ductal systems during hepaticojejunostomy. The stents are used to maintain biliary flow even in the face of tumour recurrence in the hope that survival will be prolonged until death occurs from tumour dissemination rather than liver failure and sepsis.

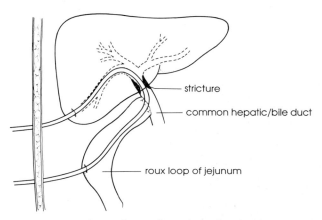

— stricture

— common hepatic/bile duct

— roux loop of jejunum

Figure 3.4 Use of a U-tube to relieve obstruction due to cholangiocarcinoma. If the tube blocks, a new tube can be 'railroaded' into position using the old tube

While the issue remains controversial, it seems logical to try to tailor the treatment of cholangiocarcinoma to the particular needs of the individual rather than attempt to treat all patients in the same way. Resection should be attempted for potentially curable lesions if feasible and if the patient is sufficiently fit, but the risks of surgery should not be underestimated and the case for referral to a specialist centre is overwhelming. Surgical bypass is the next option to consider in patients with unresectable tumours. While bypass using hepaticojejunostomy-en-Y should not pose significant technical problems for patients with cancer in the lower biliary tree, the problems increase as one deals with tumours higher in the extrahepatic bile ducts. Splitting the liver to gain access to the ducts above an unresectable tumour at the confluence carries a prohibitive mortality, and is no longer popular. The use of the left hepatic duct for hepaticojejunostomy-en-Y as popularized by Blumgart and Kelly (1984) is a very useful technique for benign stricture but with hilar cholangiocarcinoma, tumour often extends along the left duct so preventing its use (Figure 3.5). The various cholangio–enteric anastomoses

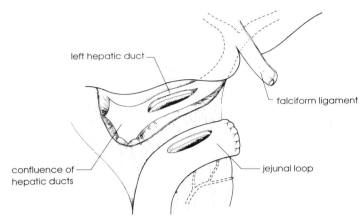

left hepatic duct

falciform ligament

confluence of
hepatic ducts

jejunal loop

Figure 3.5 Use of the left hepatic duct for relief of high bile duct obstruction. The proximity of the anastomosis to the confluence is shown. Use of the segment III duct to the left of the fissure of the falciform ligament allows more effective longstanding relief of obstruction

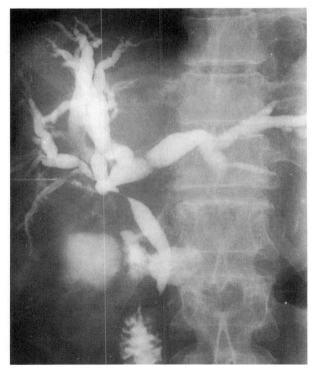

Figure 3.6 Percutaneous transhepatic cholangiogram showing a cholangiocarcinoma close to the confluence of the bile ducts. A long length of left hepatic duct is seen. A biliary-enteric anastomosis was eventually performed away from the confluence using the bile duct passing to segment III of the liver

described by Bismuth and Corlette (1975) have been used increasingly for bypass and the duct draining segment III is usually most suitable (Figure 3.6). Intra-operative ultrasonography is an invaluable aid to localizing the duct within the liver substance and an ultrasonic surgical aspirator allows dissection of the liver with minimal blood loss. It is important to appreciate that the operative mortality can be high in patients undergoing palliative surgery for cholangiocarcinoma and in many series approximates to 30% (Blumgart *et al.*, 1984). Previous intervention, either in the form of surgery or intubation, can increase both the morbidity and mortality of palliative and curative surgery in these patients and there is a strong argument against preoperative cholangiography to avoid introducing infection to part of the biliary tree which may be left undrained by the palliative bypass procedure.

There is debate regarding the use of stenting as an alternative to surgical bypass in the palliation of cholangiocarcinoma. Many reports of stenting fail to distinguish between different types of malignant obstruction or define the height of the obstruction in the biliary tree. As already emphasized, in many of these patients histological or cytological confirmation of the diagnosis is lacking. However, it seems certain that endoscopically inserted biliary prostheses which allow internal biliary drainage will establish a place in the palliative treatment of selected patients with cholangiocarcinoma.

Chemotherapy appears to have little to offer in the treatment of cholangiocarcinoma but there is evidence that radiotherapy merits further evaluation as an alternative to surgery or as adjuvant treatment in some patients. Both external irradiation (Langer *et al.*, 1985) and internal irradiation using 192-iridium wire passed down a biliary drainage tube (Fletcher *et al.*, 1983) appear to be well tolerated, but controlled data are required before effects on palliation and survival can be fully assessed.

Conclusion

Malignant obstructive jaundice remains a major diagnostic and therapeutic challenge. Recent advances in radiological asessment and tissue sampling techniques should now allow more precise diagnosis and staging. The vast majority of patients with pancreatic cancer will not be suitable for resection and the choice lies between surgical and endoscopic means of palliation. Periampullary cancer should be dealt with by pancreaticoduodenectomy whenever possible and transduodenal excision or palliative endoscopic procedures reserved for those deemed unfit for resection. Cholangiocarcinoma involving the lower and middle reaches of the extrahepatic biliary tree should be resected where possible. Hilar cholangiocarcinoma may be resectable (with or without associated liver resection) in some patients but in the majority, palliative surgical bypass or intubation may be all that is feasible. With the possible exception of periampullary cancer, malignant obstructive jaundice carries a grim prognc•is. Significant improvement will await the advent of earlier diagnosis or more effective chemotherapy and/or radiotherapy.

References

Allen-Mersh, T. G. and Earlam, R. J. (1986) Pancreatic cancer in England and Wales: surgeons look at epidemiology. *Annals of the Royal College of Surgeons of England*, **68**, 154–158

Andren-Sandberg, A. and Ihse, I. (1983) Factors influencing survival after total pancreatectomy in patients with pancreatic cancer. *Annals of Surgery*, **198**, 605–610

Aoki, K. and Ogawa, H. (1978) Cancer of the pancreas; international mortality trends. *World Health Statistics Quarterly*, **31**, 2–27

Bengmark, S. Blumgart, L. H. and Launois, B. (1986) Liver resection in high bile duct tumours. In *Liver Surgery* (eds S. Bengmark and L. H. Blumgart), Churchill Livingstone, London, pp. 81–87

Bismuth, H., Castaing, D. and Traynor, O. (1988) Resection or palliation: Priority of surgery in the treatment of hilar cancer. *World Journal of Surgery*, **12**, 39–47

Bismuth, H. and Corlette, M. B. (1975) Intrahepatic cholangioenteric anastomosis in carcinoma of the hilus of the liver. *Surgery, Gynecology and Obstetrics*, **140**, 170–178

Blamey, S. L., Fearon, K. C. H., Gilmour, W. H. *et al.* (1983) Prediction of risk in biliary surgery. *British Journal of Surgery*, **70**, 535–538

Blumgart, L. H., Benjamin, I. S., Hadjis, N. S. and Beazley, R. (1984) Surgical approaches to cholangiocarcinoma at confluence of hepatic ducts. *Lancet*, **i**, 66–70

Blumgart, L. H. and Kelly, C. J. (1984) Hepaticojejunostomy in benign and malignant high bile duct stricture: approaches to the left hepatic ducts. *British Journal of Surgery*, **71**, 257–261

Bornman, P. C., Harries-Jones, E. P., Tobias, R. *et al.* (1986) Prospective controlled trial of transhepatic biliary endoprosthesis versus bypass surgery for incurable carcinoma of head of pancreas. *Lancet*, **i**, 69–71

Cameron, J. L., Broe, P. and Zuidema, G. D. (1982) Proximal bile duct tumours. Surgical management with silastic transhepatic biliary stents. *Annals of Surgery*, **196**, 412–419

Chiappetta, A., Sperti, C., Bonadimani, B. *et al.* (1986) Surgical experience with adenocarcinoma of the ampulla of Vater. *American Journal of Surgery*, **52**, 603–605

Cohen, L., Woodruff, K. H., Hendrickson, F. R. *et al.* (1985) Response of pancreatic cancer to local irradiation with high-energy neutrons. *Cancer*, **56**, 1235–1241

Crist, D. W., Sitzmann, J. V. and Cameron, J. L. (1987) Improved hospital morbidity, mortality and survival after the Whipple procedure. *Annals of Surgery*, **206**, 358–365

Cubilla, A. L., Fortner, J. and Fitzgerald, P. J. (1978) Lymph node involvement in carcinoma of the head of the pancreas area. *Cancer*, **41**, 880–887

Cullinan, S. A. Moertel, C. G., Fleming, T. R. *et al.* (1985) A comparison of three chemotherapeutic regimes in the treatment of advanced pancreatic and gastric carcinoma. *Journal of the American Medical Association*, **253**, 2061–2967

Doberneck, R. C. and Berndt, G. A. (1987) Delayed gastric emptying after palliative gastrojejunostomy for carcinoma of the pancreas. *Archives of Surgery*, **122**, 827–829

Fletcher, M. S., Brinkley, D., Dawson, J. L. *et al.* (1983) Treatment of hilar carcinoma by bile drainage combined with internal radiotherapy using 192-iridium wire. *British Journal of Surgery*, **70**, 733–735

Fortner, J. G. (1984) Regional pancreatectomy for cancer of the pancreas, ampulla and other related sites. Tumour staging and results. *Annals of Surgery*, **199**, 418–425

Grace, P. A., Pitt, H. and Longmire, W. P. (1986) Pancreaticoduodenectomy with pylorus preservation for adenocarcinoma of the head of the pancreas. *British Journal of Surgery*, **73**, 647–650

Greenway, B. A. (1987) Carcinoma of the exocrine pancreas: a sex hormone responsive tumour. *British Journal of Surgery*, **74**, 441–442

Gudjonsson, B. (1987) Cancer of the pancreas: 50 years of surgery. *Cancer*, **60**, 2284–2303

Harvey, J. H. and Schein, P. S. (1984) Chemotherapy of pancreatic carcinoma. *World Journal of Surgery*, **8**, 935–939

Howatson, A. G. and Carter, D. C. (1985) Pancreatic carcinogenesis—enhancement by cholecystokinin in the hamster-nitrosamine model. *British Journal of Cancer*, **51**, 107–114

Ihse, I. Lilja, P., Arnesjo, B. and Bengmark, S. (1977) Total pancreatectomy for cancer. An appraisal of 65 cases. *Annals of Surgery*, **186**, 675–680

Kairaluoma, M. I., Myllylä, V., Partio, E. *et al.* (1985) Impact of new imaging techniques on survival in cancer of the head of the pancreas and periampullary region. *Acta Chirurgica Scandinavica*, **151**, 69–72

Kapur, B. M. L. (1986) Pancreaticogastrostomy in pancreaticoduodenal resection for ampullary carcinoma—experience in 31 cases. *Surgery*, **100**, 489–493

Knox, R. A. and Kingston, R. D. (1986) Carcinoma of the ampulla of Vater. *British Journal of Surgery*, **73**, 72–73

Langer, J. C., Langer, B., Taylor, B. R. *et al.* (1985) Carcinoma of the extrahepatic bile ducts: results of an aggressive surgical approach. *Surgery*, **98**, 752–759

McLoughlin, M. J. Ho., C. S., Langer, B. *et al.* (1978) Fine needle aspiration biopsy of malignant lesions in and around the pancreas. *Cancer*, **41**, 2413–2419

McPherson, G. A. D., Benjamin, I. S., Hodgson, H. J. F. *et al.* (1984) Pre-operative percutaneous transhepatic biliary drainage: the results of a controlled trial. *British Journal of Surgery*, **71**, 371–375

Mallinson, C. N., Rake, M. O., Cocking, J. B. *et al.* (1980) Chemotherapy in pancreatic cancer: results of a controlled, prospective, randomised, multicentre trial. *British Medical Journal*, **281**, 1589–1591

Mitsuyuki, M., Shibamoto, Y., Takhashi, M. *et al.* (1987) Intraoperative radiotherapy in carcinoma of the stomach and pancreas. *World Journal of Surgery*, **11**, 459–464

Mizumoto, R., Kawarada, Y. and Suzuki, H. (1986) Surgical treatment of hilar carcinoma of the bile duct. *Surgery, Gynecology and Obstetrics*, **162**, 153

Moertel, C. G., Frytak, S., Hahn, R. G. *et al.* (1981) Therapy of locally unresectable pancreatic carcinoma: a randomised comparison of high dose (6000 rads) radiation alone, moderate dose radiation (4000 rads + 5-fluorouracil), and high dose radiation + 5-fluorouracil. *Cancer*, **48**, 1705–1710

Morgan, R. G. H. and Wormsley, K. G. (1977) Progress report: Cancer of the pancreas. *Gut*, **18**, 580–596

Morrow, M., Hilaris, B. and Brennan, M. F. (1984) Comparison of conventional surgical resection, radioactive implantation and bypass procedures for exocrine carcinoma of the pancreas 1975–1980. *Annals of Surgery*, **199**, 1–5

Nix, G. A. J. J., Schmitz, P. I. M., Wilson, J. H. P. *et al.* (1984) Carcinoma of the head of the pancreas. Therapeutic implications of endoscopic retrograde cholangiopancreatography findings. *Gastroenterology*, **87**, 37–43

Pichlmayr, R., Ringe, B., Lauchart, W. *et al.* (1988) Radical resection and liver graftings as the two main components of surgical strategy in the treatment of proximal bile duct cancer. *World Journal of Surgery*, **12**, 68–77

Pitt, H. A., Gomes, A. S., Lois, J. F. *et al.* (1985) Does preoperative percutaneous biliary drainage reduce operative risk or increase hospital cost? *Annals of Surgery*, **201**, 545–552

Pour, P., Althoff, J., Kruger, F. W. and Mohr, U. (1977) A potent pancreatic carcinogen in Syrian hamsters: N-nitrosobis (2-oxopropyl) amine. *Journal of the National Cancer Institute*, **58**, 1449

Reubi, J. C., Horisberger, U., Essed, C. E. *et al.* (1988) Absence of somatostatin receptors in human exocrine pancreatic adenocarcinomas. *Gastroenterology*, **95**, 760–763

Robertson, J. F. R., Imrie, C. W., Hole, D. J. *et al.* (1987) Periampullary carcinoma–what is the prognosis? *British Journal of Surgery*, **74**, 816–819

Roldan, G. E., Gunderson, L. L., Nagorney, D. M. *et al.* (1988) External beam versus intraoperative and external beam irradiation for locally advanced pancreatic cancer. *Cancer*, **61**, 1110–1116

Ross, C. B., Sharp, K. W., Kaufman, A. *et al.* (1988) Efficacy of computerized tomography in the preoperative staging of pancreatic carcinoma. *American Journal of Surgery*, **54**, 221–225

Sarr, M. G. and Cameron, J. L. (1982) Surgical management of unresectable carcinoma of the pancreas. *Surgery*, **91**, 123–133

Shapiro, T. M. (1975) Adenocarcinoma of the pancreas: a statistical analysis of biliary bypass vs Whipple resection in good risk patients. *Annals of Surgery*, **182**, 715–721

Speer, A. G., Cotton, P. B., Russell, R. C. G. *et al.* (1987) Randomised trial of endoscopic versus percutaneous stent insertion in malignant obstructive jaundice. *Lancet*, **i**, 57–62

Terblanche, J. (1979) Carcinoma of the proximal extrahepatic biliary tree–definitive and palliative treatment. *Surgery Annual*, **11**, 249–265

Todoroki, T., Okamura, T., Fukao, K. *et al.* (1980) Gross appearance of carcinoma of the main hepatic duct and its prognosis. *Surgery, Gynecology and Obstetrics*, **150**, 33–40

Tompkins, R. K. (1982) Carcinoma of the gallbladder and biliary ducts. In *The Biliary Tract* (ed. L. H. Blumgart), Churchill Livingstone, Edinburgh, pp. 183–196

Tompkins, R. K., Thomas, D., Wile, A. and Longmire, W. P. Jr (1981) Prognostic factors in bile duct carcinoma. *Annals of Surgery*, **194**, 447–457

Trede, M. (1985) The surgical treatment of pancreatic carcinoma.`*Surgery*, **97**, 28–35

Trede, M. and Schwall, G. (1988) The complication of pancreatectomy. *Annals of Surgery*, **207**, 39–47

Tsuchiya, R., Noda, T. and Harada, N. *et al.* (1986) Collective review of small carcinomas of the pancreas. *Annals of Surgery*, **203**, 77–81

Tsunoda, T., Tsuchiya, R., Harada, N. *et al.* (1985) Surgical treatment for carcinoma of the extrahepatic bile ducts. *Japanese Journal of Surgery*, **15**, 123–129

Warshaw, A. L., Tepper, J. E. and Shipley, W. U. (1986) Laparoscopy in the staging and planning of therapy for pancreatic cancer. *American Journal of Surgery*, **151**, 76–80

Weaver, D. W., Wieneck, R. G., Bouwman, D. L. and Walt, A. J. (1987) Gastrojejunostomy – is it helpful for patients with pancreatic cancer? *Surgery*, **102**, 608–613

Wise, L., Pizzimbono, C. and Dehner, L. P. (1976) Peri-ampullary cancer: A clinicopathologic study of sixty-two patients. *American Journal of Surgery*, **131**, 141–148

Yamamoto, R., Tatsuta, M., Noguchi, S. *et al.* (1985) Histocytologic diagnosis of pancreatic cancer by percutaneous aspiration biopsy under ultrasonic guidance. *American Journal of Clinical Pathology*, **83**, 409–414

Yasuda, K., Mukai, H., Fujimoto, S. *et al.* (1988) The diagnosis of pancreatic cancer by endoscopic ultrasonography. *Gastrointestinal Endoscopy*, **34**, 1–8

Chapter 4

Colorectal cancer

C. S. McArdle

Introduction

Colorectal cancer is the second commonest cause of death from malignancy in the UK; each year there are approximately 27 000 new cases and 19 000 deaths attributable to the disease. Surgery remains the only effective method of achieving cure. Unfortunately the overall results today are not significantly better than those of the early 1960s; only 35–40% of patients survive five years.

The incidence of colon cancer is high in Northern and Western Europe, North America and New Zealand, intermediate in Central Europe and low in Africa, Asia and South America (Waterhouse *et al.*, 1976). Studies of migrants from countries at low risk have shown that, within one or two generations, the incidence of colorectal cancer rises to that of their adopted country. This has been observed among Japanese migrants to Hawaii (Haenszell *et al.*, 1973) and among Polish migrants to the United States and Australia. The subsequent risk of colorectal cancer appears to be directly related to the socio-economic level achieved.

Countries with high rates of colorectal cancer also have high rates of cancer of the ovary, endometrium, breast and prostate; breast and colorectal cancer show a particularly close association. High rates of colorectal cancer are associated with high rates of coronary heart disease. Finland, with a high incidence of coronary heart disease and low colorectal cancer rates, is an exception.

It is clear from the above that although hereditary factors may be important in some patients, the majority of cases appear to be related to environmental influences. Dietary factors, in particular a low-fibre, high-fat diet, have been shown to correlate well with known geographical variations of colorectal cancer.

The fibre hypothesis was based on the observation that people in Third World countries had a higher intake of dietary fibre and a low incidence of colorectal cancer. Burkitt proposed that a high-fibre intake increased stool bulk and reduced transit time through the large bowel thereby reducing the exposure of the colonic mucosa to potential carcinogens (Burkitt, 1971). There is, however, no clear evidence to show that a high-fibre intake consistently shortens transit time. Furthermore, two major international surveys found no correlation between dietary fibre and the geographical incidence of large bowel cancer (Drasar and Irving, 1973; Armstrong and Doll, 1975).

An alternative explanation for the apparent benefit of dietary fibre might be simultaneous ingestion of cruciferous vegetables such as cabbage (Graham *et al.*, 1978). Wattenberg showed that these vegetables increased aryl hydrocarbon hydroxylase activity which acts as a barrier to noxious chemicals in the gastrointestinal tract. He also showed that these vegetables could prevent experimentally induced tumours in rats (Wattenberg and Loub, 1978).

The alternative hypothesis, that the risk of developing colorectal cancer is directly related to animal fat intake, was based on a study of 21 countries which demonstrated a close relationship between mortality for colorectal cancer and ingestion of animal fats (Wynder, 1975). According to this hypothesis a high dietary fat intake is associated with an increase in faecal bile acids and neutral steroids. Significantly higher concentrations of bile acids and neutral steroids have been found in the faeces of omnivorous people compared with vegetarians and cancer patients compared with controls (Reddy and Wynder, 1977). The suggestion that surgical manipulations, e.g. cholecystectomy, which increase the faecal bile acid concentration also increases the incidence of colorectal cancers remains contentious (Moorehead and McKelvey, 1989). The presence of anaerobic bacteria, particularly *Clostridium paraputrificum*, is important (Hill *et al.*, 1975); this organism is known to dehydrogenate the steroid nucleus thereby producing carcinogens.

Possible links between coffee consumption, vitamin D intake and colorectal cancer remain unproven (Garland *et al.*, 1985; Jacobsen and Thelle, 1987).

Adenoma–carcinoma sequence

Apart from the uncommon situation where a carcinoma occurs in the patient with longstanding ulcerative colitis, it is now generally accepted that the majority, if not all, adenocarcinomas of the large bowel arise from neoplastic polyps or adenomas, the so called adenoma–carcinoma sequence. Large bowel adenomas can, therefore, be regarded as premalignant lesions and increasingly the attention of clinicians has focused on the detection and removal of polyps in the hope that this would reduce the subsequent development of cancer.

In countries with a high or intermediate risk for colorectal cancer, adenomas are very common. In autopsy studies, the prevalence of adenomas ranges from 24 to 61% depending on age. Thus, in one study from the USA, adenomas were present in 58% of males and 47% of females over the age of 55 (Rickert *et al.*, 1979); in most studies, an excess of males has been noted. In contrast, where the incidence of colorectal cancer is low, adenomas are infrequent.

The mere presence of adenomas, however, does not necessarily imply a proportionately greater risk of large bowel cancer. This may be related to differences in the size of adenomas. Only 5% of adenomas in Japan and 2% in Colombia are greater than 1 cm in diameter; the low incidence of cancer in these countries may, therefore, be directly related to the small numbers of large adenomas.

Approximately 50% of adenomas are found in the rectum and sigmoid colon, approximately 15% on the right side and the remainder scattered throughout. Approximately 66% are within reach of the 60 cm fibreoptic sigmoidoscope whereas only 9% lie within 25 cm, generally regarded as the upper limit for rigid sigmoidoscopy.

The WHO classification is based on the histological structure and divides adenomas into tubular, villous and an intermediate tubulovillous type. The typical tubular adenoma is a small, spherical polyp with a stalk, its smooth surface being broken into lobules by intercommunicating clefts. Histologically it consists of closely packed branching epithelial tubules, the stalk being composed of normal mucosa and submucosa. In contrast, the villous adenoma is usually large and sessile with a shaggy surface composed of numerous fronds. On histology, finger-like projections of neoplastic epithelium with a core of normal lamina propria project towards the bowel lumen, the epithelium dipping down between the processes to abut on the muscularis mucosae.

Approximately 60–70% of adenomas are tubular, 10% are villous and 20–30% belong to an intermediate tubulovillous category. Multiple polyps are present in 35–50% of patients; approximately 15% of patients have more than two adenomas. The likelihood of multiple polyps increases with age; for instance, Rickert found the prevalence of multiple lesions to be three-fold higher in patients aged over 75 compared to those aged under 60.

Evidence that adenomas are premalignant is based on a number of observations. Studies of operative specimens removed for colorectal cancer have shown that in about one-third of patients one or more adenomas are present. Furthermore, the risk of developing a second or metachronous tumour is twice as high in patients with coexistent adenomas. Adenomas are also present in 75% of patients with two or more synchronous tumours.

In addition, it is sometimes obvious on histology that the tumour is partly benign and partly malignant. Of 1961 tumours examined at St Mark's Hospital, 14.2% contained varying proportions of adenomatous tissue (Muto, Bussey and Morson, 1975). Sixty percent of tumours limited to the submucosa had an adenomatous component compared to 20% of those confined to the bowel wall and 7% of tumours extending into the extramural fat. These results suggest that the majority of large bowel cancers arise from previously benign adenomas and that as the carcinoma enlarges more of the adenomatous tissue is destroyed by or is transformed into malignant tissue.

If carcinomas develop from adenomas then it would be expected that they would occur in an older age group. Results from screening clinics where asymptomatic individuals are examined confirm this, the average age for adenomas and carcinomas being 50 and 58 years respectively.

Four factors, probably inter-related, have been shown to be important in the development of carcinomas:

Size. Large adenomas are more likely to develop malignancy. 60% of adenomas are less than 1 cm in size, about 20–25% are between 1 and 2 cm in size and only 15–20% greater than 2 cm in diameter. In a series from St Mark's Hospital of 2489 adenomas, 1.3% of adenomas less than 1 cm in diameter were malignant compared with 9.5% of those between 1 and 2 cm and 46% of those over 2 cm in diameter (Muto et al., 1977).

Histological Type. Villous adenomas are more likely to develop carcinomas. In the St Mark's series the malignancy rate was 5% for tubular adenomas, 22% for tubulovillous adenomas and 40% for villous adenomas. In different series the malignant potential varies, probably because the grading of adenomas is highly subjective. A villous growth pattern occurs more often in large adenomas, and this may suggest that as an adenoma enlarges, there is a greater tendency for a villous pattern to emerge. On the basis of size and histological type, therefore, the common small tubular adenoma has a malignant potential of approximately 1% whereas in villous tumours over 2 cm in diameter the malignant potential is considerable.

Epithelial Dysplasia. Irrespective of the histological pattern, the malignant potential of adenomas increases with the degree of dysplasia. The majority of small adenomas usually show mild dysplasia only and have a low malignant potential. The incidence of dysplasia increases with size; severe dysplasia is rare, but when it occurs the incidence of malignancy rises to 27%.

Number of Polyps. After 15 years, 50% of patients presenting with a solitary adenoma develop a second adenoma; the risk of developing invasive cancer is one in twenty (Table 4.1). In contrast, after 15 years 80% of patients presenting with multiple adenomas develop further adenomas and one in eight an invasive cancer (Morson and Bussey, 1985).

Table 4.1 Risk of further adenomas and cancer

	Adenoma			Cancer		
Years of observation	5	10	15	5	10	15
Single adenoma	14%	33%	50%	1%	2%	5%
Multiple adenomas	33%	67%	80%	7%	12%	12%

Pathology

Historically most systems of classification have initially been developed to apply to rectal cancer, and subsequently extended as a convenient method of classifying colorectal cancer in general. The first clinically applicable classification was originally described by Dukes in 1932 and subsequently modified by Dukes and Bussey (1958). Colorectal tumours were divided into three stages:

A. where the tumour was confined to the mucosa.
B. where the tumour had invaded muscle.
C. where lymph node metastases were present.

Further modifications were described by Kirklin, Dockerty and Waugh (1949) and Astler and Coller (1954). It is also conventional to add a D category which implies the presence of distant metastases. Although TNM classifications have been described they have not gained widespread acceptance and Dukes' classification or one of its modifications remains the most widely used method of pathological staging.

Ideally, a prognostic classification for patients undergoing apparently curative resection would clearly separate those with a high probability of survival from those with a high probability of dying. At best Dukes' staging or its modifications can only identify a small proportion of patients (Dukes' A) with a good prognosis. In order to improve upon the prognostic value of Dukes' staging, a number of other clinical and pathological variables have been evaluated. Factors considered to have prognostic significance independent of stage, include histological grade, the presence of venous invasion, the number of nodes involved and the presence or absence of apical lymph node metastases (Freedman, Macaskill and Smith, 1984; Phillips et al., 1984b; Chapuis et al., 1985). Unfortunately, some of these factors are dependent on subjective assessment and inter-observer variation is high. For instance, in one multicentre study the percentage of colorectal cancers considered to be well differentiated varied from 3 to 93% (Blenkinsopp *et al.*, 1981). Such discrepancies clearly limit their clinical use.

Fielding and his colleagues (1986) analysed clinical and pathological factors affecting outcome in 2524 patients who had undergone 'curative' resection. In the first group, statistical weightings were established for each prognostic factor. These, in order of importance, were lymph node status, tumour mobility, number of positive lymph nodes, presence of obstruction and depth of primary tumour penetration. These mathematical weightings were then applied to the second group of patients. However, despite the complexity of the methods used, only 23% of patients could be predicted as having an excellent prognosis with any degree of certainty.

Recently, Jass, Love and Northover (1987) have described a new prognostic classification based on four variables shown to have independent influence upon survival — the number of lymph nodes with metastatic deposits, character of invasive margin, peritumoural lymphocytic infiltration and local spread. Each of these four variables was then awarded an appropriately weighted score and on the basis of these scores the patients were divided into four groups. Survival ranged from 27 to 96% at five years. When the scoring system was applied prospectively to a second set of patients similar results were obtained.

Screening

The average delay from the onset of symptoms to surgery in the UK is approximately 8–9 months. Most of this delay is due either to the patient failing to report symptoms to the family doctor, through fear of cancer or lack of insight, or delay in referral to hospital because the symptoms attributable to colorectal cancer are very common and often non-specific. For example, recent studies have shown that 6.6% of a population had recent rectal bleeding and 12% reported alteration of bowel habit (Farrands and Hardcastle, 1984).

It is tempting to think that earlier diagnosis of symptomatic colorectal cancer would increase the proportion of early cancers. However, although the use of faecal occult blood testing to select patients for urgent fibreoptic sigmoidoscopy resulted in a reduction of the median time to diagnosis from 91 days in a control group to 17 days in a test group, the pathological stage of tumours detected in both groups was similar (Armitage *et al.*, 1984). Thus it would appear that by the time the patient reports to his family doctor, the tumour is well advanced and a reduction in the delay to diagnosis at this stage will have little effect on ultimate survival.

Attention has, therefore, focused on the detection of tumours in asymptomatic patients. Although endoscopic screening may be appropriate in high-risk patients, such as patients previously treated for adenomas, those with a family history of colorectal cancer or patients with a long history of inflammatory bowel disease, the only practical method of population screening available at the present time is by the detection of occult blood in the faeces. Haemoccult, a relatively insensitive test based upon the guaiac reagent, has a false negative rate of approximately 20%. The false negative rate can be reduced by increasing the number of tests but any increase in sensitivity results in an unacceptably high false positive rate. Immunological investigations such as the HemoQuant assay which measures stool porphyrins are more sensitive and more specific than the chemical tests, but they are expensive and complex to perform and have not yet been shown to be more cost effective in population screening.

The success of any screening programme depends on patient acceptability. In the UK the compliance rate varies from 27 to 45%. Involvement of the family doctor and a preliminary explanatory letter has been shown to improve cooperation. Unfortunately, the elderly are least likely to comply even although the likelihood of detecting a neoplasm is highest in this group.

In the Nottingham study, individuals aged over 50 years were randomized to a group offered FOB testing or a control group. Of the 52 258 individuals offered screening, 27 651 (53%) completed the tests and 2.3% had a positive result; 63 large bowel cancers and 367 adenomas were diagnosed. Of the 63 cancers detected, 52% were Dukes' A. In addition, 76 adenomas with a diameter over 2 cm, lesions with a high risk of malignancy, were detected. A further 13 cancers were detected on re-screening at two years; of these 7 were Dukes' A. This compares with a total of 123 cancers detected in the control group, 11% of which were Dukes' Stage A (Hardcastle et al., 1989).

It may, however, be premature to conclude that the detection of a high percentage of Dukes' A tumours is synonymous with a more favourable outcome. Earlier detection by definition means that the tumour has been discovered at an earlier stage in the natural history of the disease and ensures that observed patient survival will be longer. Furthermore, screening will detect a statistically disproportionate number of biologically favourable slow growing tumours; this also contributes to more favourable staging. Whether screening can genuinely improve outcome, independent of these biological biases, can only be determined by prospective randomized clinical trials such as those currently being undertaken in Nottingham.

At the moment, therefore, there is no conclusive evidence that screening decreases mortality from colorectal cancer; the prognosis of patients who develop colorectal cancer may be much more dependent upon its inherent biological behaviour than on the precise time of detection. Moreover, although FOB testing is cheap, the subsequent radiological and endoscopic investigations of those patients with a positive FOB are costly and most people with a positive FOB test will suffer inconvenience, fear and unnecessary investigation and yet ultimately prove not to have cancer.

Results of treatment

The results of treatment are disappointing, largely as a result of the advanced nature of the disease at the time of presentation. Of 645 patients admitted to the Royal Infirmary in Glasgow over a 6-year period, almost 45% had evidence of local tumour fixation and over 25% had distant metastases; 23% were admitted as an emergency (McArdle et al., 1990). The overall resectability rate was 70%, of which 52% were regarded as curative. Palliative diversion was performed in 21% of patients and 8% underwent laparotomy only or had no surgical treatment.

Approximately 70% of patients undergoing apparently curative resection survived 2 years and 50% survived 5 years. Survival was directly related to stage, 81% of patients with Dukes' A tumours surviving 5 years compared with 56% of Dukes' B and 33% of Dukes' C patients. Approximately 80% of patients

Table 4.2 Survival (UK studies)

Centre (authors)	Type of study	No. of patients	Operative mortality (%)	Curative resections (%)	5-year survival (%)	5-year survival curative resection (%)
Birmingham (Slaney, 1971)	Population-based	12494	–	49	21	42
Aberdeen (Clarke and Needham, 1980)	Population-based	433	17	50	29	50
Oxford (Gill and Morris, 1978)	Hospital-based	335	6	57	26	37
Bristol (Umbleby and Williamson, 1984)	Hospital-based	727	17	60	27	–
Glasgow (GRI series)	Hospital-based	645	13	52	27	50
St Mark's (Lockhart-Mummery et al., 1976)	Specialist Centre	3163	2	80	47	57
Leeds (Whittaker and Goligher, 1976)	Specialist Centre	550	11	74	43	49

undergoing palliative resection and virtually all patients undergoing palliative diversion died within 2 years.

These results are similar to previous population-based studies, but are worse than those achieved in specialist centres (Table 4.2). This apparent discrepancy in outcome is largely, although not entirely, accounted for by the marked difference in patient population. In the Royal Infirmary series, a large proportion of patients presented as emergencies, with local tumour fixity or distant metastases; less than 3% of patients had Dukes' A tumours. In contrast, specialist centres tend to deal with younger, fitter patients on a non-urgent basis; there is also a significantly higher proportion of early tumours. Analysis of survival stage by stage for population based and specialist centres studies have shown remarkably little difference (Stewart et al., 1979; Goligher, 1981).

Clearly the outlook for patients with unresectable disease or evidence of dissemination at the time of laparotomy is extremely poor. Moreover, in most series, 40–50% of patients undergoing apparently curative resection also die within 5 years. At necropsy 70% of these patients have evidence of dissemination (Gilbert et al., 1984).

Death from disseminated disease following apparently curative resection has, in the past, been attributed to the dissemination of tumour at the time of surgery. It is now know, however, that the majority of patients who ultimately die of liver metastases have occult hepatic metastases, not detected by the surgeon at the time of laparotomy.

The existence of occult hepatic metastases was first described in 1941 by Goligher. In a study of 790 patients considered to have a disease-free liver at surgery, 31 died during the immediate postoperative period; post-mortem examination demonstrated the presence of hepatic metastases in 5 (16%) patients. Recently, Gray (1980) analysed 116 patients with gastrointestinal cancer who had died within one month of surgery. At laparotomy, the liver was considered to be disease free in 78 patients, and in 38 it was considered to contain metastases. These assessments proved to be incorrect at post-mortem examination in 9 of the 116 cases. In 6 of the 78 patients considered to be disease free, post-mortem examination revealed the presence of metastases; in contrast, 3 of the 38 patients thought to have metastases were shown to have benign lesions. These findings emphasize the inadequacies of palpation of the liver at the time of laparotomy. Clearly, the surgeon may miss metastases; furthermore, he may mistake benign lesions for secondary deposits.

More recently, Finlay and McArdle (1986) assessed the effect of occult hepatic metastases on survival following apparently curative resection for colorectal cancer. They followed 71 patients for 5 years after apparently curative resection. One of the 71 patients undergoing 'curative' surgery died postoperatively and at post-mortem examination small hepatic metastases were found. Hepatic ultrasonography and/or computed tomography performed during the immediate postoperative period in the remaining 70 patients suggested the presence of hepatic metastases in 16. All developed clinically obvious hepatic metastases; 15 died within 5 years. Occult hepatic metastases were therefore detected in 17 (24%) of the 71 patients. The majority of these occult hepatic metastases were located within the inaccessible posterior aspect of the right lobe of liver. They ranged from 0.4 cm to 3.0 cm in diameter; only 3 patients had metastases less than 1 cm in size. Only 6 patients with occult hepatic metastases had metastases confined to the liver at the time of death. Ten of the 46 patients with negative scans at the time of surgery died of loco-regional recurrence.

One of the patients with occult hepatic metastases survived 5 years; in contrast, only 5 of 54 patients without evidence of occult hepatic metastases at the time of surgery died of disseminated disease. The presence or absence of occult hepatic metastases at the time of surgery therefore predicted the majority of deaths from disseminated disease following apparently curative resection for colorectal cancer.

Studies of the rate of growth of these occult hepatic metastases showed that the tumour doubling time was approximately 86 days (Finlay et al., 1988). Assuming a single cell origin and Gompertzian growth, these results suggest that the occult hepatic metastases had been present for more than 2 years prior to clinical presentation and that their overall lifespan was approximately 4 years.

Similarly, in the past, local recurrence has been attributed to the implantation of tumour cells at the time of resection, spread from adjacent lymph node metastases or the development of a metachronous tumour. By undertaking meticulous examination of the operative specimen, however, Quirke and his colleagues (1986) demonstrated tumour involvement of the lateral resection margin in 14 of 52 (27%) patients; 12 of these subsequently developed local recurrence. The situation is therefore analogous to the relationship between occult hepatic metastases and the subsequent development of overt disease. In rectal, and probably colonic, cancer local recurrence is mainly due to inadequate resection of the primary tumour.

Clearly these observations have major implications for the management of patients undergoing resection for colorectal cancer. Patients with occult hepatic metastases at surgery have a poor prognosis and might benefit from adjuvant therapy. In contrast, those patients who truly do have a disease-free liver at the time of surgery are predominantly at risk of dying from loco-regional recurrence. The incidence of local recurrence varies widely among surgeons; attention to surgical technique in this group might therefore improve survival (Heald and Ryall, 1986). In patients in whom adequate clearance is not possible, radiotherapy might be used to control local disease.

Staging

Hepatic metastases

In view of the profound effect of hepatic metastases on survival it is clearly important to establish the presence or absence of hepatic metastases prior to or during surgery.

Liver function tests are of limited value. In early studies, alkaline phosphatase and gammaglutamyl transpeptidase was found to be elevated in over 70% of patients with liver metastases; the majority of these patients, however, had hepatic enlargement and the presence of metastases was suspected clinically. In a recent study in patients with known metastases, liver function tests failed to detect more than half the liver metastases, most of which were greater than 2 cm in diameter (Huguier and Lacaine, 1981).

Similarly, early reports in patients with known hepatic matastases suggested that up to 90% of lesions could be detected using liver scintigraphy, ultrasonography or computed tomography (Schreve *et al.*, 1984). However, these conclusions were based on the premise that the findings at laparotomy are the 'gold standard' with which other investigative techniques should be compared; it makes the assumption that the surgeon can detect the presence of liver metastases with unerring accuracy. Yet, clearly, this is not so.

Although the relative value of imaging techniques has been well established in patients with overt hepatic metastases, the value of these techniques in the detection of occult disease has only recently been assessed. In the study described by Finlay and McArdle (1986), the majority of patients with occult hepatic metastases were identified by a combination of carefully employed ultrasonography and computed tomography. It remains to be seen whether these results can be reproduced in routine clinical practice; computed tomography is time consuming and in the above study had a high false positive rate. Clearly there is a need to develop alternative methods of detecting occult hepatic metastases.

Dynamic hepatic scintigraphy is a method of enhancing the diagnostic accuracy of isotopic hepatic imaging. The liver receives approximately 20–30% of its blood supply via the hepatic artery, the remainder coming from the portal vein. Dynamic hepatic scintigraphy is based on the premise that because liver metastases have an arterial blood supply the increased proportion of arterial blood perfusing the liver produces an altered pattern of flow. The ratio of arterial to total liver blood flow is expressed as the hepatic perfusion index (HPI).

In the Leeds study, 47 of 50 patients with overt hepatic metastases at laparotomy had elevated HPI indices (Leveson *et al.*, 1985). Of the remaining 100 patients thought to have disease-free livers, 43 had elevated HPI values. Fifty patients with ostensibly normal livers at laparotomy were reviewed after 1 year. Of these, 18 had developed hepatic metastases; all had elevated HPI values at the time of initial laparotomy. The remaining 32 patients remained disease free; of these, 11 had elevated HPI values at the time of surgery. Overall, therefore, no patients with a normal HPI developed hepatic metastases and 18 of 29 patients with elevated HPI values at the time of initial laparotomy subsequently developed clinically overt hepatic metastases. The disadvantage of dynamic hepatic scintigraphy remains that it is unable to provide information about the number and anatomical site of metastases. Furthermore, doubts about its reliability have been expressed (Laird, Williams and Williams, 1987).

An alternative approach is the use of intraoperative ultrasound probes. *In vitro* studies have shown these probes are capable of detecting 95% of metastases 1 cm in diameter or greater and 67% of those 0.5 to 1.0 cm in diameter (Thomas, Morris and Hardcastle, 1987).

Machi and his colleagues (1987) have evaluated intraoperative ultrasonography in 84 patients undergoing surgery for colorectal cancer; all patients had undergone preoperative ultrasonography and computed tomography. Thirty-one of 32 metastases diagnosed by preoperative investigations and/or surgical exploration were also identified by intraoperative ultrasonography. In addition, however, intraoperative ultrasonography detected a further 14 metastatic lesions in 10 (11.9%) patients. Six of these were already known to have metastatic disease, but the remaining 4 were considered to be disease free on the basis of preoperative investigations and laparotomy findings. All the metastases were less than 2 cm in diameter, were situated deep in the liver substance and were non-palpable.

On the basis of these findings intraoperative ultrasonography would currently appear to be the best available method of detecting 'occult' hepatic metastases. The technique has the capacity to detect, with a reasonable degree of accuracy, metastases as small as 0.5 cm lying deep within the liver substance. The detection of such lesions at operation would facilitate resection or placement of a hepatic artery catheter for subsequent chemotherapy. Furthermore, the ability of intraoperative ultrasonography to demonstrate the relationship between tumours and intrahepatic vascular structures suggests that it has an important role during the planning of hepatic resection.

Surveillance

Carcinoembryonic antigen (CEA) has been used as a tumour marker in colorectal cancer for over two decades, despite this its value remains uncertain. Elevated levels of CEA in patients with colorectal cancer tend to be indicators of advanced or progressive disease, and hence are associated with a poor prognosis. CEA is not specific for colorectal cancer and elevated levels may also occur in patients with cancer of non-colorectal origin, especially gastric and breast cancer, and in patients with functional hepatic impairment or inflammatory bowel disease.

Previous studies have suggested that elevated levels of CEA prior to surgery reflected the extent of disease and predicted the likelihood of subsequent tumour recurrence. Recent studies have failed to confirm this. Lewi and his colleagues (1984) showed that, although preoperative CEA levels reflected the extent of the underlying disease process, elevated levels failed to predict patients with a poor prognosis following apparently curative resection. Approximately 75% of patients undergoing apparently curative resection survived 2 years and 45% survived 5 years irrespective of preoperative CEA levels.

The role of CEA in the early detection of recurrent disease has also been extensively evaluated. In general, although grossly elevated levels of CEA are found in patients with advanced metastatic disease, the ability to identify local recurrence or hepatic metastases at a potentially curable stage is disappointing. The test is limited by the observation that approximately one-third of patients do not have abnormal serum concentrations of CEA at any stage of the disease whereas others who are disease free may show transient rises (Northover, 1986). Nevertheless, a recent review concluded that serial estimations of CEA was the best non-invasive method for detecting asymptomatic recurrence following apparently curative resection (NIH Consensus Statement, 1981).

The rate of rise of CEA may be important. Two distinct patterns of CEA rise have been described: a fast rise in which serum concentrations quadruple within 6 months and a slow rise in which concentrations do not reach three times normal values for at least 12 months (Wood *et al.*, 1980). The majority of patients with a fast rise had distant metastases with or without local recurrence, whereas the majority of those with a slow rise had local recurrence alone. Survival was significantly worse in patients with rapidly rising CEA levels. Boey and his colleagues (1984) reached similar conclusions. In contrast, Hine and Dykes (1984a) failed to confirm that the pattern in rise in CEA was of practical value in distinguishing localized from distant recurrence. Furthermore, valuable time may be lost while plotting the rate of rise of CEA.

Whether CEA-initiated early detection and second-look laparotomy in asymptomatic patients influences survival remains controversial. The Columbus group have consistently claimed that this is so. Martin and his colleagues (1977) performed CEA-initiated second-look laparotomy in 25 patients. Of the 22 patients with proven tumour recurrence, 16 (73%) had distant metastases and 6 (27%) had localized tumours; 1 patient survived 3 years. They subsequently reported that 61% of patients re-explored on the basis of an elevated CEA had resectable disease compared with only 27% of a group of patients in whom second-look laparotomies were undertaken for clinically apparent recurrence (Martin *et al.*, 1980).

Attiyeh and Stearns (1981) performed 37 second-look laparotomies in 32 asymptomatic patients who had significant CEA elevations following curative resection for colorectal cancer. Recurrence was confirmed in 33 (89%) patients; 4 patients underwent negative laparotomy. Liver metastases were present in 18 patients, 7 of whom underwent resection; loco-regional recurrence was found in 15 patients, 9 of whom underwent resection. The overall resectability rate was therefore 43%. Lower CEA levels, shorter time delays to surgery and slower rates of CEA rise were related to the resectability rate. Eight patients were alive and well at a median follow-up of 15 months.

Staab and his associates (1985) described 40 patients with colorectal cancer who underwent second-look laparotomy. In 25 patients the decision to re-operate was based on elevated levels of CEA alone; 11 underwent curative or palliative resection. Survival appeared to be better than a comparable group of patients who had refused re-operation.

Nevertheless, the suggestion that some patients undergoing CEA-initiated re-operation survive significantly longer than those coming to surgery as a result of routine clinical surveillance remains unproven. If, as suggested by Quirke and his colleagues (1986) the majority of local recurrences result from inadequate clearance of the primary tumour at the time of initial surgery it seems unlikely that 'cure' could be achieved at a second-look laparotomy.

It also seems unlikely that many patients with hepatic metastases will benefit. Finlay and McArdle (1983) showed that the overall lifespan of hepatic metastases was approximately 4 years, whereas the interval between the initial CEA rise and death was only 5 months. Perhaps it is therefore not surprising that attempts to treat patients with chemotherapy on the basis of elevated postoperative CEA levels have proved unsuccessful (Hine and Dykes, 1984b). For similar reasons CEA-initiated second-look laparotomy may fail to improve survival. Only a large scale prospective study in which CEA-initiated laparotomy was compared with a conventional clinically based regime will answer this question (Northover, 1986).

Surgery

The surgery of colorectal cancer is based on the following principles:

1. Colorectal cancer spreads in a predictable fashion to the adjacent mesenteric lymph nodes.
2. Survival after apparently curative resection is directly related to the stage of the disease, e.g. the depth of tumour penetration and/or the presence of lymph node metastases at the time of surgery.
3. While other factors, e.g. venous and lymphatic invasion, influence long-term survival, these findings are only apparent on examination of the resected specimen.
4. Unlike solid tumours of other organs, e.g. lung and breast, radical as opposed to localized resection may play a crucial role in determining survival (Enker, 1981).

The clinicopathological assessment and staging of patients with colorectal cancer has recently been reviewed (Williams, Jass and Hardcastle, 1988). Prior to surgery the nature of the tumour and the extent of disease should be established. For patients with rectal cancer, the degree of fixity (mobile, tethered or fixed) and the extent of circumferential involvement should be established by palpation. The height of the tumour should be determined using a rigid sigmoidoscope. Wherever possible a biopsy should be obtained, if necessary by colonoscopy, to confirm the presence of tumour and establish the degree of differentiation. In some centres, further information may be obtained about the degree of local spread, the distance of the tumour from the anal sphincter and the presence of enlarged lymph nodes by computed tomography or endoanal ultrasonography (Beynon, 1989).

The presence or absence of hepatic metastases should be established by ultrasound or, if available, computed tomography. Synchronous lesions, either adenomas or a second tumour should be excluded by double-contrast barium enema or colonoscopy. Preoperative intravenous pyelography is not routinely required (Phillips et al., 1983), but may be useful in certain patients, for example those with fixed masses in the sigmoid colon or caecum.

At the time of laparotomy particular attention should be paid to the degree of fixity of the primary tumour and the extent of spread, in particular the presence or absence of enlarged nodes, peritoneal seedlings and liver metastases. The number of liver metastases should be noted and biopsy taken wherever possible. Enlarged lymph nodes not included in the resection specimen or suspected peritoneal metastases should also be biopsied. If there is any doubt as to the completeness of excision the tumour bed should be biopsied.

The fixity of the primary tumour will determine resectability and the extent of spread, and ultimate survival. As a general rule, mobile tumours should always be resected, irrespective of the presence or absence of liver metastases. If the tumour is free and easily mobile, this should present no problem. However, if the tumour is tethered to surrounding structures e.g. uterus, bladder or small bowel, resection of these organs may also be necessary. In patients with locally advanced tumours, direct tumour infiltration is present in only one-third of patients and survival following extended radical surgery is similar to that obtained after standard excision of tumours of the same stage (Pittam et al., 1984). In patients in whom the primary tumour is fixed and resection is not feasible the tumour should be bypassed. In fixed tumours of the sigmoid and rectosigmoid, however, it may not be possible to gain access distal to the tumour and in these circumstances colostomy may be required.

Nevertheless, despite apparently adequate surgery many patients die of hepatic metastases. Based on the premise that these metastases were due to the dissemination of malignant cells by tumour manipulation, Turnbull popularized the so called 'no-touch' isolation technique whereby the lymphovascular pedicles were ligated and the colon divided before the cancer bearing segment was mobilized. In his study the 5-year survival of 460 patients undergoing apparently curative resection, undertaken by Turnbull personally using the 'no-touch' technique, was 69% compared with 52% in 128 similar patients undergoing conventional surgery by other surgeons at the same institution (Turnbull *et al.*, 1967).

Opponents of this technique, however, attributed his results to better patient selection; they noted that similar results had been achieved by extended resection alone. Recently, the 'no-touch' isolation technique has been compared with conventional surgery in a large prospective randomized study. Although fewer liver metastases occurred in the 'no-touch' isolation group, this fell far short of significance (Wiggers *et al.*, 1988). Perhaps this is not surprising in view of the observation that the majority of liver metastases developing following apparently curative resection are present but undetected by the surgeon at the time of laparotomy.

Obstruction

Traditionally, patients presenting with acute large bowel obstruction due to left-sided colonic lesions were managed by a three-stage approach: initial transverse colostomy to provide decompression, subsequent resection of the primary lesion with anastomosis of the colon, followed eventually by closure of the colostomy. This approach is associated with a high cumulative morbidity and mortality and is associated with a prolonged period of hospitalization. Frequently the planned sequence of surgical procedures is not completed leaving the patient with an unsatisfactory permanent stoma. Hartmann's procedure with resection of the primary lesion, formation of a proximal end colostomy and closure of the rectal stump has gained widespread acceptance. Analysis of the results of the two-stage procedure in 122 patients showed the cumulative mortality rate to be 9% (Koruth *et al.*, 1985). The use of intraoperative colonic irrigation may facilitate primary resection and anastomosis in the hands of experienced colorectal surgeons (Koruth *et al.*).

Carcinoma of rectum

Conventionally cancers of the upper rectum were treated by low anterior resection whereas tumours below this level were treated by abdominoperineal resection. Two recent developments, however, have radically altered this approach. The first of these has been the development of the circular stapling device which has facilitated the performance of low rectal anastomosis. The second was the reappraisal of the so-called 5 cm rule. Until recently it was believed that failure to resect 5 cm of rectum distal to the tumour would compromise recurrence and survival (Enker, 1981).

However, these assumptions have recently been challenged. The Leeds group examined specimens obtained from 50 patients undergoing potentially curative abdominoperineal resection for rectal tumours situated 5–10 cm from the anal verge (Williams, Dixon and Johnston, 1983). In only 5 patients (10%) had the tumour spread more than 1 cm distally; each of these patients had a poorly differentiated Dukes' C tumour and each was dead or dying of distant metastases within 3 years of surgery. They also compared survival in 48 patients with a distant margin of less than 5 cm with 31 patients with a distal margin greater than 5 cm. Despite a higher proportion of unfavourable tumours in patients with a small distal resection margin, the incidence of recurrence and survival was similar in both groups.

Pollett and Nicholls (1983) also assessed the extent of distal clearance in 334 patients undergoing curative anterior resection for carcinoma of the rectum. The length of rectum below the tumour was 2 cm or less in 55 patients, 2–5 cm in 177 patients and 5 cm or more in 102 patients. There was no difference in local recurrence rates or overall survival (Table 4.3). These results also suggested that a margin less than 2 cm distal to a rectal cancer does not adversely affect local recurrence or survival. Encouraged by these findings many surgeons now would perform sphincter-saving surgery for tumours of the middle third of rectum.

Table 4.3 Five-year survival

	No.	%
<2 cm	55	69.1
2–5 cm	177	68.4
>5 cm	102	69.6

The increasing use of sphincter-saving surgery is, however, not without its drawbacks. It has long been recognized that anastomotic leakage can be demonstrated radiologically in up to 70% of low and 40% of high anastomoses. Clinically significant leaks, as judged by faecal fistula and local abscess formation occurred less frequently. There is little difference in clinical leakage rate between careful hand-held suture techniques and the use of stapling devices (McGinn et al., 1985; Everett, Friend and Forty, 1986). Indeed the type of anastomosis is of less importance than the site and who performs it. Fielding and his colleagues (1978) have shown that the leak rate among surgeons varied from less than 5% to almost 30%. Traditionally, in difficult anastomosis temporary defunctioning colostomy has been performed in the hope that this will prevent anastomotic leakage; there is, however, little evidence that defunctioning colostomy is beneficial in this context (Fielding et al., 1984). Temporary colostomy is now seldom performed.

The development of local recurrence has more sinister implications. Using data derived from a collaborative study of colorectal cancer in the large bowel cancer project, Phillips and his colleagues (1984a) examined those factors which influenced local recurrence following apparently curative abdominoperineal excision or anterior resection. More patients developed local recurrence following anterior resection than after abdominoperineal resection (Table 4.4). These results might suggest that anterior resection should be abandoned; many surgeons would feel that a 50% increase in the incidence of local recurrence which clearly prejudices the patient's survival outweighs the disadvantages of a permanent colostomy. However, the results obtained in the large bowel cancer project are

Table 4.4 Local recurrence

	AR	AP
No.	370	478
Recurrence	67	57
%	18	12*

* $P < 0.02$.

representative of a wide range of surgeons of varying technical ability and interests. There was a wide variation in local recurrence rate amongst surgeons, varying from less than 5% to over 20%. This clearly strengthens the argument that colorectal surgery, particularly surgery for carcinoma of the rectum should be undertaken by specialist surgeons. In single centres, the results achieved with an anterior resection and abdominoperineal excision are similar (Williams and Johnston, 1984; McDermott *et al.*, 1985; Williams, Durdey and Johnston, 1985).

Radiotherapy

Despite apparently curative resection, approximately one-third of patients with rectal carcinoma develop pelvic recurrence (Gunderson and Sosin, 1974; Gilbert *et al.*, 1984); the median time to recurrence is approximately 12 months. The likelihood of pelvic recurrence increases with stage, histological grade and the presence of microscopic tumour involvement of the lateral resection margins. Although there is substantial evidence that radiotherapy is useful in advanced disease, the value of adjuvant treatment remains unclear.

Preoperative radiotherapy (Table 4.5)

Early non-randomized studies from New York using preoperative low-dose radiotherapy showed an increase in survival from 23% to 37% in patients with involved lymph nodes; there was no improvement in survival for the group as a whole (Stearns *et al.*, 1959). A subsequent study from the same institution failed to confirm these findings (Stearns *et al.*, 1974).

In the Veterans Administration Surgical Adjuvant Group study, 700 patients were randomized to surgery alone or to receive a short course of preoperative

Table 4.5 Preoperative radiotherapy

Centre	Authors	Dose	No. of patients	5-year survival (%)	
				RT	Control
New York	Stearns *et al.* (1974)	2000	790	57	58
VASAG	Higgins *et al.* (1975)	2000	700	35	29
Toronto	Rider *et al.* (1977)	500	125	36	38
MRC	MRC (1984)	500 v. 2000	824	40	38
VASOG	Higgins *et al.* (1986)	3150	361	50	50
EORTC	Gerard *et al.* (1985)	3450	410	60	58

low-dose irradiation which included a perineal boost for patients with low-lying tumours (Higgins *et al.*, 1975). Of irradiated patients undergoing abdominoperineal resection 41% survived 5 years compared with 28% of controls; there also appeared to be a reduction in the number of lymph nodes involved and in the incidence of pelvic recurrence after irradiation. There was no difference in survival for any other subgroup.

In the Toronto study, patients were randomized to a single low dose prior to surgery or surgery alone. Although there was no difference in overall survival, a significant benefit was found in patients with involved nodes (Rider *et al.*, 1977).

The Medical Research Council (MRC) subsequently compared both the short course and single dose of preoperative radiotherapy, as advocated by the Veterans and the Toronto group, with surgery alone (Second Report of a Medical Research Council Working Party, 1984). They found a decrease in tumour size and in the number of involved lymph nodes in patients who had received preoperative radiotherapy but no improvement in overall survival in any subgroup and no decrease in pelvic tumour recurrence following irradiation.

The Veterans Administration have since initiated a second study comparing preoperative intermediate dose radiotherapy with surgery alone in patients undergoing abdominoperineal resection (Higgins *et al.*, 1986). Analysis showed no difference in survival between the groups.

Similar results were obtained in the EORTC and Stockholm studies (Gerard *et al.*, 1985); Stockholm Rectal Cancer Study Group, 1987). There was no difference in survival between the irradiated and control groups. In both these studies, however, there was a significant decrease in pelvic recurrence rates. For example, in the EORTC study, 95% of patients receiving radiotherapy were disease free at 5 years compared with 65% of patients treated by surgery alone. Furthermore, preliminary results from a number of unpublished studies currently underway show significant reductions in local recurrence rates.

There also have been reports of benefit following high-dose, preoperative radiotherapy in patients with fixed or inoperable tumours (Dosoretz *et al.*, 1983; Mohiuddin and Marks, 1987). It is claimed that up to 80% of these tumours may be rendered operable; indeed in 5–6% of patients no residual tumour was demonstrated in the resection specimen. High-dose radiotherapy does not appear to make subsequent surgery hazardous and, perhaps surprisingly, there appears to be no adverse effect on anastomotic healing. The value of high dose preoperative radiotherapy for fixed tumours is currently being assessed in a MRC study.

Postoperative radiotherapy

Preoperative radiotherapy has the advantage of being given over a short time with negligible morbidity. However, without accurate staging, it is difficult to identify which patients require treatment; for instance, unnecessary treatment with its attendant morbidity may be given to patients with Dukes' A tumours, the majority of whom will have been cured by surgery.

In contrast, although postoperative radiotherapy does result in significant morbidity, it can be confined to patients with more advanced tumours. Postoperative radiotherapy requires a more prolonged period of treatment, typically 4 or 5 weeks, and may be delayed by surgical complications. Owing to the development of small bowel adhesions following surgery high-dose radiotherapy may result in significant morbidity (Hoskins *et al.*, 1985). Careful planning, the use of multiple fields and surgical exclusion of small bowel from the pelvis may reduce morbidity (Bakare, Shafir and McElhinney, 1987).

Preliminary results have been obtained from 3 randomized studies of postoperative radiotherapy for resected Dukes' B and C rectal cancers; all these trials use similar radiotherapy doses (4000–5000 rads in 4–5 weeks). In the Gastrointestinal Tumor Study Group (GITSG) trial (1985) recruitment was terminated prematurely when preliminary analysis suggested that adjuvant therapy was beneficial. Subsequent analysis, however, showed no difference in survival. In the Danish study, there were also no significant differences in local recurrence rates or overall survival (Balslev *et al.*, 1986). In contrast, in the NSABP study (Fisher *et al.*, 1988) 16% of patients receiving radiotherapy developed local recurrence compared with 25% of patients in the control group. Some of these apparent differences may be resolved when the results of the third MRC trial on rectal cancer are analysed.

Despite the information generated by these studies, the true value of perioperative radiotherapy remains in doubt. It seems likely that both pre- and postoperative radiotherapy reduce local recurrence rates but the effect on survival is less clear. However, a recent analysis of 3000 patients included in randomized studies worldwide suggested that radiotherapy might reduce the odds of death by about 9% (Buyse, Zeleniuch-Jacquotte and Chalmers, 1988). The effect of radiotherapy might be more pronounced, although still small and not statistically significant, in patients undergoing apparently curative resection. In these patients the reduction in the odds of death was approximately 18%, equivalent to a 4% survival benefit at 5 years.

Palliative radiotherapy

The main symptom of recurrent rectal cancer following surgery is pain. Radiotherapy provides complete pain relief in approximately half the patients and partial pain relief in two-thirds (Taylor, Kerr and Arnott, 1987); 5% may survive 3 years.

Radiotherapy may also provide useful symptom control in patients with inoperable tumours. Pain relief can be achieved in approximately 80% and the control of blood or mucous discharge in approximately two-thirds; unfortunately, control of diarrhoea is less satisfactory (Taylor, Kerr and Arnott, 1987). Ten percent of these patients may survive 3 years.

The endocavitary technique for early lesions has been pioneered by Papillon (1975). Of 186 patients treated in his series, 26 failed of which 12 were salvaged by surgery. Of the group followed for 5 years only 9% died of cancer. Similar results have been achieved by Sischy and his colleagues (Sischy, Hinson and Wilkinson, 1988). The technique, however, is suitable only for a small minority of carefully selected lesions and is not widely available.

Chemotherapy

Adjuvant systemic therapy

Since its introduction almost 30 years ago, 5-fluorouracil has been extensively investigated in patients with colorectal cancer. Early studies in the 1970s, administering 5-fluorouracil as adjuvant therapy by a variety of routes and using different dosage schedules failed to show any benefit in relapse-free or overall survival in treated patients.

Recent large-scale studies have confirmed the inability of adjuvant cytotoxic therapy to prolong survival. In the Gastrointestinal Tumor Study Group (GITSG) study, 572 patients who had undergone 'curative' resection of a Dukes' Stage B2 or C colonic cancer were randomized to: (a) no further treatment; (b) chemotherapy with 5-fluorouracil and methyl-CCNU; (c) non-specific immunostimulation with BCG, or (d) a combination of the two (Gastrointestinal Tumor Study Group, 1984). At a median interval of 5½ years, there was no significant difference in disease-free or overall survival amongst the four study arms. Leukaemia developed in 7 patients receiving chemotherapy.

In contrast, in the GITSG rectal cancer study, patients who received both radiotherapy and chemotherapy had lower recurrence rates than surgery only controls (Gastrointestinal Tumor Study Group, 1985). There was also a trend towards improved survival in this group. Non-haematological side-effects were recorded in 35% of patients who had received combined radiotherapy and chemotherapy.

The Veterans Administration Surgical Oncology Group (VASOG) have recently updated their results. In the first study patients undergoing curative resection were randomized to receive either no adjuvant therapy or 5-fluorouracil and methyl-CCNU (Higgins et al., 1984a). Treated patients appeared to have a slightly more favourable survival than did controls; however, this difference appeared to be confined to patients with 1 to 4 positive lymph nodes in the resected specimen (51% v. 31% 5-year survival). In the second study, patients with incomplete resection were randomized to 5-fluorouracil and methyl-CCNU + immunotherapy. No difference in survival was noted (Higgins et al., 1984b).

Despite more than 6000 randomized patients in published trials, the effect of adjuvant systemic chemotherapy upon mortality remains unclear. A recent overview suggests that 5-fluorouracil containing regimens administered over an extended period of time may reduce the odds of death by about 17% resulting in an increase in 5-year survival of approximately 3% (Buyse, Zeleniuch-Jacquotte and Chalmers, 1988).

Since then, the results of the NSABP studies have been reported (Fisher et al., 1988; Wolmark et al., 1988). Both studies show significant reductions in mortality in the chemotherapy-treated groups. However, as in the previous studies, the toxicity associated with the use of systemic chemotherapy is substantial. Partly because of toxicity and partly because of the equivocal results obtained in the above studies, adjuvant systemic chemotherapy for colorectal cancer is rarely used outside clinical trials.

Portal vein perfusion

Based on the premise that metastases released by handling of the primary tumour reached the liver via the portal vein and that these micrometastases subsequently developed into overt macroscopic liver metastases, Taylor and his colleagues (1985) undertook a randomized trial of adjuvant cytotoxic liver perfusion. Two hundred and forty-four patients undergoing 'curative' resection for colorectal cancer were randomized to receive either no further treatment or 5-fluorouracil (1 g), administered as a continuous infusion into the portal venous system for the first 7 postoperative days. After a median follow-up of 4 years, there were 54 deaths in the control group and 26 in the perfusion group. Twenty-two patients in the control group and 5 in the perfused group developed objective evidence of liver metastases. The benefit appeared to be limited to patients with Dukes' B colon cancer.

In the Australian and New Zealand cancer trial, 232 patients with Stage B or C colorectal cancer were randomized to receive no further treatment, systemic 5-fluorouracil, or 5-fluorouracil by portal vein infusion (Gray *et al.*, 1987). Initial analysis suggested that there was a significant improvement in overall survival in patients with Dukes' C tumours. A similar study using a postoperative infusion of 5-fluorouracil and mitomycin showed a non-significant reduction in hepatic metastases in the perfused group (Metzger *et al.*, 1984). There is clearly a need for further studies to confirm or refute these findings and identify the patients most likely to benefit.

Hepatic metastases

The median survival for untreated patients with overt hepatic metastases at laparotomy is approximately 6 months; virtually all are dead within 2 years of diagnosis although the occasional patient may survive 5 years. Survival is closely related to the extent of liver involvement. For instance, in a retrospective study of 113 patients with clinically diagnosed hepatic metastases the mean survival time for patients with widespread liver metastases was 3.1 months compared with 10.6 months for patients with metastases confined to one lobe and 16.7 months for those with solitary metastases (Wood, Gillis and Blumgart, 1976). All patients with multiple metastases were dead by 3 years, whereas 13% of patients with solitary lesions survived more than 3 years.

The management of hepatic metastases has recently been reviewed by Taylor (1985). Hepatic resection may be indicated in patients with liver metastases involving a single lobe without invasion of the inferior vena cava or portal vein, where the primary tumour has been adequately excised and there is no evidence of distant metastases elsewhere. Operative mortality in most series has now fallen to acceptable levels; between 25 and 40% survive 5 years (Greenway, 1988). To what extent these results reflect the selection of fit patients with slow growing tumours and favourable biological characteristics remains debatable. In most studies some patients, especially those with solitary metastases, survive long term without treatment. Nevertheless, despite the absence of an appropriate control group the results of resection do appear to offer hope for some patients.

However, although surgical resection in selected patients may be appropriate, the majority of patients are not suitable as multiple metastases are present. Alternative forms of treatment have been singularly unsuccessful. Systemic therapy with single agent 5-fluorouracil or 5-fluorouracil combinations has a response rate of approximately 15%; hepatic irradiation is associated with unacceptable morbidity; various combinations of hepatic artery ligation and devascularization and portal vein infusion may relieve pain, but do not influence survival (Taylor, 1985).

It is now well recognized that the majority of liver metastases depend on an arterial blood supply for continuing growth. The continuing failure of systemic chemotherapy to influence survival and the development of indwelling catheters has revived interest in the concept of regional chemotherapy. Regional chemotherapy is based on the premise that by delivering the cytotoxic drug direct to the target organ via the arterial supply, high levels of cytotoxic drug can be achieved within the target organ with minimal systemic toxicity.

Most commonly the common hepatic artery arises from the coeliac axis, gives off the gastroduodenal, right gastric and cystic arteries before dividing into right and left hepatic arteries. Access to the arterial supply of the liver can be obtained by implanting a catheter in the gastroduodenal artery so that the catheter tip lies at the origin of the gastroduodenal artery; in this way hepatic blood flow is not impeded. Vascular anomalies are common, for instance the right hepatic artery not uncommonly arises from the superior mesenteric artery, and preoperative angiography is mandatory (Goldberg et al., 1989). The hepatic artery catheter may be connected either to a refillable implantable pump designed to administer a slow infusion or a subcutaneous portal for intermittent administration of cytotoxic drugs.

The development of a refillable implantable pump (Infusaid) has attracted considerable interest. The pump delivers a continuous infusion of FUDR (a 5-fluorouracil analogue which has similar cytotoxic properties). Preliminary studies suggest that a ten-fold increase in tumour FUDR concentration compared to systemic adminstration can be achieved. Partial response rates of over 80% and possible prolongation of survival when treated patients were compared to historical controls have been reported (Balch et al., 1983; Niederhuber et al., 1984; Cohen, Kaufman and Wood, 1985). Despite the absence of conclusive data confirming the benefit of this approach, over 8000 pumps have been inserted in the USA. A prospective randomized study comparing survival and quality of life in patients with unresectable hepatic metastases treated by implanted pump with that of patients receiving conventional palliation has recently been set up in the UK (Allen-Mersh, 1989). Hopefully, the results of this study will in time clarify the benefits or otherwise of this technique.

The intermittent administration of 5-fluorouracil alone via a hepatic artery catheter has been shown to be ineffective, and an alternative method of improving the delivery of cytotoxic agents to tumour tissue is required. Ensminger and his colleagues (1985) have suggested that the use of biodegradable starch microspheres to 'dam-back' hepatic blood flow may increase the extraction of cytotoxic drugs. Our initial experience suggests that this may be so (Goldberg et al., 1990).

A further development is the use of cytotoxic-loaded biodegradable or radioactive microspheres. Preliminary studies have shown that cytotoxic loaded microspheres administered via the renal or hepatic arteries are trapped in the target organ, releasing the cytotoxic drug locally (Kerr et al., 1988; McArdle et al., 1988). Similar results have been obtained with radioactive microspheres (Mantravadi et al., 1982).

Such techniques, however, would not be expected to significantly benefit patients with liver metastases unless there was some way to target the cytotoxic or radioactive microspheres towards tumour tissue, thereby protecting normal liver substance from unwanted side-effects.

Tumour blood vessels tend to be deficient in smooth muscle and have, therefore, an attenuated response to vasoactive agents. Recent studies have shown that the use of an angiotensin II infusion can significantly increase tumour blood flow relative to normal liver thereby diverting the therapeutic microspheres towards the tumour tissue (Sasaki et al., 1985; Goldberg et al., 1987).

In the past, few patients with colorectal liver metastases received any form of treatment. A number of potential therapeutic options are now available and cautious optimism may be justified. Although encouraging, however, these results were achieved in a highly selected patient population and the benefits have still to be confirmed in randomized prospective clinical trials.

References

Allen-Mersh, T. G. (1989) Colorectal liver metastases: is no treatment still best ? *Journal of the Royal Society of Medicine*, **82**, 2–3

Armitage, N. C., Farrands, P. A., Vellacott, K. D. and Hardcastle, J. D. (1984) Faecal occult blood screening in symptomatic patients in general practice. *Gut*, **25**, A 1171–1172

Armstrong, B. K. and Doll, R. (1975) Environmental factors and cancer incidence and mortality in different countries, with special reference to dietary practice. *International Journal of Cancer*, **15**, 616–631

Astler, V. B. and Coller, F. A. (1954) The prognostic significance of direct extension of carcinoma of the colon and rectum. *Annals of Surgery*, **139**, 846–852

Attiyeh, F. F. and Stearns, M. W. (1981) Second-look laparotomy based on CEA elevations in colorectal cancer, *Cancer*, **47**, 2119–2125

Bakare, S. C., Shafir, M. and McElhinney, A. J. (1987) Exclusion of small bowel from pelvis for postoperative radiotherapy of rectal cancer. *Journal of Surgical Oncology*, **35**, 55–58

Balch, C. M., Urist, M. M., Seng-Jaw, S. and McGregor, M. (1983) A prospective phase II clinical trial of continuous FUDR regional chemotherapy for colorectal metastases to the liver using a totally implantable drug infusion pump. *Annals of Surgery*, **198**, 567–573

Balslev, I., Pedersen, M., Teglbjaerg, P. S. *et al.* (1986) Postoperative radiotherapy in Dukes' B and C carcinoma of the rectum and rectosigmoid. *Cancer*, **58**, 22–28

Beynon, J. (1989) An evaluation of the role of rectal endosonography in rectal cancer. *Annals of the Royal College of Surgeons of England*, **71**, 131–139.

Blenkinsopp, W. K., Stewart-Brown, S., Blesovsky, L. *et al.* (1981) Histopathology reporting in large bowel cancer. *Journal of Clinical Pathology*, **34**, 509–513

Boey, J., Cheung, H. C., Lai, C. K. and Wong, J. (1984) A prospective evaluation of serum carcinoembryonic antigen (CEA) levels in the management of colorectal carcinoma. *World Journal of Surgery*, **8**, 279–286

Burkitt, D. P. (1971) Epidemiology of cancer of the colon and rectum. *Cancer*, **28**, 3–13.

Buyse, M., Zeleniuch-Jacquotte, A. and Chalmers, T. C. (1988) Adjuvant therapy of colorectal cancer. Why we still don't know. *Journal of the American Medical Association*, **259**, 3571–3578

Chapuis, P. H., Dent, O. F., Fisher, R. *et al.* (1985) A multivariate analysis of clinical and pathological variables in prognosis after resection of large bowel cancer. *British Journal of Surgery*, **72**, 698–702

Clarke, D. V., Jones, P. F. and Needham, C. D. (1980) Outcome in colorectal carcinoma: seven-year study of a population. *British Medical Journal*, **1**, 431–435

Cohen, A. M., Kaufman, S. D. and Wood, W. C. (1985) Treatment of colorectal cancer hepatic metastases by hepatic artery chemotherapy. *Diseases of Colon and Rectum*, **28**, 389–393

Dosoretz, D. E., Gunderson, L. L., Hedberg, S. *et al.* (1983) Preoperative irradiation for unresectable rectal and rectosigmoid carcinomas. *Cancer*, **52**, 814–818

Drasar, B. S. and Irving, D. (1973) Environmental factors in cancer of the colon and breast. *British Journal of Cancer*, **27**, 167–172

Dukes, C. E. (1932) The classification of cancer of the rectum. *Journal of Pathology and Bacteriology*, **35**, 323–332

Dukes, C. E. and Bussey, H. J. R. (1958) The spread of rectal cancer and its effects on prognosis. *British Journal of Cancer*, **12**, 309–320

Enker, W. E. (1981) Extent of operations for large bowel cancer. In *Clinical Surgery International 1. Large Bowel Cancer* (ed. J. J. DeCosse), Edinburgh, Churchill-Livingstone, 78–93

Ensminger, W. D., Gyres, J. W., Stetson, P. and Walker-Andrews, S. (1985) Phase 1 study of hepatic arterial degradable starch microspheres and mitomycin. *Cancer Research*, **45**, 4464–4467

Everett, W. G., Friend, P. J. and Forty, J. (1986) Comparison of stapling and hand-suture for left-sided large bowel anastomosis. *British Journal of Surgery*, **73**, 345–348

Farrands, P. A. and Hardcastle, J. D. (1984) Colorectal screening by a self-completion questionnaire. *Gut*, **25**, 445–447

Fielding, L. P., Phillips, R. K. S., Fry, J. S. and Hittinger, R. (1986) Prediction of outcome after curative resection for large bowel cancer. *Lancet*, **ii**, 904–907

Fielding, L. P., Stewart-Brown, S. and Dudley, H. A. F. (1978) Surgeon-related variables and the clinical trial. *Lancet*, **ii**, 778–779

Fielding, L. P., Stewart-Brown, S., Hittinger, R. and Blesovsky, L. (1984) Covering stoma for elective anterior resection of the rectum: an outmoded operation? *American Journal of Surgery*, **147**, 524–530

Finlay, I. G. and McArdle, C. S. (1983) Role of carcinoembryonic antigen in detection of asymptomatic disseminated disease in colorectal carcinoma. *British Medical Journal*, **286**, 1242–1244

Finlay, I. G. and McArdle, C. S. (1986) Occult hepatic metastases in colorectal carcinoma. *British Journal of Surgery*, **73**, 732–735

Finlay, I. G., Meek, D., Brunton, F. and McArdle, C. S. (1988) Growth rate of hepatic metastases in colorectal carcinoma. *British Journal of Surgery*, **75**, 641–644.

Fisher, B., Wolmark, N., Rochette, H. *et al.* (1988) Postoperative adjuvant chemotherapy or radiation therapy for rectal cancer: results from NSABP protocol R-01. *Journal of the National Cancer Institute*, **80**, 21–29

Freedman, L. S., Macaskill, P. and Smith, A. N. (1984) Multivariate analysis of prognostic factors for operable rectal cancer. *Lancet*, **ii**, 733–736

Garland, C., Shekelle, R. B., Barrett-Connor, E. *et al.* (1985) Dietary vitamin D and calcium and risk of colorectal cancer: A 9-year prospective study in men. *Lancet*, **i**, 307–309

Gastrointestinal Tumour Study Group (1984) Adjuvant therapy of colon cancer – results of a prospectively randomized trial. *New England Journal of Medicine*, **310**, 737–743

Gastrointestinal Tumour Study Group (1985) Prolongation of the disease-free interval in surgically treated rectal carcinoma. *New England Journal of Medicine*, **312**, 1465–1472

Gerard, A., Berrod, J. L., Pene, F. *et al.* (1985) Interim analysis of a phase III study on preoperative radiation therapy in resectable rectal carcinoma. *Cancer*, **55**, 2373–2379

Gilbert, J. M., Jeffrey, I., Evans, M. and Kark, A. E. (1984) Sites of recurrent tumour after curative colorectal surgery: implications for adjuvant therapy. *British Journal of Surgery*, **71**, 203–205

Gill, P. G. and Morris, P. J. (1978) The survival of patients with colorectal cancer treated in a regional hospital. *British Journal of Surgery*, **65**, 17–20

Goldberg, J. A., Bradnam, M. S., Kerr, D. J. *et al.* (1987) Single photon emission computed tomographic studies (SPECT) of hepatic arterial perfusion sintigraphy (HAPS) in patients with colorectal liver metastases: improved tumour targetting by microspheres with angiotensin II. *Nuclear Medicine Communications*, **8**, 1025–1032

Goldberg, J. A., Kerr, D. J., Stewart, I. and McArdle, C. S. (1990) A comparison of regional and systemic chemotherapy for hepatic metastases. *European Journal of Surgical Oncology* (in press)

Goldberg, J. A., Leiberman, D. P. and McArdle, C. S. (1989) A useful maneuver for hepatic arterial catheterization in patients with metastatic hepatic disease and abnormal vascular anatomy. *Surgery, Gynecology and Obstetrics*, **169**, 71–72

Goldberg, J. A., Morran, C., Leiberman, P. *et al.* (1990c) Regional therapy for liver metastases: experience with hepatic artery catheters. *British Journal of Surgery* (in press)

Goligher, J. C. (1941) The operability of carcinoma of the rectum. *British Medical Journal*, **ii**, 393–397

Goligher, J. C. (1981) Results of operations for large bowel cancer. In *Clinical Surgery International 1. Large Bowel Cancer* (ed. J. J. DeCosse), Edinburgh, Churchill-Livingstone, pp. 154–165

Graham, S., Dayal, H. S., Swanson, M. *et al.* (1978) Diet in the epidemiology of cancer of the colon and rectum. *Journal of the National Cancer Institute*, **61**, 709–714

Gray, B. N. (1980) Surgeon accuracy in the diagnosis of liver metastases at laparotomy. *Australia and New Zealand Journal of Surgery*, **50**, 524–526

Gray, B. N., deZwart, J., Fisher, R. *et al.* (1987) The Australian and New Zealand trial of adjuvant chemotherapy in colon cancer. In *Adjuvant Therapy of Cancer V* (ed. S. E. Salmon), New York, Grune and Stratton, pp. 537–546

Greenway, B. (1988) Hepatic metastases from colorectal cancer: resection or not? *British Journal of Surgery*, **75**, 513–519

Gunderson, L. L. and Sosin, H. (1974) Areas of failure found at reoperation (second or symptomatic look) following 'curative surgery' for adenocarcinoma of the rectum. Clinicopathological correlation and implications for adjuvant therapy. *Cancer*, **34**, 1278–1292

Haenszell, W., Berg, J. W., Segi, M. *et al.* (1973) Large bowel cancer in Hawaiian Japanese. *Journal of the National Cancer Institute*, **51**, 1765–1779

Hardcastle, J. D., Thomas, W. M., Chamberlain, J. *et al.* (1989) Randomized controlled trial by faecal occult blood screening for colorectal cancer. *Lancet,* **i**, 1160–1164

Heald, R. J. and Ryall, R. D. H. (1986) Recurrence and survival after total mesorectal excision for rectal cancer. *Lancet,* **i**, 1479–1482

Higgins, G. A., Amadeo, J. H., McElhinney, J. *et al.* (1984a) Efficacy of prolonged intermittent therapy with combined 5-fluorouracil and methyl – CCNU following resection for carcinoma of the large bowel. A Veterans Administration Surgical Oncology Group report. *Cancer,* **53**, 1–8

Higgins, G. A., Conn, G. H., Jordan, P. H. *et al.* (1975) Prospective radiotherapy for colorectal cancer. *Annals of Surgery,* **181**, 624–631

Higgins, G. A., Donaldson, R. C., Rodgers, L. S. *et al.* (1984b) Efficacy of MER immunotherapy when added to a regimen of 5-fluorouracil and methyl – CCNU following resection for carcinoma of the large bowel. A Veterans Administration Surgical Oncology Group report. *Cancer,* **54**, 193–198

Higgins, G. A., Humphrey, E. W., Dwight, R. W. *et al.* (1986) Preoperative radiation and surgery for cancer of the rectum. *Cancer,* **58**, 352–359

Hill, M. J., Drasar, B. S., Williams, R. E. O., *et al.* (1975) Faecal bile-acids and clostridia in patients with cancer of the large bowel. *Lancet,* **i**, 535–538

Hine, K. R. and Dykes, P. W. (1984a) Serum CEA testing in the post-operative surveillance of colorectal carcinoma. *British Journal of Cancer,* **49**, 689–693

Hine, K. R. and Dykes, P. W. (1984b) Prospective randomised trial of early cytotoxic therapy for recurrent colorectal carcinoma detected by serum CEA. *Gut,* **25**, 682–688

Hoskins, R. B., Gunderson, L. L., Dosoretz, D. E. *et al.* (1985) Adjuvant postoperative radiotherapy in carcinoma of the rectum and rectosigmoid. *Cancer,* **55**, 61–71

Huguier, M. and Lacaine, F. (1981) Hepatic metastases in gastrointestinal cancer. *Archives of Surgery,* **116**, 399–402

Jacobsen, B. K. and Thelle, D. S. (1987) Coffee, cholesterol, and colon cancer: is there a link? *British Medical Journal,* **294**, 4–5

Jass, J. R., Love, S. B. and Northover, J. M. A. (1987) A new prognostic classification of rectal cancer. *Lancet,* **i**, 1303–1306

Kerr, D. J., Willmott, N., Lewi, H. and McArdle, C. S. (1988) The pharmacokinetics and distribution of Adriamycin-loaded albumin microspheres following intra-arterial administration. *Cancer,* **62**, 878–882

Kirklin, J. W., Dockerty, M. B. and Waugh, J. M. (1949) The role of the peritoneal reflexion in the prognosis of carcinoma of the rectum and sigmoid colon. *Surgery, Gynecology and Obstetrics,* **88**, 326–331

Koruth, N. M., Krukowski, Z. H., Youngson, G. G. *et al.* (1985) Intra-operative colonic irrigation in the management of left-sided large bowel emergencies. *British Journal of Surgery,* **72**, 708–711

Laird, E. E., Williams, D. and Williams, E. D. (1987) Can the hepatic perfusion index improve routine diagnosis of liver disease? *Nuclear Medicine Communications,* **8**, 959

Leveson, S. H., Wiggins, P. A., Giles, G. R. *et al.* (1985) Deranged liver blood flow patterns in detection of liver metastases. *British Journal of Surgery,* **72**, 128–130

Lewi, H., Blumgart, L. H., Carter, D. C. *et al.* (1984) Pre-operative carcino-embryonic antigen and survival in patients with colorectal cancer. *British Journal of Surgery,* **71**, 206–208

Lockhart-Mummery, H. E., Ritchie, J. K. and Hawley, P. R. (1976) The results of surgical treatment of carcinoma of the rectum at St Mark's Hospital from 1948 to 1972. *British Journal of Surgery,* **63**, 673–677

McArdle, C. S., Hole, D., Hansell, D. *et al.* (1990) A prospective study of colorectal cancer in the West of Scotland: a ten year follow-up. *British Journal of Surgery,* **77**, 280–282

McArdle, C. S., Lewi, H., Hansell, D. *et al.* (1988) Cytotoxic-loaded albumin microspheres: a novel approach to regional chemotherapy. *British Journal of Surgery,* **75**, 132–134

McDermott, F. T., Hughes, E. S. R., Pihl, E. *et al.* (1985) Local recurrence after potentially curative resection for rectal cancer in a series of 1008 patients. *British Journal of Surgery,* **72**, 31–37

McGinn, F. P., Gartell, P. C., Clifford, P. C. and Brunton, F. J. (1985) Staples or sutures for low colorectal anastomoses: a prospective randomized trial. *British Journal of Surgery,* **72**, 603–605

Machi, J., Isomoto, H., Yamashita, Y. *et al.* (1987) Intraoperative ultrasonography in screening for liver metastases from colorectal cancer: Comparative accuracy with traditional procedures. *Surgery,* **101**, 678–684

Mantravadi, R. V. P., Spigos, D. G., Tan, W. S. and Felix, El. (1982) Intra-arterial yttrium 90 in the treatment of hepatic malignancy. *Radiology*, **142**, 783–786

Martin, E. W., Cooperman, M., Carey, L. C. and Minton, J. P. (1980) Sixty second-look procedures indicated primarily by rise in serial carcinoembryonic antigen. *Journal of Surgical Research*, **28**, 389–394

Martin, E. W., James, K. K., Hurtubise, P. E. *et al.* (1977) The use of CEA as an early indicator for gastrointestinal tumour recurrence and second-look procedures. *Cancer*, **39**, 440–446

Metzger, U., Mermillod, B., Aeberhard, P. *et al.* (1984) Adjuvant portal liver infusion with 5-fluorouracil and mitomycin-C following curative large bowel cancer surgery. In *Adjuvant Therapy of Cancer IV* (ed. S. E. Jones and S. E. Salmon), New York, Grune and Stratton, pp. 471–478

Mohuiddin, M. and Marks, G. J. (1987) High dose preoperative radiation and sphincter preservation in the treatment of rectal cancer. *International Journal of Radiation Oncology, Biology and Physics*, **13**, 839–842

Moorehead, R. J. and McKelvey, S. T. D. (1989) Cholecystectomy and colorectal cancer. *British Journal of Surgery*, **76**, 250–253

Morson, B. C. and Bussey, H. J. R. (1985) Magnitude of risk for cancer in patients with colorectal adenomas. *British Journal of Surgery*, **72**, S23–S25

Muto, T., Bussey, H. J. R. and Morson, B. C. (1975) The evolution of cancer of the colon and rectum. *Cancer*, **36**, 2251–2270

Muto, T., Ishikawa, K. and Kino, I. *et al.* (1977) Comparative histologic study of adenomas of the large intestine in Japan and England, with special reference to malignant potential. *Diseases of the Colon and Rectum*, **20**, 11–16

Niederhuber, J., Ensminger, W., Gyves, J. *et al.* (1984) Regional chemotherapy of colorectal cancer metastatic to the liver. *Cancer*, **53**, 1336–1343

NIH Consensus Statement (1981) Carcinoembryonic antigen: its role as a marker in the management of cancer. *British Medical Journal*, **282**, 373–375

Northover, J. (1986) Carcinoembryonic antigen and recurrent colorectal cancer. *Gut*, **27**, 117–122

Papillon, J. (1975) Intracavity irradiation of early rectal cancer for cure. *Cancer*, **36**, 696–701

Phillips, R., Hittinger, R., Saunders, V. *et al.* (1983) Preoperative urography in large bowel cancer: a useless investigation? *British Journal of Surgery*, **70**, 425–427

Phillips, R. K. S., Hittinger, R., Blesovsky, L. *et al.* (1984a) Local recurrence following curative surgery for large bowel cancer: II. The rectum and rectosigmoid. *British Journal of Surgery*, **71**, 17–20

Phillips, R. K. S., Hittinger, R., Blesovsky, L. *et al.* (1984b) Large bowel cancer: surgical pathology and its relationship to survival. *British Journal of Surgery*, **71**, 604–610

Pittam, M. R., Thornton, H. and Ellis, H. (1984) Survival after extended resection for locally advanced carcinomas of the colon and rectum. *Annals of the Royal College of Surgeons of England*, **66**, 81–84

Pollett, W. G. and Nicholls, R. J. (1983) The relationship between the extent of distal clearance and survival and local recurrence rates after curative anterior resection for carcinoma of the rectum. *Annals of Surgery*, **198**, 159–163

Quirke, P., Durdey, P., Dixon, M. F. and Williams, N. S. (1986) Local recurrence of rectal adenocarcinoma due to inadequate surgical resection. Histopathological study of lateral tumour spread and surgical excision. *Lancet*, **ii**, 996–998

Reddy, B. S. and Wynder, E. L. (1977) Metabolic epidemiology of colon cancer. Faecal bile-acids and neutral steroids in colon cancer patients and patients with adenomatous polyps. *Cancer*, **39**, 2533–2539

Rickert, R. R., Auerbach, O., Garfinkel, L. *et al.* (1979) Adenomatous lesions of the large bowel: an autopsy survey. *Cancer*, **43**, 1847–1857

Rider, W. D., Palmer, J. A., Mahoney, L. J. and Robertson, C. T. (1977) Preoperative irradiation in operable cancer of the rectum: report of the Toronto trial. *Canadian Journal of Surgery*, **20**, 335–338

Roswit, B., Higgins, G. A. and Keehn, R. J. (1975) Preoperative irradiation for carcinoma of the rectum and rectosigmoid colon: report of a National Veterans Administration randomised study. *Cancer*, **35**, 1597–1602

Sasaki, Y., Imaoka, S., Hasegawa, Y. *et al.* (1985) Changes in distribution of hepatic blood flow induced by intra-arterial infusion of angiotensin II in human hepatic cancer. *Cancer*, **55**, 311–316

Schreve, R. H., Terpstra, O. T., Ausema, L. *et al.* (1984) Detection of liver metastases. A prospective study comparing liver enzymes, scintigraphy, ultrasonography and computed tomography. *British Journal of Surgery*, **71**, 947–949

Second Report of a Medical Research Council Working Party (1984) The evaluation of low dose preoperative X-ray therapy in the management of operable rectal cancer; results of a randomly controlled trial. *British Journal of Surgery,* **71**, 21–25

Sischy, B., Hinson, E. J. and Wilkinson, D. R. (1988) Definitive radiation therapy for selected cancers of the rectum. *British Journal of Surgery,* **75**, 901–903

Slaney, G. (1971) Results of treatment of carcinoma of the colon and rectum. In *Modern Trends in Surgery*–3 (ed. W. T. Irvine), London, Butterworths, pp. 69–89

Staab, H. J., Anderer, F. A., Stumpf, E. *et al.* (1985) Eighty-four potential second-look operations based on sequential carcinoembryonic antigen determinations and clinical investigations in patients with recurrent gastrointestinal cancer. *American Journal of Surgery,* **149**, 198–204

Stearns, M. W., Deddish, M. R., Quan, S. H. Q. and Leaming, R. H. (1974) Preoperative roentgen therapy for cancer of the rectum and rectosigmoid. *Surgery, Gynecology and Obstetrics,* **138**, 584–586

Stearns, M. W., Quan, S. H. Q. and Deddish, M. R. (1959) Preoperative roentgen therapy for cancer of the rectum. *Surgery, Gynecology and Obstetrics,* **109**, 225–229

Stewart, R. J., Robson, R. A., Stewart, A. W. *et al.* (1979) Cancer of the large bowel in the defined population: Canterbury, New Zealand, 1970–4. *British Journal of Surgery,* **66**, 309–314

Stockholm Rectal Cancer Study Group (1987) Short-term preoperative radiotherapy for colorectal cancer. *American Journal of Clinical Oncology,* **10**, 369–375

Taylor, I. (1985) Colorectal liver metastases – to treat or not to treat? *British Journal of Surgery,* **72**, 511–516

Taylor, I., Machin, D., Mullee, M. *et al.* (1985) Randomized controlled trial of adjuvant portal vein cytotoxic perfusion in colorectal cancer. *British Journal of Surgery,* **72**, 359–363

Taylor, R. E., Kerr, G. R. and Arnott, S. J. (1987) External beam radiotherapy for rectal adenocarcinoma. *British Journal of Surgery,* **74**, 455–459

Thomas, W. M., Morris, D. L. and Hardcastle, J. D. (1987) Contact ultrasonography in the detection of liver metastases from colorectal cancer: an *in vitro* study. *British Journal of Surgery,* **74**, 955–956

Turnbull, R. B., Kyle, K., Watson, F. R. and Spratt, J. (1967) Cancer of the colon: The influence of the no-touch isolation technic on survival rates. *Annals of Surgery,* **166**, 420–425

Umpleby, H. C. and Williamson, R. C. N. (1984) Carcinoma of the large bowel in the first four decades. *British Journal of Surgery,* **71**, 272–277

Waterhouse, J., Muir, C., Correa, P. and Powell, J. (1976) *Cancer Incidence in Five Continents,* Vol 3, International Agency for Research on Cancer, Lyons

Wattenberg, L. W. and Loub, W. D. (1978) Inhibition of polycyclic aromatic hydrocarbon induced neoplasia by naturally occurring indoles. *Cancer Research,* **38**, 1410–1413

Whittaker, M. and Goligher, J. C. (1976) The prognosis after surgical treatment for carcinoma of the rectum. *British Journal of Surgery,* **63**, 384–388

Wiggers, T., Jeekel, J., Arends, J. W. *et al.* (1988) No-touch isolation technique in colon cancer: a controlled prospective trial. *British Journal of Surgery,* **75**, 409–415

Williams, N. S., Dixon, M. F. and Johnston, D. (1983) Reappraisal of the 5 centimetre rule of distal excision for carcinoma of the rectum: a study of distal intramural spread and of patients' survival. *British Journal of Surgery,* **70**, 150–154

Williams, N. S., Durdey, P. and Johnston, D. (1985) The outcome following sphincter saving resection and abdominoperineal resection for low rectal cancer. *British Journal of Surgery,* **72**, 595–598

Williams, N. S., Jass, J. R. and Hardcastle, J. D. (1988) Clinicopathological assessment and staging of colorectal cancer. *British Journal of Surgery,* **75**, 649–652

Williams, N. S. and Johnston, D. (1984) Survival and recurrence after sphincter saving resection and abdominoperineal resection for carcinoma of the middle third of the rectum. *British Journal of Surgery,* **71**, 278–282

Wolmark, N., Fisher, B., Rochette, H. *et al.* (1988) Postoperative adjuvant chemotherapy or BCG for colon cancer: results from NSABP protocol C-01. *Journal of the National Cancer Institute,* **80**, 30–36

Wood, C. B., Gillis, C. R. and Blumgart, L. H. (1976) A retrospective study of the natural history of patients with liver metastases from colorectal cancer. *Clinical Oncology,* **2**, 285–288.

Wood, C. B., Ratcliffe, J. G., Burt, R. W. *et al.* (1980) The clinical significance of the pattern of elevated serum carcinoembryonic antigen (CEA) levels in recurrent colorectal cancer. *British Journal of Surgery,* **67**, 46–48

Wynder, E. L. (1975) The epidemiology of large bowel cancer. *Cancer Research,* **35**, 3388–3394

Chapter 5

Endocrine tumours

J. R. Farndon

Introduction

Two pivotal developments have allowed better understanding and classification of endocrine tumours:

1. Radio-immunoassay techniques were described by Berson and Yalow and the hormonal products of endocrine tumours could then be readily measured (Berson and Yalow, 1973). It is the retained capacity of most endocrine tumours to produce their hormonal products in excess (with physiological consequences) that allows effective diagnosis and monitoring of therapy.
2. All endocrine tumours can be better understood through their common embryological origins and many structural and functional similarities character-ized by the APUD descriptives (Pearse, 1966; 1968): Fluorogenic Amino content (e.g. catecholamines) and/or amine Precursor Uptake (e.g. Dopa) and amino acid Decarboxylase with high content of side-chain carboxyl groups, non-specific esterases and/or cholinesterases, and alpha-glycerophosphate dehydrogenase with demonstration of specific immunofluorescence (Pearse, 1974).

The cells of this series are likely to originate from the neural tube, neural ridges or crest. The hypothalamo–hypophyseal complex is wholly neuroectodermal and, in the amphibian, the parathyroids come from this source. Dispersion of neural crest cells could account for the APUD contributions to foregut and pulmonary systems. Placodal ectoderm makes important contributions to the pharyngeal pouch endocrine derivatives of birds and mammals (Pearse and Takor, 1976).

The amount of interest generated by endocrine tumours far outweighs their importance in terms of frequency and malignant potential. Thyroid malignancy — the commonest endocrine tumour — occurs at a rate of 9 per million males and 24 per million females each year. These are the 26th and 20th commonest malignancies in males and females respectively (Cancer Research Campaign, 1987). Most endocrine tumours are benign neoplasms and even those which are truly malignant are often associated with an indolent course allowing prolonged survival after treatment. Only 4 men and 10 women per million population, for example, die each year from thyroid cancer (overall mortality for all neoplasms is 3029 males and 2616 females per million per year) (Cancer Research Campaign).

This chapter will attempt to review endocrine neoplasms, giving priority to those truly malignant tumours occurring more frequently and those associated with morbidity which requires an understanding of their pathophysiology to allow implementation of effective therapy.

The thyroid

Although derived embryologically from endoderm and neuroectoderm many cell types exist within the thyroid, each of which can give rise to specific tumours and the follicular cell, itself, may produce two or three forms of differentiated thyroid cancer which may be the progenitor of the undifferentiated form (Figure 5.1).

Classification of thyroid neoplasms

Differentiated tumours comprise papillary, follicular and Hürthle types

Papillary carcinoma occurs at any age but is more frequent between the ages of 30 and 50 years with a marked female preponderance (Mazaferri et al., 1977). The lesions are often cystic and histologically characterized by the presence of papillary fronds although rarely is this the only architectural form. Follicles and trabeculae occur and mixed follicular/papillary variants are described. Spread is usually to regional lymph nodes and at least 50% of patients will have nodal metastases at presentation. The tumours are frequently multifocal. They can be small and solitary — the so-called occult papillary carcinoma — often found coincidentally or during screening procedures (Hubert et al., 1980).

Follicular thyroid carcinoma is less common than the papillary type, occurs in an older age group, usually presents as a solitary nodule, metastasizes mainly through vascular channels and as many as 50% of patients can have metastases when first seen (Taylor, 1980). Lymph node metastases are rare. Oxyphilic cells — Hürthle or Azkanazy cells — may comprise the majority of these tumours and many now distinguish the Hürthle cell tumour as a separate entity.

Hürthle cell carcinoma might comprise less than 5% of all thyroid malignancies but one-third of patients will die of their disease — a degree of moderate malignancy (Har-el et al., 1986). Benign variants occur but these are not easily distinguished by specific immunohistochemical markers. Classification has to depend upon traditional histological features such as invasion and metastasis (Johnson et al., 1987). The disease again occurs with a female preponderance between the fourth and eighth decades.

Tumours of the parafollicular cell

Medullary thyroid carcinoma (MTC) is also considered to be a differentiated neoplasm arising from the C-cells or parafollicular cells which occurs infrequently — accounting for less than 10% of all thyroid neoplasms. It occurs in four different clinical settings:

1. MTC associated with multiple endocrine neoplasia type IIa (familial autosomal dominant).
2. MTC associated with multiple endocrine neoplasia type IIb (probably familial autosomal dominant).
3. Familial MTC without associated endocrinopathies.
4. Sporadic MTC.

The tumour has characteristic microscopic appearances with sheets of uniform

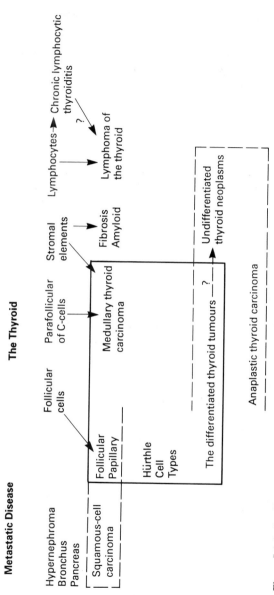

Figure 5.1 A classification of thyroid malignancy

polygonal cells with variable amounts of fibrous stroma. Amyloid may occur in larger lesions.

C-cell hyperplasia is described as the precursor of familial MTC (Block *et al.*, 1980) and unilateral single focus disease characterizes the sporadic tumour. The disease metastasizes to lymph nodes, viscera and skeleton and is variably aggressive depending upon the clinical setting. Treatment is made more effective by the use of measurements of calcitonin — the hormonal product of the C-cell — which acts as a tumour marker. Screening programmes using calcitonin measurement allow more effective therapy of the familial syndromes but this disease is still associated with a measurable mortality. The spectrum of aggression ranges from MTC in MEN IIb, to sporadic MTC, to MTC in MEN IIa to pure familial MTC without other endocrinopathies which appears to be totally indolent (Wells *et al.*, 1985; Farndon *et al.*, 1986).

Undifferentiated or anaplastic thyroid cancer
This may arise from a pre-existing differentiated tumour. Patients will often describe the presence of a longstanding thyroid swelling which suddenly changes character. Areas of differentiated tumour can often be found on histological examination. The cellular pattern is bizarre and metastases occur to lymph nodes, skeleton and lungs. The tumour occurs in patients over 60 years of age and more frequently in females and is associated with poor survival.

A proportion of thyroid tumours arise from non-thyroid cells
Lymphomas of the thyroid gland occur in patients with a median age of about 60 years with an almost 2:1 female to male ratio. The disease occurs in patients with thyroids demonstrating a background of chronic lymphocytic thyroiditis and in whom antithyroid antibodies are detected in a majority. Care must be taken in making the diagnosis and distinguishing this condition from Hashimoto's thyroiditis. The disease can be aggressive with 5-year survival rates as low as 13% for those with immunoblastic tumours but may be indolent and responsive with 5-year rates of 92% for those with low-grade tumours (Aozasa *et al.*, 1986).

Squamous-cell carcinoma can occur as a primary neoplasm within the thyroid but often occurs in middle-aged or elderly persons with a past history of goitre which proves to be a well-differentiated carcinoma (Mahoney, Saffos and Rhatigan, 1980). The squamous element is aggressive and the outlook is usually poor. The tumour is often mistaken for metastases from a primary elsewhere, such as a lesion in the oropharynx or larynx.

Metastases within the thyroid masquerade as primary tumours and occur from lesions exhibiting spread by the blood-borne route and with an often occult primary, e.g. hypernephroma, bronchial carcinoma, melanoma and pancreatic carcinoma. Diagnosis can be made by fine-needle biopsy and there is little or no value in surgical treatment since the outlook is usually so poor (Lennard, Wadhera and Farndon, 1984). The distribution of thyroid neoplasms is summarized in Table 5.1.

The biology of thyroid neoplasms

TSH activates the adenylate cyclase and the phosphoinositide turnover–protein kinase C–calcium systems in thyroid cells and appears to have some role in the growth of normal and neoplastic thyroid cells. TSH may work in concert with

Table 5.1 Distribution of thyroid tumours by histological type-II.
Adapted from the data of Har-el *(1986)*

Type	Number	(%)
Mixed follicular and papillary	197	(35.9)
Papillary	144	(26.2)
Follicular	122	(22.2)
Medullary	11	(2.0)
Anaplastic	49	(8.9)
Hürthle	17	(3.1)
Squamous	6	(1.1)

growth factors such as epidermal growth factor. Some growth factors influence thyroid growth through TSH (Duh and Clark, 1987).

Graves' disease and thyroid cancer occur together with unexpected frequency (Farbota *et al.*, 1985). Thyroid-stimulating antibodies may, therefore, play a part in the pathogenesis of thyroid cancer. Filetti *et al.* (1988) recently reported patients in whom this phenomenon may have been implicated. Suppressive therapy with exogenous hormone in this situation may have an adverse effect since this does not inhibit, and might enhance, the synthesis of thyroid-stimulating antibodies (Wenzel and Lente, 1984). If thyroid-stimulating antibodies are present and the patient is unresponsive to thyroxine then attempts to reduce antibody levels might allow control, e.g. high-dosage steroids (Werner and Platman, 1965).

By making a careful examination of very small thyroid carcinomas from 78 patients Kasai and Sakamoto (1987) found that the papillary:follicular carcinoma ratio increased as the size of the carcinoma increased. They felt that the follicular neoplasm could be the 'seed' or initial tumour, that there was no sex difference in carcinogenesis but that the probability of cancer development was higher in females. These findings might explain the papillary/follicular variants which are described and the lack of certainty on histopathological diagnosis might account for the sometimes conflicting survival data for different tumours.

Verhagen *et al.* (1985) looked at hexokinase and its isoenzymes activity in thyroid glands to see if this allowed better differentiation of tumour types. Lower proportions of hexokinase were found in the cytosol from papillary carcinomas compared with follicular and undifferentiated neoplasms. Isoenzyme patterns were different between carcinomas and normal tissues but these differences were not apparent between adenomas and normal thyroid tissue.

Since the histological type of a tumour might influence the operative strategy others have attempted to refine peroperative frozen section diagnostic techniques. It has now been shown that 'ground glass' nuclei and 'orphan Annie eye' nuclei can be identified by frozen section or imprint cytology to allow the confident diagnosis of papillary carcinoma peroperatively (Dominguez-Malagon, Szymanski-Gomez and Gaytan-Garcia, 1988).

Applications of newer technologies, such as flow cytometry to archival histological material does not always allow better understanding. Patients with aneuploid tumours have less favourable cumulative survival but for those with papillary and follicular neoplasms, multivariate analysis using the Cox model showed age at diagnosis, follicular type and extent of invasion beyond the capsule were more important independent prognostic factors. Increasing probability of

DNA aneuploidy with increasing age partially explains the poorer prognosis from differentiated thyroid cancers in older patients (Joensuu *et al.*, 1986).

Bacourt *et al.* (1986) found that the most significant prognostic variable was clinical stage (classified as 'nodule within a lobe', 'lobar' — involving a whole lobe and 'massive' — involving the whole thyroid). Hannequin, Liehn and Delisle (1986) urged caution in the application of the results obtained from one group to another population. It would appear that a personalized multifactorial analysis on one's own patients would be the only way to determine a prognostic index.

The diagnosis of thyroid cancer

The corner stone of diagnostic methods in the diagnosis of thyroid tumours must be fine-needle aspiration biopsy for cytology (FNABC). If combined with flow cytometry for DNA analysis and measurement of other cellular parameters other prognostic indices may be evaluated (Bäckdahl *et al.*, 1987). The technique must no longer be thought of as controversial or unreliable. There is no requirement to seek corroborative histology by drill or cutting needle biopsy.

Silverman *et al.* (1986) found the sensitivity to be 93%, specificity 95.1% with positive and negative predictive values being 88.9% cent and 96.5% respectively. The complication rate was low and the technique of FNABC was proposed as *the* initial diagnostic test of thyroid nodules. Savings accrued from non-requested isotope or ultrasound scans can be considerable. Decision-making based on cytology can reduce the incidence of operations on benign disease and increase the proportion of surgery for neoplasia (Al-Sayer *et al.*, 1985).

Most cytologists cannot and will not distinguish between follicular adenoma and follicular carcinoma which imposes a strategy to operate upon patients in whom this cytological diagnosis is reached (Harsoulis *et al.*, 1986). The combination of FNABC and selective surgery, however, allows better patient survival with reduced morbidity than a policy of resection for all patients with cold nodules (Molitch *et al.*, 1984).

Cystic lesions can usually be aspirated to resolution and this provides immediate mental relief for the patient. The caveat concerning possible malignant change in a cyst wall must be remembered (Anon., 1977).

Operative strategy for thyroid cancer

Since objective data is lacking to allow agreement on the classification, prognostic markers and survival characteristics of thyroid cancer it is impossible to make categorical statements on the optimal surgical procedure. Indeed, a debate can be readily constructed within the same volume between those advocating more conservative procedures — 'Individualizing the extent of surgery for thyroid cancer' (Esselstyn, 1983) and those with a more radical approach — 'Total thyroidectomy in the treatment of thyroid carcinoma' (Thompson, 1983a). An attempt will be made to suggest rationalized procedures for each tumour.

Papillary carcinoma

This tumour is usually readily diagnosed preoperatively by fine-needle biopsy. For tumours of 1.5 cm diameter or less it has been shown that conservative surgery (never bilateral lobectomy) and if involved nodes — lymphadenectomy or modified neck dissection — allowed no operative deaths and all patients followed were alive and free of disease. Subsequent surgical intervention was necessary in less than 10% of cases and modified neck dissection in 3% (Hubert *et al.*, 1980).

In a large series of patients (731) from Norway only 12% developed metastases outside regional nodes and one-third of these had this extent of disease at presentation. Seventy percent of the others developed distant metastases despite a total thyroidectomy. Male sex, advanced age and advanced local tumour stage were associated with occurrence of distant metastases but better prognostic determinants were required if individual treatment was to be prescribed (Hoie *et al.*, 1988) — a further reflection of the difficulties in being objective in this disease despite 700 patients observed over 30 years!

Vickery, Wang and Walker (1987) had reached similar conclusions and stated: 'Minimization of the complications of these modalities (total thyroidectomy and radioactive iodine), however laudable, does not constitute a justification for their use. Because of the low morbidity and long survival with this tumour, it is unlikely that a properly randomized prospective evaluation of papillary thyroid carcinoma will be completed'.

Follicular carcinoma

Preoperative cytology will identify a follicular neoplasm but will not distinguish between an adenoma and a carcinoma. Operative strategy is, therefore, less easily planned. Follicular carcinoma is rarely diagnosed, however, in lesions less than 2 cm in diameter and after total thyroidectomy intraglandular spread and multicentricity are rare. Total thyroidectomy allows ^{131}I treatment of bone metastases, however, and although some patients survive beyond 20 years, cure is unlikely (Thompson, 1983b). There are no objective data to suggest that total lobectomy, followed by completion thyroidectomy for local relapse or to allow ^{131}I treatment for distant metastases, would produce significantly different results.

Serum thyroglobulin is a more reliable marker for tumour recurrence in follicular carcinoma than papillary carcinoma (Müller-Gärtner and Schneider, 1988). Since this tumour is usually more aggressive than papillary carcinoma, since thyroid replacement is easy and since ^{131}I is effective therapy there is a better case for advocating total thyroidectomy for this lesion.

Hürthle cell carcinoma

This tumour is associated with a significant mortality and radioactive iodine therapy is of little use. The greatest difficulty in deciding operative strategy is knowing whether the lesion is benign or malignant. Recent cytophotometric studies suggests that those tumours associated with invasion were largely aneuploid but the percentage of cycling tumour cells, and nuclear size and shape were not useful in separating benign from malignant neoplasms (Flint *et al.*, 1988). The combination of fine-needle biopsy with an ability to carry out cytophotometric measurement might allow the identification of those patients who would most benefit from total thyroidectomy.

Medullary thyroid carcinoma

Apart from familial disease without associated endocrinopathies it is recommended that patients with this tumour should undergo total thyroidectomy and central compartment dissection. MTC occurring as an autosomal dominant trait without associated endocrinopathies appears to be such an indolent disease that surgery *might* not have any part to play (Farndon *et al.*, 1986). Thyroidectomy in patients in either of the other settings will show multicentric disease in 90% and nodal metastases in 20% (Russell *et al.*, 1983). It has been demonstrated that the application of screening programmes (once the disease has been characterized as familial, MEN IIa or b) will allow very early resection of premalignant disease and better disease-free survival (Stjernholm *et al.*, 1980; Brunt and Wells, 1987).

Measurement of plasma calcitonin concentrations following surgery allows a biochemical detection of recurrent disease. Measurement of basal and provoked calcitonin concentrations with selective venous sampling might demonstrate recurrent disease in resectable areas (Norton, Doppman and Brennan, 1980). Prolonged reoperation (up to 12 hours) with extensive neck and mediastinal node dissections might achieve normalization of plasma calcitonin but this procedure has yet to be shown to provide prolonged survival in this condition (Tisell *et al.*, 1986).

Lymphoma of the thyroid

It is less clear, with this tumour, of the part played by surgical excision. A 20-year experience in one centre might accrue 70 or 80 patients and within this group will be differing proportions of tumour type and stage. Surgery should consist of an adequate biopsy which might be a lobectomy with lymph node sampling. This should allow histological characterization and will provide evidence of extra-thyroidal and nodal involvement. Two-thirds of the tumours are likely to be germinal centre cell type with a follicular or follicular/diffuse pattern in one-fifth. The 5-year survival (13%) of the immunoblastic types will be much poorer than those of intermediate (79%) and low grade (92%) categories despite therapy with radiation and chemotherapy (Aozasa *et al.*, 1986).

Anaplastic thyroid tumours

These cancers are amongst the most aggressive afflicting man and median survival from diagnosis is often only 3–6 months. Surgery alone does little to influence these results and death would often be from unpleasant local regrowths often requiring tracheostomy as a final burden in the weeks before an inevitable death. At the Karolinska Hospital in Stockholm a combination of chemotherapy and radiother-apy allowed debulking of tumour in 50% of patients. A combination of preoperative and postoperative radiotherapy with chemotherapy (bleomycin, cyclophosphamide and 5-fluorouracil) during remission gave a 12% survival beyond 3 years (Talroth *et al.*, 1987). This aggressive but tolerable therapy might allow patients some extension of life of better quality without the unpleasant death of suffocation. Surgery can only be palliative and debulking in nature because of the pernicious and highly infiltrative nature of these tumours.

Once biopsy or surgical debulking has taken place then careful immunohistoche-mical examination of apparent anaplastic tumours should be undertaken. Stains against thyroglobulin, calcitonin and leucocyte common antigen might allow reclassification of tumours as lymphomas, MTC or haemangioendothelioma in up to 20% of cases and thereby redirect more appropriate therapy (Shevro *et al.*, 1988).

The parathyroid glands

The incidence of hyperparathyroidism has probably not changed over the years but is being diagnosed more frequently since the advent of health examinations associated with multichannel blood autoanalysis. Heath and his colleagues (1980) showed that these patients might have few, if any symptoms — vague muscle weakness or mild psychiatric disturbance such as depression. Akerström *et al.* (1986) similarly demonstrated, in a Swedish population, that primary hyperparathyroidism was being diagnosed and treated more frequently especially in old women without symptoms or with vague neuromuscular or psychiatric impairment. A less abnormal serum calcium was associated with a higher incidence of chief-cell hyperplasia found at surgery in this group. They felt that chief-cell hyperplasia might represent an early form of the disease before the development of a single autonomous adenoma. Earlier workers had noted this higher incidence of hyperplasia (Esselstyn *et al.*, 1974) with almost 50% of patients demonstrating primary hyperplasia.

Parathyroid carcinoma

Against this changing background of mainly benign disease the incidence of parathyroid carcinoma remains very low and accounts for about 1% of patients with primary hyperparathyroidism. There are no obvious clinical or biochemical markers which distinguish patients with parathyroid carcinoma. Histological studies do not always help because they lack diagnostic predictability. The presence of a rim of normal or atrophic parathyroid, nuclear characteristics, the presence of fibrous bands, stromal and intracytoplasmic fat content, mitotic figures and vascular and capsular invasion are all parameters which have been used to help distinguish hyperplasia from adenoma and from carcinoma. Carcinoma, however, is usually confirmed on subsequent development of local recurrence or metastases at a later date (Roth, 1983).

Chief cells predominate but oxyphil and transitional oxyphil cells may also be found. The cell arrangement varies from a more solid to a trabecular pattern but it might be difficult to distinguish between an adenoma and cancer (Grimelius, Akerström and Johansson, 1981).

Parathyroid carcinoma of the oxyphil cell type has been reported (Obara *et al.*, 1985) but the diagnosis was only made in each patient when metastases developed 5 and 8 years after the initial surgery. Initial diagnoses had been of parathyroid adenoma but metastases eventually showed oxyphil cells and electron microscopy demonstrated the typical cell type packed with numerous mitochondria.

Flow cytometric analysis of DNA content in parathyroid lesions did little to enhance the distinction between benign and malignant lesions. It suggested that tetraploid and near-triploid aneuploid patterns in adenomas and some chief-cell hyperplasias might be early markers of malignant potential (Bowlby, De Bault and Abraham, 1987).

Parathyroid carcinomas usually remain functional and troublesome hypercalcaemia can add to the patient's suffering. Occasionally these tumours are non-secretory and although they have light and electron microscopic features of parathyroid carcinomas and immunoreactivity demonstrated in sections there might be *no* clinical or laboratory evidence of primary hyperparathyroidism (Murphy *et al.*, 1986).

Treatment of parathyroid carcinoma

If the condition is recognized peroperatively *en-bloc* resections offer the best results with neck dissection when there is evidence of regional node metastases. Postoperative markers of tumour recurrence are serum calcium and PTH measurements and if the disease recurs in the neck or lungs then *en-bloc* radical dissection, mediastinal dissection for lymph nodes and pulmonary resection are recomended (Fujimoto and Obara, 1987). The surgery is rarely curative but palliation can be obtained by reducing hypercalcaemia. Radiotherapy is of little use.

Mithramycin produces a potent hypocalcaemic effect which might be effective for many months (Trigonis *et al.*, 1984) and Jüngst (1984) reported symptomatic relief using disodium clodronate. As with many other endocrine neoplasms some patients survive for many years with known metastases (Van Heerden *et al.*, 1979).

Gastrointestinal endocrine tumours

The carcinoid syndrome

The enterochromaffin cells are to be found throughout the length of the gastrointestinal system and assume a rightful place in the APUD system as they synthesize, store and secrete amines, notably serotonin and those in the small intestine motilin — a 22 amino acid peptide. The tumours can be particularly indolent but usually do metastasize to the liver when the syndrome develops — in part because of the liver's capacity to inactivate hormones released into the portal circulation. The rare carcinoid in extraportal sites (e.g. ovarian teratoma, lungs) releases endocrine mediators directly into the systemic circulation and can cause the syndrome before metastasizing. Some carcinoid tumours, especially those of the appendix, can be associated with a very favourable outlook — simple appendicectomy for tumours up to 2 cm in diameter can be associated with no evidence of local or distant recurrence in over 80% of such patients studied to a median time of more than 26 years (Moertel *et al.*, 1987).

In a study of over 400 patients with carcinoid tumours Greenberg and his colleagues (1987) showed that 5-year survival figures for surgically treated carcinoids varied according to site: 85.6% appendix, 66% small intestine and 37.7% for large intestine. The likelihood of death was related independently to increasing age, advanced stage, location within the large intestine and occurrence of another malignancy. The overall 5-year survival for bronchopulmonary carcinoids, for comparison, was 87.6%.

Photographic cytophotometric DNA patterns in ileal carcinoid tumours showed an increased incidence of non-diploidy in patients surviving less than 3–4 years when histology and immunohistochemistry demonstrated no clear cut differences. Nobin and his colleagues (1987) felt, therefore, that this determination might help in assessing the malignant potential of ileal carcinoids. Kujari *et al.* (1988) using flow cytometric methods demonstrated a higher incidence of aneuploid tumours which appeared to be associated with a poorer prognosis but did not preclude tumour-secreting biogenic amines.

Treatment options

Resection of obvious primary tumours especially if symptomatic can bring some relief. Excision or enucleation of hepatic metastases can be undertaken but it has recently been suggested that symptom control with simple blocking drugs is the best first-line therapy. Thereafter somatostatin can be used and hepatic artery embolization or chemotherapy should be used as a third-line therapy (Hodgson, 1988).

Kvols et al. (1986) showed that a long-acting somatostatin analogue (SMS 201–995, Sandoz) could produce symptomatic relief in all patients and would produce at least 50% decrease in urinary 5-HIAA levels in over 70% of patients.

Actual tumour regression has been documented in 2 patients by Harris and Smith (1982) who used the serotonin antagonist cyproheptadine. They felt that the hepatic deposits may have regressed by modulation of their blood supply through the blocking effects of cyproheptadine on serotonin-1, serotonin-2 and histamine-1 receptors.

Other agents may prove effective in symptomatic and biochemical control of the syndrome; salmon calcitonin appears to mimic somatostatin in its effects (Antonelli et al., 1987), H_2-receptor blockers may exert their beneficial effects not through inhibition of the action of histamine but through reducing serum serotonin concentrations (Noppen et al., 1988) and new 5-hydroxytryptamine M-receptor blocking drugs (ICS 205–930, Sandoz), although not influencing urinary 5-HIAA excretion, markedly improve the frequency and severity of the diarrhoea (Anderson et al., 1987).

More 'vigorous' therapies might also have a part to play in therapy of the carcinoid syndrome. Although associated with side-effects and some morbidity human leucocyte interferon has been shown to be effective in producing clinical and biochemical evidence of tumour regression (Oberg et al., 1986). Cis-platinum has been demonstrated to be effective in producing marked tumour regression in a patient with metastatic ovarian carcinoid tumour (Porter and Ostrowski, 1988).

Pancreatic endocrine tumours

Each of the 5 cell types within the islets can give rise to a tumour associated with production of its specific polypeptide or amine: alpha cells — glucagon, beta cells — insulin, delta cells — somatostatin, F (or D_2 or PP) cells — pancreatic polypeptide and enterochromaffin cells — serotonin. Other 'ectopic' cells reside in the pancreas and many produce specific tumours, e.g. gastrinoma (gastrin), vipoma (vasoactive intestinal peptide). The ectopically functioning tumours have a higher potential for malignant behaviour. Most of the tumours can produce potentially dangerous functional disturbance and timely therapy (including surgery) might allow years of symptom free survival (Carter, 1987).

Insulinoma

Proye and Boissel (1988) in a review of nearly 400 patients found that 79% had benign tumours and only 11% had carcinoma. Ninety per cent of those with malignant insulinomas have metastases at presentation and, therefore, surgery cannot be curative. Other therapies can give good symptomatic relief and the beta cell toxin streptozotocin can be used effectively, especially if care is taken to reduce nephrotoxicity (Tobin, Warenius and Morris, 1987).

Gastrinoma

As many as 60% of gastrinomas are malignant but their size and histological appearance does not accurately reflect their biological behaviour (Wolfe, Alexander and McGuigan, 1982). No tumour will be found in a proportion of patients and in others the tumour and/or its metastases will be unresectable (Deveney and Deveney, 1987). Others report a favourable outcome from conservative surgery for the extrapancreatic tumour with lymph node metastases (Bornman *et al.*, 1987) or prolonged survival even with documented hepatic metastases (Davis and Vansant, 1979).

There should be little need to resort to total gastrectomy to treat gastrinomas since acid secretion can be so effectively reduced by the use of H_2-receptor blocking drugs or H^+-K^+-ATPase inhibitors such as omeprazole. Somatostatin analogues (such as SMS 201–995, Sandoz) can arrest tumour growth in those patients in whom it produces a reduction in gastrin or gastric acid secretion. It appears ineffective in those with very high basal gastrin levels (Vinik *et al.*, 1988).

Pancreatic endocrine tumour and multiple endocrine neoplasia type I syndrome

Gastrinomas are the second commonest endocrine tumour after hyperparathyroidism to form the clustering of multiple endocrine neoplasia, type I(MEN 1). Farndon *et al.* (1987) showed, however, that there was little value screening patients for gastrinomas if parathyroid pathology was established. Lamers *et al.* (1988) have similarly demonstrated that serum pepsinogen I is not a marker for gastrinomas, is not inherited as a genetic trait and appears to be elevated secondary to the chronic hypergastrinaemia.

In the MEN I setting, however, there is a case to be made for total pancreatectomy at presentation since the disease produces significant morbidity and mortality. The tumours are often multiple and can occur asynchronously with a common malignant component (Tisell *et al.*, 1988).

Other pancreatic tumours

Our knowledge about the biology of the other endocrine pancreatic tumours is increasing slowly because of their rarity. It is known that pancreatic polypeptide is a useful adjunctive marker of these tumours and an atropine suppression test can distinguish normal from tumour-related secretion but measurement of other specific hormones is still required (Adrian *et al.*, 1986). Pancreatic polypeptide need not be associated with any functional abnormality.

Pilato *et al.* (1988) showed that in multiple pancreatic tumours from one patient with the MEN I syndrome there was a non-random expression of the tumoral phenotype — demonstrated by immunohistochemical methods. The tumour and its metastases can, however, manifest multiple clinical syndromes simultaneously with secretion of gastrin, glucagon, ACTH and serotonin (Lokich *et al.*, 1987). It is, perhaps, by studying these fascinating but rare tumours with their multipotential functional capacity, their biochemical markers and frequent genetic component, that we will understand the more general process of neoplasia.

The adrenal gland

This organ, perhaps more than any other, demonstrates the complex relationships which can occur due to diverse embryological origins, the medulla coming from ectoderm and the cortex from mesoderm. It has more tangible neural connections, especially to the medulla, than other APUD glands. Tumours are occasionally described with bizarre hormonal complements which demonstrate the multipotential of some of these tumour cells and their common embryological origin. Sparagana, Feldman and Molnar (1987) described a phaeochromocytoma which produced mainly adrenalin but also contained cells producing vasoactive intestinal peptide and serotonin.

Adrenocortical neoplasms

Approximately one-half of clinically detected adrenocortical neoplasms are benign and functioning and most will demonstrate signs and symptoms of glucocorticoid (Cushing's syndrome) or mineralocorticoid (Conn's syndrome) excess. The other 50% will be adrenocortical carcinomas about half of which will retain functional capacity. The greater application of CT scanning and, to a lesser extent, ultrasonography, has led to the discovery of unexpected adrenal masses — the so-called 'incidentalomas'. Sometimes no evidence of function or symptoms can be ascribed to these coincidentally uncovered tumours. They might, however, be adrenocortical carcinomas (especially if greater than 3 cm in diameter) or metastases from occult primary neoplasms. Thompson and Cheung (1987) recommend operative exploration in all patients with 'incidentalomas' of 3 cm or more in diameter except in those over the age of 60 with normal biochemistry and imaging characteristics.

Conn's syndrome

Scott *et al.* (1986) in studies on over 300 patients with the syndrome showed that 72% of patients will have a solitary benign cortical adenoma, 27% bilateral cortical hyperplasia and 1% multiple and/or bilateral adenomas. Carcinoma-producing Conn's syndrome is exceedingly rare. As with other endocrine tumours diagnosis of malignancy on histological grounds is not easy and the smallest tumour might metastasize widely.

Cushing's syndrome

Watson and his colleagues (1986) have shown that perhaps 17% of patients presenting for surgery of this syndrome will have an adrenocortical carcinoma. Although functional the carcinomas have less efficient steroidogenic enzyme systems. Survival, interestingly, was reduced in those with adenomas for the first 2 years but was very poor for those with carcinomas (only one-third alive at 2 years).

Recently, more encouraging results have been described by the use of chemotherapeutic regimens. Van Slooten *et al.* (1984) using Op′-DDD, Eriksson *et al.* (1987) using Op′-DDD in combination with streptozotocin and Schlumberger *et al.* (1988) using 5-fluorouracil, doxorubicin and cisplatin for patients with too large a tumour burden for treatment with Op′-DDD.

The adrenal medulla — phaeochromocytoma

The incidence of malignant phaeochromocytomas varies from 1 to 13% depending upon the series and Dow *et al.* (1982) suggest that this variation might be accounted for by the difficulty in deciding malignant features on histology and the possibility that the incidence of malignancy is higher in extra-adrenal tumours.

A further APUD link proves of value in these rare tumours; neuron-specific enolase has been found to be elevated in those patients with malignant phaeochromocytomas when compared with circulating levels in those patients with benign tumours. Neuron-specific enolase is found in other APUD tumours, e.g. islet-cell carcinoma and some in MTC but it does appear to be specific for marking the malignant phaeochromocytoma (Oishi and Sato, 1987).

Surgery can often do little more than debulk these malignant lesions. Alpha- and beta- adrenergic blockade can then provide some symptom control. Other treatment options have recently been developed. Sutton *et al.* (1982) were some of the first to demonstrate that ^{131}I-labelled meta-iodobenzylguanidine is taken up specifically by metastases of a malignant phaeochromocytoma. Thompson *et al.* (1984) showed that increasing the dose of ^{131}I loaded on this guanethidine analogue allows delivery of therapeutic doses of radiation to the tumour and its metastases. Some patients demonstrated objective responses with diminution of size of primary and metastatic tumours and a corresponding decrease in the secretion of catecholamines. The tumour is notoriously difficult to treat and it is pleasing to read of other reports suggesting that combination therapy (cyclophosphamide, vincristine and decarbazime) and high-voltage irradiation can produce objective responses (Siddiqui *et al.*, 1988). They report decreased plasma catecholamines, reduced dose of antihypertensives and partial response of bone metastases.

Conclusions

The pituitary, ectopic hormone producing tumours and the majority of benign endocrine tumours have been neglected! It is hoped that this glimpse of malignant endocrine tumours explains some of the fascination engendered by these rare lesions. By studying their unique relationships, functionally and embryologically, we might be afforded better understanding of the process of neoplasia at large.

References

Adrian, T. E., Uttenthal, L. O., Williams, S. J. and Bloom, S. R. (1986) Secretion of pancreatic polypeptide in patients with pancreatic endocrine tumours. *New England Journal of Medicine*, **315**, 287–291

Akerström, G., Bergström, R., Grimelius, L. *et al.* (1986) Relation between changes in clinical and histopathological features of primary hyperparathyroidism. *World Journal of Surgery*, **10**, 696–702

Al-Sayer, H. M., Krukowski, Z. H., Williams, V. M. M. and Matheson, N. A. (1985) Fine needle aspiration cytology in isolated thyroid swellings: a prospective two year evaluation. *British Medical Journal*, **290**, 1490–1492

Anderson, J. V., Coupe, M. O., Morris, J. A. *et al.* (1987) Remission of symptoms in carcinoid syndrome with a new 5-hydroxytryptamine M receptor antagonist. *British Medical Journal*, **294**, 1129

Anon. (1977) Diagonosing thyroid nodules. *Lancet*, ii, 1268

Antonelli, A., Del Guerra, P., Fierabracci, A. *et al.* (1987) Effect of salmon calcitonin on symptoms and urinary excretion of 5-hydroxyindoleacetic acid in the carcinoid syndrome. *British Medical Journal*, **295**, 961

Aozasa, K., Inoue, A., Kazuo, T. K. *et al.* (1986) Malignant lymphomas of the thyroid gland. *Cancer* **58**, 100–104

Bäckdahl, M., Wallin, G., Löwhagen, T. *et al.* (1987) Fine needle biopsy cytology and DNA analysis. *Surgical Clinics of North America*, **67**, 197–211

Bacourt, F., Asselain, B., Savoie, J.C. *et al.* (1986) Multifactorial study of prognostic factors in differentiated thyroid carcinoma and a re-evaluation of the importance of age. *British Journal of Surgery*, **73**, 274–277

Berson, S. A. and Yalow, R. S. (1973) General Radioimmunoassay. In *Methods in Investigative and Diagnostic Endocrinology. Peptide Hormones* (ed. S. A. Berson and R. S. Yalow), New York, American Elsevier, pp. 84–120

Block, M. A., Jackson, C. E., Greenawald, K. A. *et al.* (1980) Clinical characteristics distinguishing hereditary from sporadic medullary thyroid carcinoma: treatment implications. *Archives of Surgery*, **115**, 142–148

Bornman, P. C., Marks, I. N., Mee, A. S. and Price, S. (1987) Favourable response to conservative surgery for extra pancreatic gastrinoma with lymph node metastases. *British Journal of Surgery*, **74**, 198–201

Bowlby, L., De Bault, L. E. and Abraham, S. R. (1987) Flow cytometric DNA analysis of parathyroid glands. *American Journal of Pathology*, **128**, 338–344

Brunt, L. M. and Wells, S. A. (1987) Advances in the diagnosis and treatment of medullary thyroid carcinoma. *Surgical Clinics of North America*, **67**, 263–279

Cancer Research Campaign (1987) *Facts on Cancer*, Factsheet 1.2, 1.3, 3.2 and 3.3

Carter, D. C. (1987) Pancreatic endocrine tumours. *British Medical Journal*, **294**, 593–594

Davis, C. E. and Vansant, J. H. (1979) Zollinger–Ellison syndrome. *Annals of Surgery*, **189**, 620–626

Deveney, C. W. and Deveney, K. E. (1987) Zollinger–Ellison syndrome (Gastrinoma). *Surgical Clinics of North America*, **67**, 411–422

Dominguez-Malagon, H. R., Szymanski-Gomez, J. J. and Gaytan-Garcia, S. R. (1988) Optically clear and vacuolated nuclei. *Cancer*, **62**, 105–108

Dow, C. J., Palmer, M. K., O'Sullivan, J. P. and Kirkham, J. S. (1982) Malignant phaeochromocytoma: report of a case and a critical review. *British Journal of Surgery*, **69**, 338–340

Duh, Q. and Clark, O. H. (1987) Factors influencing the growth of normal and neoplastic thyroid tissue. *Surgical Clinics of North America*, **67**, 281–298

Eriksson, B., Öberg, K., Curstedt, T. *et al.* (1987) Treatment of hormone-producing adrenocortical cancer with O, p'-DDD and streptozocin. *Cancer*, **59**, 1398–1403

Esselstyn, C. B. (1983) Individualizing the extent of surgery for thyroid cancer: a re-appraisal. In *Endocrine Surgery Uptake* (ed. N. W. Thompson and A. J. Vinik), Grune and Stratton, New York, pp. 67–70

Esselstyn, C. B., Levin, H. S., Eversman, J. J. *et al.* (1974) Re-appraisal of parathyroid pathology in hyperparathyroidism. *Surgical Clinics of North America*, **54**, 443–447

Farbota, L. M., Calandra, D. B., Lawrence, A. M. and Paloyan, E. (1985) Thyroid carcinoma in Graves' disease. *Surgery*, **98**, 1148–1152

Farndon, J. R., Geraghty, J. M., Dilley, W. G. (1987) Serum gastrin, calcitonin and prolactin as markers of Multiple Endocrine Neoplasia Syndromes in patients with primary hyperparathyroidism. *World Journal of Surgery*, **11**, 252–257

Farndon, J. R., Leight, G. S., Dilley, W. G. *et al.* (1986) Familial medullary thyroid carcinoma without associated endocrinopathies: a distinct clinical entity. *British Journal of Surgery*, **73**, 278–281

Filetti, S., Belfiore, A., Daniels, G. H. *et al.* (1988) The role of thyroid-stimulating antibodies of Graves' disease in differentiated thyroid cancer. *New England Journal of Medicine*, **318**, 753–759

Flint, A., Davenport, R. D., Lloyd, R. V. *et al.* (1988) Cytophotometric measurements of Hürthle cell tumours of the thyroid gland. *Cancer*, **61**, 110–113

Fujimoto, Y. and Obara, T. (1987) How to recognize and treat parathyroid carcinoma. *Surgical Clinics of North America*, **67**, 343–357

Greenberg, R. S., Baumgarten, D. A., Clark, W. S. *et al.* (1987) Prognostic factors for gastrointestinal and bronchopulmonary carcinoid tumours. *Cancer*, **60**, 2476–2483

Grimelius, L., Akerström, G. and Johansson, H. (1981) *The Parathyroids — Location and Histopathological Diagnosis*. Uppsala, USA: Institute of Pathology and Department of Surgery, University Hospital

Hannequin, P., Liehn, J. C. and Delisle, M. J. (1986) Multifactorial analysis of survival in thyroid cancer. *Cancer*, **58**, 1749–1755

Har-el, G., Hadar, T., Segal, K. *et al.* (1986) Hürthle cell carcinoma of the thyroid gland. *Cancer*, **57**, 1613–1617

Harris, A. L. and Smith, I. E. (1982) Regression of carcinoid tumour with cyproheptadine. *British Medical Journal*, **285**, 475

Harsoulis, P., Leontsini, M., Economou, A. *et al.* (1986) Fine needle aspiration biopsy cytology in the diagnosis of thyroid cancer: comparative study of 213 operated patients. *British Journal of Surgery*, **73**, 461–464

Heath, H., Hodgson, S. F. and Kennedy, M. A. (1980) Primary hyperparathyroidism. *New England Journal of Medicine*, **302**, 189–193

Hodgson, H. J. F. (1988) Controlling the carcinoid syndrome. *British Medical Journal*, **297**, 1213–1214

Hoie, J., Stenwig, A. E., Kullman, G. and Lindegaard, M. (1988) Distant metastases in papillary thyroid cancer. *Cancer*, **61**, 1–6

Hubert, J. P., Kiernan, P. D., Beahrs, O. H. *et al.* (1980) Occult papillary carcinoma of the thyroid. *Archives of Surgery*, **115**, 394–398

Joensuu, H., Klemi, P., Eerola, E. and Tuominen, J. (1986) Influence of cellular DNA content on survival in differentiated thyroid cancer. *Cancer*, **58**, 2462–2467

Johnson, T. L., Lloyd, R., Burney, R. E. and Thompson, N. W. (1987) Hürthle cell thyroid tumours. *Cancer*, **59**, 107–112

Jüngst, D. (1984) Disodium clodronate effective in management of severe hypercalcaemia caused by parathyroid carcinoma. *Lancet*, **ii**, 1043

Kasai, N. and Sakamoto, A. (1987) New subgroupings of small thyroid carcinomas. *Cancer*, **60**, 1767–1770

Kujari, H., Joensuu, H., Klemi, P. *et al.* (1988) A flow cytometric analysis of 23 carcinoid tumours. *Cancer*, **61**, 2517–2520

Kvols, L. K., Moertel, C. G., O'Connell, M. J. *et al.* (1986) Treatment of the malignant carcinoid syndrome. Evaluation of a long-acting somatostatin analogue. *New England Journal of Medicine*, **315**, 663–666

Lamers, C. B. H. W., Rotter, J. I., Jansen, J. B. M. J. and Samloff, I. M. (1988) Serum pepsinogen I in familial Multiple Endocrine Neoplasia type I. *Digestive Diseases and Sciences*, **33**, 1274–1276

Lennard, T. W. J., Wadhera, V. and Farndon, J. R. (1984) Fine needle aspiration biopsy in diagnosis of metastases to the thyroid gland. *Journal of the Royal Society of Medicine*, **77**, 196–197

Lokich, J., Bothe, A., O'Hara, C. and Federman, M. (1987) Metastatic islet cell tumour with ACTH, gastrin and glucagon secretion. *Cancer*, **59**, 2053–2058

Mahoney, J. P., Saffos, R. O. and Rhatigan, R. M. (1980) Follicular adenocarcinoma of the thyroid gland. *Histopathology*, **4**, 547–557

Mazaferri, E. L., Young, R. L., Oertel, J. E. *et al.* (1977) Papillary thyroid carcinoma: the impact of therapy in 576 patients. *Medicine (Baltimore)*, **56**, 171–196

Moertel, C. G., Weiland, L. H., Nagorney, D. M. and Dockerty, M. B. (1987) Carcinoid tumours of the appendix: treatment and prognosis. *New England Journal of Medicine*, **317**, 1699–1701

Molitch, M. E., Beck, J. R., Dreisman, M. *et al.* (1984) The cold thyroid nodule: an analysis of diagnostic and therapeutic options. *Endocrine Review*, **5**, 185–189

Müller-Gärtner, H. and Schneider, C. (1988) Clinical evaluation of tumour characteristics predisposing serum thyroglobulin to be undetected in patients with differentiated thyroid cancer. *Cancer*, **61**, 976–981

Murphy, L. N., Glennon, P. G., Diocee, M. S. *et al.* (1986) Nonsecretory parathyroid carcinoma of the mediastinum. *Cancer*, **58**, 2468–2476

Nobin, A., Erhardt, K., Auer, G. *et al.* (1987) Nuclear DNA patterns and survival in metastasizing ileal carcinoids. *World Journal of Surgery*, **11**, 372–377

Noppen, M., Jacobs, A., Van Belle, S. *et al.* (1988) Inhibitory effects of ranitidine on flushing and serum serotonin concentrations in carcinoid syndrome. *British Medical Journal*, **296**, 682–683

Norton, J. A., Doppman, J. L. and Brennan, M. F. (1980) Localization and resection of clinically inapparent medullary carcinoma of the thyroid. *Surgery*, **87**, 616–622

Obara, T., Fujimoto, Y., Yamaguchi, K. *et al.* (1985) Parathyroid carcinoma of the oxyphil cell type. *Cancer*, **55**, 1482–1489

Oberg, K., Norhelm, I., Lind, E. *et al.* (1986) Treatment of malignant carcinoid tumors with human leukocyte interferon: long-term results. *Cancer Treatment Reports*, **70**, 1297–1304

Oishi, S. I. and Sato, T. (1987) Elevated serum neuron-specific enolase in patients with malignant pheochromocytoma. *Cancer*, **61**, 1167–1170

Pearse, A. G. E. (1966) Common cytochemical properties of cells producing polypeptide hormones with particular reference to calcitonin and the thyroid C cell. *Veterinary Record*, **79**, 587–590

Pearse, A. G. E. (1968) Common cytochemical and ultrastructural characteristics of cells producing polypeptide hormones (the APUD series) and their relevance to thyroid and ultimobronchial C cells and calcitonin. *Proceedings of the Royal Society, B*, **170**, 71–80

Pearse, A. G. E. (1974) The APUD cell concept and its implications in pathology. *Pathology Annual*, **9**, 27–41

Pearse, A. G. E. and Takor, T. (1976) Neuroendocrine embryology and the APUD concept. *Clinical Endocrinology*, **5**, 2295–2445

Pilato, F. P., D'Adda, T., Banchini, E. and Bordi, C. (1988) Nonrandom expression of polypeptide hormones in pancreatic endocrine tumors. *Cancer*, **61**, 1815–1820

Porter, A. T. and Ostrowski, M. J. (1988) Successful treatment of malignant carcinoid tumour with intravenous Cis-Platinum. *European Journal of Surgical Oncology*, **14**, 703–704

Proye, C. and Boissel, P. (1988) Preoperative imaging versus intraoperative localization of tumours in adult surgical patients with hyperinsulinemia: a multicenter study of 338 patients. *World Journal of Surgery*, **12**, 685–690

Roth, S. (1983) The parathyroid gland. In *Principles and Practise of Surgical Pathology* (ed. S. G. Silverberg), Wiley, New York, pp. 1443–1466

Russell, C. F., Van Heerden, J., Sizemore, G. W. *et al.* (1983). The surgical management of medullary thyroid carcinoma. *Annals of Surgery*, **197**, 42–48

Schlumberger, M., Ostronoff, M., Bellaiche, M. *et al.* (1988) 5-fluorouracil, Doxorubicin and Cisplatin regimen in adrenal cortical carcinoma. *Cancer*, **61**, 1492–1494

Scott, W. H., Sussman, C R., Page, D. L. *et al.* (1986) Primary aldosteronism caused by adrenocortical carcinoma. *World Journal of Surgery*, **10**, 646–653

Shevro, J., Gal, R., Avidor, I. *et al.* (1988) Anaplastic thyroid carcinoma; a clinical, histologic and immunohistochemical study. *Cancer*, **62**, 319–325

Siddiqui, M. Z., Finn, E., Von Eyben, F. and Spanos, G. (1988) High-voltage irradiation and combination chemotherapy for malignant pheochromocytoma. *Cancer*, **62**, 686–690

Silverman, J. F., West, L., Larkin, E. W. *et al.* (1986) The role of fine needle aspiration biopsy in the rapid diagnosis and management of thyroid neoplasms. *Cancer*, **57**, 1164–1170

Sparagana, M., Feldman, J. M. and Molnar, Z. (1987) An unusual pheochromocytoma associated with an androgen secreting adrenocortical adenoma. *Cancer*, **60**, 223–231

Stjernholm, M. R., Freudenbourg, J. C., Mooney, H. S. *et al.* (1980) Medullary carcinoma of the thyroid before age 2 years. *Journal of Clinical Endocrinology and Metabolism*, **51**, 252–253

Sutton, H., Wyeth, P., Allen, A. P. *et al.* (1982) Disseminated malignant phaeochromocytoma: localisation with iodine-131-labelled meta-iodobenzylguanidine. *British Medical Journal*, **285**, 1153–1154

Talroth, E., Wallin, G., Lundell, G. *et al.* (1987) Multimodality treatment in anaplastic giant cell thyroid carcinoma. *Cancer*, **60**, 1428–1431

Taylor, S. (1980) Thyroid tumours. In *The Thyroid Gland* (ed. M. De Visscher), Raven Press, New York, pp. 257–278

Thompson, N. W. (1983a) Total thyroidectomy in the treatment of thyroid carcinoma. In *Endocrine Surgery Update* (ed. N. W. Thompson and A. J. Vinik), Grune and Stratton, New York, pp. 71–84

Thompson, N. W. (1983b) The thyroid nodule — surgical management. In *Endocrine Surgery* (ed. I. D. A. Johnston and N. W. Thompson), Butterworths, London, pp. 14–24

Thompson, N. W., Allo, M. D., Shapiro, B. *et al.* (1984) Extra-adrenal and metastatic pheochromocytoma: the role of 131-I Metaiodobenzylguanidine (^{131}IMIBG) in localization and management. *World Journal of Surgery*, **8**, 605–611

Thompson, N. W. and Cheung, P. S. Y. (1987) Diagnosis and treatment of functioning and nonfunctioning adrenocortical neoplasms including incidentalomas. *Surgical Clinics of North America*, **67**, 423–436

Tisell, L., Hansson, G., Jansson, S. and Salander, H. (1986) Reoperation in the treatment of asymptomatic metastasizing medullary thyroid carcinoma. *Surgery*, **99**, 60–66

Tissel, L. E., Ahlman, H., Jansson, S. and Grimelius, L. (1988) Total pancreatectomy in the MEN I syndrome. *British Journal of Surgery*, **75**, 154–157

Tobin, M. V., Warenius, H. M. and Morris, A. I. (1987) Forced diuresis to reduce nephrotoxicity of streptozotocin in the treatment of advanced metastatic insulinoma. *British Medical Journal*, **294**, 1128

Trigonis, C., Cedermark, B., Willems J. *et al.* (1984) Parathyroid carcinoma. Problems in diagnosis and treatment. *Clinical Oncology*, **10**, 11–19

Van Heerden, J. A., Weiland, L. H., Remine, W. H. *et al.* (1979) Cancer of the parathyroid gland. *Archives of Surgery*, **114**, 475–480

Van Slooten, H., Moolenaar, A. J., Van Seters, A. P. and Smeenk, D. (1984) The treatment of adrenocortical carcinoma with O,p'-DDD: prognostic simplifications of serum level monitoring. *European Journal of Cancer and Clinical Oncology*, **20**, 47–53

Verhagen, J. N., Van Der Heijden, M. C. M., Rijksen, G. *et al.* (1985) Determination and characterization of hexokinase in thyroid cancer and benign neoplasms. *Cancer*, **55**, 1519–1524

Vickery, A. L., Wang, C. and Walker, A. M. (1987) Treatment of intrathyroidal papillary carcinoma of the thyroid. *Cancer*, **60**, 2587–2595

Vinik, A. I., Tsai, S., Moattari, A. R. and Cheung, P. (1988) Somatostatin analogue (SMS 201–995) in patients with gastrinomas. *Surgery*, **104**, 834–842

Watson, R. G. G., Van Heerden, J. A., Northcutt, R. C. *et al.* (1986) Results of adrenal surgery for Cushing's syndrome: 10 years' experience. *World Journal of Surgery*, **10**, 531–538

Wells, S. A., Dilley, W. G., Farndon, J. R. *et al.* (1985) Early diagnosis and treatment of medullary thyroid carcinoma. *Archives of Internal Medicine*, **145**, 1248–1252

Wenzel, K. W. and Lente, J. R. (1984) Similar effects of thionamide drugs and perchlorate on thyroid stimulating immunoglobulins in Graves' disease: evidence against an immunosuppressive action in thionamide drugs. *Journal of Clinical Endocrinology and Metabolism*, **58**, 62–69

Werner, S. C. and Platman, S. R. (1965) Remission of hyperthyroidism (Graves' disease) and altered pattern of serum-thyroxine binding induced by prednisone. *Lancet*, **ii**, 751–756

Wolfe, M. M., Alexander, R. W. and McGuigan, J. E. (1982) Extrapancreatic, extraintestinal gastrinoma: effective treatment by surgery. *New England Journal of Medicine*, **306**, 1533–1536

Chapter 6

Breast cancer

C. S. McArdle

Breast cancer is the commonest malignancy in women in North America and Western Europe. The average Western woman has a 1:16 chance of developing breast cancer during her lifetime; it is the commonest cause of death in middle-aged women. In the UK 21 000 new cases are diagnosed annually; worldwide over 0.25 million cases occur each year. Less than 1% of cases occur in males.

There is a steep rise in incidence above the age of 30 years with a slight plateau between 45 and 55 years and a slower but steady rise thereafter. There is marked variation in the incidence of breast cancer between different countries, the rates in the USA being six times higher than Asia or Africa. Countries currently with low incidence rates are, however, experiencing the greatest increase in the number of new cases.

Risk factors

Several factors are associated with increased risk (Table 6.1).

Table 6.1 Risk factors in breast cancer

Age	>45
Geographic	N. America/Europe
Age at menarche	Early
Age at natural menopause	Late
Parity	Nulliparous
Age at first full-term pregnancy	>30
Family history	First-degree relative
Dietary	Increased fat consumption
Previous benign breast disease	Epitheliosis
Contraceptive pill	Duration of use prior to first pregnancy

Age at menarche and menopause

The risk of developing breast cancer for women whose menarche occurred before 12 years of age is approximately twice that of those whose periods commenced after 13 years. Furthermore, the risk in women who menstruated until 55 years is approximately twice that of women undergoing the menopause before the age of 45 years (Henderson, Pike and Ross, 1984). The suggestion that there might be a link between oestrogen replacement therapy and post-menopausal women and breast cancer has not been confirmed (Armstrong, 1988; Bergkvist *et al.*, 1989).

Age at first full-term pregnancy

The increased breast cancer risk in nulliparous women has long been recognized. The protective effect of pregnancy, however, is related to age at first full-term pregnancy (McMahon *et al.*, 1970). The protective effect of first pregnancy decreases up to the age of about 32 years. For women with their first pregnancy above this age the risk of breast cancer is, in fact, greater than that of nulliparous women. Lactation, *per se*, has little if any effect on breast cancer risk.

Family history

Women with a family history of breast cancer have a risk 2–3 times that of the general population. This appears to be greatest for women with a first-degree relative or relatives developing breast cancer before the age of 40 years (Table 6.2) (Sattin *et al.*, 1985).

Table 6.2 Familial risk of breast cancer

Risk factor	Relative risk
First-degree relative	2.3
Second-degree relative	1.5
Mother and sister	13.6
Relative <45 years at diagnosis	2.8

Dietary factors

The relationship between dietary factors and breast cancer risk has not been clearly established. It is, however, known that there is a strong correlation between increased risk of breast cancer and fat intake. Suggestions that intake of coffee and alcohol and vitamin A deficiency may be important have not, as yet, been substantiated (Skegg, 1987).

Benign breast disease

Although fibroadenomas and fibrocystic disease do not predispose to malignancy they may be associated with features, e.g. epitheliosis, that are. Roberts and her colleagues (1984) reported that the risk of breast cancer in women initially attending a breast clinic with benign disease was 2.7 times the expected rate; nevertheless, only 1 patient in 50 with breast cancer has had previous breast surgery.

Oral contraception

The relationship between oral contraceptive usage and breast cancer risk remains inconclusive. Pike and his colleagues (1983) compared 314 women with breast cancer aged less than 37 years at diagnosis with a control group, and demonstrated that long-term use of an oral contraceptive before the age of 25 was associated with increased risk of breast cancer, particularly if a preparation with a high progestogen content had been used. Vessey and his colleagues (1983) compared 1176 breast cancer patients aged less than 50 with controls, and found no statistically significant difference in oral contraceptive use between the groups. They subsequently reported a further analysis of women aged 40 years or less; in this group there appeared to be an excess of contraceptive usage prior to first full-term pregnancy in the breast cancer group (McPherson et al., 1983).

More recently a case control study undertaken in Sweden and Norway showed a two-fold increase in risk after 12 years or if oral contraceptives were used for more than 7 years prior to first full-term pregnancy (Meirik et al., 1986). The latest studies from the UK appear to provide further support for the view that long-term use of oral contraceptives may increase the risk of breast cancer in young women (Kay and Hannaford, 1988; UK National Case Control Study Group, 1989).

In contrast, the Cancer and Steroid Hormone (CASH) study, a large multicentre population based case-control study of over 2000 American women aged 20–44 years failed to demonstrate a significant impact on risk (Stadel et al., 1985). A similar study from New Zealand also failed to support the hypothesis that use of oral contraceptives at young ages increases the risk of breast cancer (Paul et al., 1986). It may be, however, that if there is a long latent period before development of breast cancer, the effect of oral contraceptives will not become apparent for a number of years.

Stress

The suggestion that stress increases the risk of developing breast cancer remains unproven (Jones, Goldblatt and Leon, 1984).

Early diagnosis and screening

Prognosis is closely related to the clinical stage at presentation. Attention has therefore been directed towards screening programmes. Methods of screening include physical examination by a doctor or nurse, breast self-examination or mammography.

There is no evidence that physical examination alone is an effective method of screening. Breast self-examination, although widely advocated as a method of screening for cancer, has failed to prevent cancer deaths. In Nottingham, nearly 50 000 women were offered instruction in breast self-examination; about half accepted. The characteristics of the 319 cancers diagnosed during the study were compared with cancer diagnosed immediately before the study began. Although there was a significant reduction in size at presentation, the difference was not reflected in an improvement in survival (Dowle et al., 1987).

The role of mammography has been investigated in a number of randomized and non-randomized studies. The first of these, the health insurance plan (HIP) study, was started in 1963 in New York.

Health insurance plan (HIP) study

Sixty-two thousand women aged 40–64 years were randomly allocated to routine medical care or a screening programme. Two-thirds of those offered screening attended for initial assessment which consisted of physical examination and mammography. They were then offered annual screening for 3 years; all but 12% had at least one additional examination.

After 18 years 126 patients in the study population had died of breast cancer compared with 163 in the control group (Shapiro, 1989). The benefit appeared to be largely confined to women over 50 years of age.

These results, however, have not been universally accepted. It was noted that 74% of tumours detected by mammography were node negative, compared with 75% of those detected by clinical examination alone, suggesting that mammography did not pick up lesions earlier than clinical examination (Skrabanek, 1985). Furthermore, a significant percentage of those patients said to have mammographically-detected lesions were on subsequent clinical examination found to have palpable lesions.

Further studies have since been reported from Sweden, the Netherlands and the UK (Table 6.3).

Table 6.3 Relative risk of dying in patients eligible for screening

Centre	Type of study	Age (years)	No. eligible	Relative risk	95% confidence interval
Swedish Two county	Randomized	40–49 50–74	19 937 58 148	1.26 0.61	0.56–2.84 0.44–0.84
Nijmegen	Case-controlled	35–70	30 502	0.48	0.23–1.00
Utrecht	Case-controlled	50–64	20 555	0.30	0.13–0.70
UK	Non-randomized	45–64	45 841	0.80	0.64–1.01
Malmo	Randomized	45–54 55–69	7 981 13 107	1.29 0.79	0.74–2.25 0.51–1.24

Swedish two county study

In the Swedish study, almost 135 000 women aged 40–74 years were randomly allocated to screening or a control group (Tabar *et al.*, 1985). Screening consisted of a single oblique view repeated every 2 years for women under 50 years and once every 3 years for women over the age of 50. Compliance on initial screening was 89%.

There was a highly significant reduction (25%) in the number of Stage II and advanced cancers and a corresponding increase in Stage I and *in-situ* cancers in the study group.

Overall there was a 31% reduction in mortality from breast cancer in the screened population. The difference in cumulative mortality rates between the two groups emerged at 4 years, and steadily widened thereafter. The reduction in mortality was confined to those aged over 50 years; there were too few deaths in the group aged less than 50 years to allow useful analysis. Skrabanek, however, has pointed out that, despite the large numbers in the studies, there was no overall difference in survival between the screened and control population (Skrabanek, 1988).

Nijmegen project

In the Dutch study, single view mammography was offered to 30 000 women aged over 35 years living in Nijmegen (Verbeek *et al.*, 1984); screening was repeated on four occasions every 2 years. Initial compliance was 85%.

Utrecht project

In the Belgian study, physical examination and mammography was offered to over 20 000 women aged 50–64 years (Collette *et al.*, 1984) screening was repeated at 12, 18 and 24 months. Initial compliance was 72%.

In both the Nijmegen and Utrecht projects deaths from breast cancer in women offered screening, whether or not they accepted, were considered to be 'cases'. Controls were chosen from women living in the same city, the number of controls selected for each case being 5 and 3 respectively. The results suggested that the risk of dying from breast cancer in the screened patients was 50–70% less than controls.

UK studies

Preliminary results from the UK have now been reported (UK Trial of Early Detection of Breast Cancer Group, 1988). Annual physical examination with biennial mammography was provided to 45 841 women aged 45–64 years living in Edinburgh and Guildford. Initial acceptance for screening was 60% in Edinburgh and 72% in Guildford. No reduction in mortality was noted during the first five years, but thereafter the gap between the groups widened. There was a 20% reduction in breast cancer deaths in the population offered screening; these results, however, failed to reach significance.

Malmo study

In the Malmo Study over 42 000 women aged over 45 years were randomized into study and control groups (Andersson *et al.*, 1988). The women in the study group were offered mammography at intervals of 18–24 months. Five rounds of screening were completed. The mean follow-up was almost 9 years. The number of deaths in each group was almost identical. The effect of screening depended on age; there were more deaths in young women in the screened group whereas there was a 20% reduction in deaths in women aged over 55 years.

Based on the information available from the initial overseas studies, the UK working party concluded that deaths from breast cancer in women aged 50–64 years could be reduced by one-third or more by screening and that screening centres should be established throughout the UK. The recommendation of the Forrest Committee that all patients within this age group should be offered mammography every 3 years, is now being implemented (Anon., 1987).

These assumptions, however, have not gone unchallenged. As Skrabanek pointed out, although the breast cancer mortality at 7 years was reduced by 31% in the Swedish study, this represented only 7 deaths per 100 000 women per year prevented by screening. In the UK, where compliance rates have been lower, even these levels are unlikely to be achieved. Furthermore, the above proposals assume that the positive predictive value of mammography will be in the region of 35% i.e. a ratio of two benign to each malignant lesion on biopsy (Reidy and Hoskins, 1988); many centres have failed to achieve this level. Therefore, for every patient with breast cancer, several will be exposed to unnecessary anxiety and investigation. There will be a significant knock-on effect for surgical and pathological services.

It therefore remains to be seen whether breast cancer screening will ever prove cost effective. It has been estimated that the cost of saving one life by mammographic screening is approximately £80 000 (Roberts, Farrow and Charney, 1985); it may well be higher.

Histological classification

The most commonly used classification is that of the World Health Organisation (Table 6.4). Malignant epithelial tumours include non-invasive tumours, invasive tumours of various subtypes, and Paget's disease of the nipple. The great majority of carcinomas are either invasive ductal or invasive lobular, the two groups with the worst prognosis (Rilke, 1984). Medullary, papillary and colloid carcinomas are relatively uncommon, but have a better prognosis (Table 6.5).

Table 6.4 Histological classification (WHO)

1. Non-invasive
   a. Intraductal carcinoma
   b. Lobular carcinoma-in-situ

2. Invasive
   a. Invasive ductal carcinoma
   b. Invasive ductal carcinoma with a predominant intraductal component
   c. Invasive lobular carcinoma
   d. Mucinous carcinoma
   e. Medullary carcinoma
   f. Papillary carcinoma
   g. Tubular carcinoma

3. Paget's disease of the nipple

Table 6.5 Survival

Tumour type	Incidence (%)	Survival (%)
Invasive ductal	63	54
Invasive lobular	8	54
Medullary	5	63
Papillary	2	83
Colloid	2	73

Certain features of the primary tumour may be used to predict outcome. These include:

Size. In general, the smaller the primary tumour the better the prognosis; 18% of patients with tumours 1–2 cm die within 5 years compared with 43% of patients with tumours up to 6 cm in diameter (Fisher, Slack and Bross, 1969).

Tumour Grade. Tumour grade is based on a subjective assessment of the degree of tubule formation, nuclear pleomorphism, elastosis and the frequency of hyperchromatic and mitotic figures (Bloom and Field, 1971). Patients with favourable grade tumours tend to survive longer; furthermore, it has been suggested that they are more likely to respond to hormonal therapy.

Vascular and Lymphatic Invasion. The reported incidence of vascular invasion varies from 5% to 45% (Stewart and Rubens, 1984). The presence of vascular invasion is associated with poor survival; 27% of patients with vascular invasion survive 5 years. Lymphatic invasion occurs in approximately one-third of patients; these patients are generally regarded as having a poor prognosis.

Elastosis and Lymphoid Infiltration. The presence of elastosis or a lymphoid infiltrate is usually regarded as a good prognostic sign; recently, however, Fisher and his colleagues (1980) found no correlation between the presence of elastosis and prognosis.

Tumour Necrosis. In contrast the presence of tumour necrosis is associated with a poor survival (Fisher et al., 1978a).

Axillary Lymph Node Histology. Nodal factors include the presence or absence of nodal metastases, the number of nodes involved and the presence or absence of sinus histiocytosis or reactive follicular hyperplasia. Fisher and his colleagues (1978b) have shown that the absolute number of lymph nodes containing metastases is a better predictor of survival than the proportion involved. Patients with extra nodal extension of metastases show a higher relapse rate despite treatment. Several studies have shown that sinus histiocytosis is associated with a good prognosis.

Staging (TNM)

TNM staging is based on the characteristics of the primary tumour, the presence or absence of axillary lymph node metastases, and the presence or absence of metastatic disease. On the basis of TNM classification patients can be grouped into 4 stages (Table 6.6). There is a close association between the risk of recurrent disease and increasing stage.

Table 6.6 Stage

Stage I		
T0–1	N0 or N1A	M0
Stage II		
T0–1	N1b	M0
T2	N0–1	M0
Stage III		
T1–2	N2	M0
T3	N0–2	M0
Stage IV		
Any T	Any N	M1

Steroid receptors

Oestrogen and progesterone receptors have been studied extensively in breast cancer (Clark, Osborn and McGuire, 1984; Williams *et al.*, 1987). Several studies have suggested that oestrogen receptor-positive patients have a better prognosis than those who are oestrogen receptor-negative. Furthermore, it has been suggested that the pattern of distant metastases may be influenced by oestrogen receptor status, oestrogen receptor-positive tumours tending to recur in bone whereas oestrogen receptor-negative tumours spread to viscera (Campbell *et al.*, 1981).

Oestrogen receptor and nodal status can be combined to provide useful prognostic information. Node-negative patients with oestrogen receptor-positive tumours have a relatively good prognosis, whereas those with involved lymph nodes and an oestrogen receptor-negative tumour have a very poor prognosis. Patients who either have involved lymph nodes or an oestrogen receptor-negative tumour have an intermediate prognosis (Cooke *et al.*, 1979; Leake *et al.*, 1981b). These factors may, therefore, be used to predict outcome or select appropriate treatment. Progesterone receptor-positive patients are generally thought to have a better outlook than those who are progesterone receptor-negative although this belief has recently been challenged (Sutton *et al.*, 1987). Recent studies suggest that epidermal growth factor receptor status may provide further prognostic information, particularly in those who have oestrogen receptor-negative tumours (Sainsbury *et al.*, 1987).

Oestrogen receptor status may also be used in advanced disease to predict response to hormonal therapy. Less than 10% of oestrogen receptor-negative tumours respond compared with 56% of oestrogen receptor-positive tumours (McGuire *et al.*, 1977). If receptor is present in both cytoplasm and nucleus, 70% of patients will respond (Leake *et al.*, 1981a).

Diagnosis

Traditionally patients with a suspicious breast lump have been subjected to open biopsy and frozen section, mastectomy being performed if the presence of cancer was confirmed. This approach, however, precludes the possibility of informed discussion with the patient. Uncertainty about the diagnosis adds to the patient's fear and anxiety, not only in patients who subsequently are found to have breast cancers, but also in those who have benign breast disease.

Fine-needle aspiration cytology or tru-cut biopsy is now widely used. The accuracy of fine-needle aspiration is dependent upon the skill of the surgeon and the experience of the cytologist. Unsatisfactory smears are common, up to 25% in some series. For this reason it is advantageous to have the cytologist working in the clinic; if the smears are unsatisfactory further samples can then readily be obtained. Dixon and his colleagues (1984) showed that the sensitivity of fine-needle aspiration was only 66% when aspiration was performed by several doctors, rising to 99% when the aspirates were obtained by a single surgeon. Occasional false-positive diagnoses have been reported, usually in patients with fibroadenomas, and some surgeons would therefore not be prepared to undertake mastectomy in young women on the basis of fine-needle aspiration cytology alone.

Preoperative confirmation of the diagnosis allows the nature of the disease, surgery and possible postoperative treatment to be discussed with the patient.

Although it does not obviate the fear associated with the diagnosis of cancer, it does remove the anxiety that exists when the diagnosis is uncertain.

Mammography

The mammographic appearances of breast cancer are those of a dense spiculated mass with or without microcalcification, microcalcification alone or distortion of the breast architecture. With good quality mammograms and an experienced radiologist, the diagnostic accuracy in patients with cancer is approximately 90% (Cahill et al., 1981). Mammography is less accurate in premenopausal patients because of the density of breast tissue.

Paradoxically, in patients with a discrete breast lump, mammography is of limited value because biopsy will be indicated irrespective of the mammographic findings. Mammography may be more useful in patients without an obvious lesion, for example those with a nipple discharge or retraction. Mammography may also be a useful technique to maintain surveillance of the opposite breast following mastectomy or the residual breast following breast conservation surgery. Mammography is of course widely used in screening programmes.

Preoperative assessment

Early enthusiasm for extensive screening procedures prior to surgery has now waned since the yield from those investigations is extremely low. Chest X-ray should be performed prior to surgery; the value of most other investigations is limited by the high false-positive rate (Coombes et al., 1980). Less than 3% of patients with clinical Stage I and II disease have true positive isotope bone scans (McNeil, 1984); less than 2% have liver metastases. The recent development of an antibody for epithelial membrane antigen may ultimately facilitate the detection of occult marrow deposits (Mansi et al., 1987).

Primary treatment of operable breast cancer

The primary treatment of operable breast cancer remains controversial. The extent of primary surgery, the need for postoperative radiotherapy and the role of adjuvant systemic therapy require continuing evaluation.

Extent of surgery

Radical mastectomy

Radical mastectomy was based on the hypothesis that breast cancer spread in a predictable fashion, consisting of 3 phases: (1) an initial phase during which a tumour was localized to the breast; (2) a second phase during which malignant cells spread to the regional lymph nodes, and (3) finally a phase in which the tumour became widely disseminated. It would therefore seem reasonable that radical surgery would 'cure' patients with disease limited to the breast or axilla. However, although radical mastectomy provided good local control of the disease, survival rates were disappointing; less than half the patients survived 5 years.

The failure to achieve cure in patients with apparently localized disease led some surgeons to believe that the Halsted mastectomy was insufficiently radical. They claimed that dissection of the supraclavicular and internal mammary lymph nodes (super-radical mastectomy) or the use of radical postoperative radiotherapy produced superior results. These claims, however, have since been shown to be invalid (Table 6.7).

Table 6.7 Role of surgery: randomized trials comparing extended radical and radical mastectomy with simple mastectomy and radiotherapy (RT)

Centre (authors)	No. in study	Randomization	Survival (%)	Follow-up (1 yr)
Five centre (Lacour et al., 1983)	1453	Radical v. extended radical	53 56	10
Manchester (Turner et al., 1981)	534	Radical v. modified radical	70 70	5
Copenhagen (Kaae and Johansen, 1977)	559	Extended radical v. simple + RT.	37 36	15
Cambridge (Brinkley and Haybittle, 1971)	204	Radical + RT v. modified simple + RT	49 46	10
NSABP (B-04) (Fisher et al., 1985b)	727 (node negative)	Radical v. simple + RT	58 59	10
	586 (node positive)	Radical v. simple + RT	38 39	10

In a multicentre study, 1453 patients with operable breast cancer were randomized to radical or extended radical mastectomy (Lacour et al., 1983). At 10 years there was no significant difference in overall survival. Internal mammary node metastases were present in 20% of patients treated by extended surgery; however, only 4% of the radical mastectomy group developed clinically detectable parasternal metastases (Veronesi and Valagussa, 1981). Presumably, patients in the radical mastectomy group with occult internal mammary node metastases died of disseminated disease before these occult metastases became clinically apparent. Similarly no difference in survival was found when radical and modified radical (Patey) mastectomy were compared (Turner et al., 1981).

Simple mastectomy
In 1948 McWhirter suggested that treatment of the primary tumour should be limited to simple mastectomy and that the axillary, supraclavicular and internal mammary nodes should be treated by radiotherapy. The results he obtained were comparable to those achieved in other centres using radical mastectomy; of over 1500 patients treated, 62% survived 5 years and 46% 10 years (McWhirter, 1964).

The results of controlled trials comparing simple mastectomy and postoperative radiotherapy with radical mastectomy in its classical, modified or extended form, have subsequently confirmed that there is little difference in disease-free or overall survival (Table 6.7). For example, in the NSABP (B-04) study, over 1300 women with Stage I or II breast cancer were allocated to receive either radical mastectomy alone or simple mastectomy and radiotherapy. There were no differences in recurrence-free or overall survival at 5 years between the treatment groups for either Stage I or Stage II disease (Fisher et al., 1985b).

Postoperative radiotherapy

Several studies have examined the effects of postoperative radiotherapy on local disease and survival. These studies were designed to compare the results of irradiation given immediately postoperatively with those obtained when irradiation was withheld until loco-regional recurrence occurred. In general, although local recurrence rates were higher in the surgery only group, loco-regional recurrence was well controlled by delayed radiotherapy. There were no differences in survival between the radiotherapy and surgery only groups (Table 6.8).

Table 6.8 Role of radiotherapy: randomized trials of radical or simple mastectomy with or without radiotherapy (RT)

Centre (authors)	No. in study	Randomization	Survival (%)	Follow-up (yr)
Manchester (Easson, 1968)	1461	Radical mastectomy v. radical mastectomy + RT	46 44	10
NSABP (B-02) (Fisher et al., 1970)	1103	Radical mastectomy v. radical mastectomy + RT	62 56	5
Oslo (Host and Brennhord, 1977)	1090	Radical mastectomy + Ooph. v. radical mastectomy + Ooph. + RT	70 72	5
Stockholm (Wallgren et al., 1980)	644	Modified radical mastectomy v. modified radical mastectomy + RT	73 77	5
Cancer Research Campaign (CRC Working Party, 1980)	2243	Simple mastectomy v. simple mastectomy + RT	70 73	5
NSABP (B-04) (Fisher et al., 1985b)	717	Simple mastectomy v. simple mastectomy + RT	54 59	10
Manchester (Lythgoe and Palmer, 1982)	714	Simple mastectomy v. simple mastectomy + RT	55 62	10

For example, in the Manchester study, following radical mastectomy over 1400 patients were randomized to receive postoperative radiotherapy or to be watched; in the latter group radiotherapy was delayed until local recurrence developed (Easson, 1968). The incidence of local recurrence was higher in those who did not receive radiotherapy; at 10 years, 32% of the 'watched' patients had developed local recurrence compared to 19% in the treated group. However, loco-regional recurrence was well controlled by delayed radiotherapy. Approximately 30% of patients in each group survived 15 years; there were no differences in overall survival between the treated and watched groups.

Similarly, although immediate postoperative radiotherapy reduced the incidence of loco-regional recurrence following simple mastectomy, it did not affect ultimate outcome (Table 6.8). For example, in the Cancer Research Campaign Study, over 2200 patients with Stage I and Stage II disease were randomized to simple mastectomy or simple mastectomy with immediate postoperative radiotherapy. At 5 years the loco-regional recurrence rate was three times higher in the control group. At a median follow up of 8 years, there was no difference in overall survival between the groups (Cancer Research Campaign Working Party, 1980).

Breast conservation

It is clear from the above studies that although radical surgery and radiotherapy may reduce the incidence of loco-regional recurrence, they do not affect ultimate outcome. The concept that breast cancer spreads in a step-wise fashion and can therefore be 'cured' by radical treatment is no longer tenable. The logic of undertaking mastectomy, with the resultant cosmetic disfiguration and psychological sequelae in patients who are ultimately destined to die from disseminated disease, has therefore been questioned.

The concept that breast cancer could be treated by more conservative techniques is not new. In non-randomized studies, the survival rates in selected patients undergoing breast conservation were comparable to those of historical or matched controls undergoing mastectomy (Peters, 1977; Calle, 1985). The first randomized study was undertaken at Guy's Hospital (Atkins et al., 1972). Three hundred and seventy postmenopausal patients were randomized to radical mastectomy or extended local excision; both groups received postoperative radiotherapy. Although there was a higher incidence of loco-regional recurrence in Stage I patients treated by local excision, the survival rates were comparable (Hayward, 1977). In patients with clinically involved nodes there was also a higher incidence of distant relapse and consequently a somewhat lower survival rate. This study has since been criticized because of the low dose of radiotherapy used.

More recent results, however, have shown no difference in outcome.

Milan study

In the Milan study 691 women with tumours less than 2 cm in diameter without palpable axillary nodes were randomized to quadrantectomy, axillary dissection and radiotherapy or radical mastectomy (Veronesi et al., 1981). In the initial phase of the study all patients with positive axillary lymph nodes received postoperative radiotherapy; in the later stages these patients received adjuvant chemotherapy (CMF). There were no significant differences in disease-free or overall survival (Table 6.9).

Table 6.9 Survival following breast conservation

Centre (authors)	No. in study	Randomization	Survival (%)	Follow-up (Yr)
Milan (Veronesi et al., 1981)	701	Radical mastectomy v. quadrantectomy + RT	90 90	5
NSABP (B-06) (Fisher et al., 1985a)	758 (node negative)	Simple mastectomy v. segmental resection + RT	82 92	5
	453 (node positive)	Simple mastectomy v. segmental resection + RT	66 75	5

NSABP (B-06) study

In the NSABP study, 1843 patients with tumours up to 4 cm in diameter were randomized to total mastectomy, segmental resection or segmental resection with postoperative radiotherapy (Fisher et al., 1985a; 1989). The incidence of local recurrence in the residual breast following segmental mastectomy was significantly higher in those not receiving postoperative radiotherapy (39% v. 10%). There was, however, no significant difference in overall survival among the three treatment groups (Table 6.9). Similar results have been obtained in the Scottish study (Stewart, Prescott and Forrest, 1989).

It is clear that there is a significant trend towards breast conservation in the UK. Whereas in 1983 only 18% of surgeons offered conservative surgery, by 1986 almost 65% undertook breast conservation techniques (Morris, Royle and Taylor, 1989). It is important to recognize, however, that this approach should be restricted to those patients in whom it has been shown to be valid (e.g. patients with tumours less than 4 cm) otherwise it is likely that there will be unacceptably high local recurrence rates. It is of note that in the NSABP study, tumour was found in 10% of the segmental specimens necessitating total mastectomy in these patients. The local recurrence rate was lower in the Milan study presumably because the primary surgery was more extensive. In view of the high local recurrence rate following local excision alone (28% in the NSABP study) it may be that patients with histologically involved nodes should receive postoperative radiotherapy to provide adequate local control.

Adjuvant systemic therapy

The failure of radical local therapy to improve survival suggests that the hypothesis upon which radical surgery and radiotherapy was based was incorrect. Gradually it was recognized that the vast majority of women with clinically operable breast cancer already have microscopic distant metastases which are undetectable at the time of presentation using current techniques. More recently, therefore, attention has focused on the possibility of using adjuvant systemic therapy to inhibit the growth of these micrometastases.

Adjuvant hormonal therapy

Ovarian ablation
Approximately 30% of patients with advanced breast cancer respond to either additive or ablative endocrine therapy. It would therefore seem logical to expect that ovarian ablation, used as an adjunct to surgery, would improve survival. Several studies however have failed to substantiate this hypothesis (Ravdin et al., 1970; Cole 1975; Nissen-Meyer, 1975). All these studies were undertaken before methods of measuring oestrogen receptor status were available. It has, therefore, been argued that a potential benefit in oestrogen receptor-positive patients may not have been detected because of the small groups in the individual studies.

The results of the Toronto study, however, are interesting. In this study, 109 women aged 35–70 years were randomized to no further treatment or ovarian irradiation; a subgroup of premenopausal women over 45 years received prednisolone 7.5 mg/24h for five years. Although there was no significant survival benefit in the group receiving ovarian irradiation as a whole, there was a significant difference in disease-free survival and survival in the subgroup of premenopausal patients over 45 years receiving ovarian irradiation and prednisolone (Meakin *et al.*, 1977). This apparent benefit is currently being investigated by the Scottish Breast Cancer Trials Organisation.

Adjuvant tamoxifen

Despite the disappointing results from studies of prophylactic ovarian ablation, interest in adjuvant hormonal therapy was rekindled by the introduction of tamoxifen. The lack of toxicity associated with the use of tamoxifen suggested that it would be an ideal agent for prophylaxis. Results from a number of major randomized trials using tamoxifen as adjuvant therapy are now available.

NATO study

In the Nolvadex Adjuvant Trial Organisation (NATO) study 1285 patients were randomized to receive either tamoxifen 10 mg b.d. for two years or no further treatment (Baum *et al.*, 1985). At a median follow-up of 45 months, 152 patients had developed recurrence in the tamoxifen group compared with 220 in the control group ($P<0.0001$). There were also significantly fewer deaths in the tamoxifen-treated group compared with controls (113 v. 158 respectively; $P<0.002$). Subgroup analysis, according to menopausal and axillary node status showed no evidence of a differential effect in any of the subgroups.

In contrast, although there were significantly fewer recurrences in the treated group in both the Swedish and Danish studies, there were no differences in overall survival (Rose *et al.*, 1985a; Wallgren *et al.*, 1986).

Scottish study

In the Scottish trial, 1312 women were randomized to receive either adjuvant tamoxifen 20 mg daily for 5 years or tamoxifen for first relapse; 157 patients in the adjuvant tamoxifen group developed recurrence compared with 250 of those allocated to receive tamoxifen on relapse. The beneficial effect of adjuvant tamoxifen occurred irrespective of nodal status; 117 (18%) of the patients receiving adjuvant tamoxifen died; despite the fact that the majority of patients (93%) in the observation group received tamoxifen for first relapse, 151 (23%) died (Scottish Cancer Trials Office, 1987). This study is of particular interest as it is the only study comparing adjuvant systemic therapy with the same systemic therapy on relapse.

The relationship between oestrogen receptor status and response remains controversial. In the NATO study, 46% of tumours were assayed; the beneficial effect of tamoxifen was present in both receptor-positive and receptor-negative patients. In the Danish study receptor assays were available in 18% of patients. When the results for receptor-positive patients were analysed according to receptor level, apparently conflicting evidence was obtained (Rose *et al.*, 1985b). Patients with oestrogen receptor values greater than 99 fmol/mg received significantly greater benefit from tamoxifen; patients with oestrogen receptor values between 10 and 99 fmol/mg appeared to fare worse with tamoxifen. In the Scottish study, the findings were similar to those of the Danish study, in that patients with high levels of receptor benefited most from adjuvant tamoxifen. In contrast to the Danish study, however, patients with intermediate levels also benefited (Stewart and Prescott, 1985). The relationship between oestrogen receptor status and likelihood of response therefore remains uncertain.

Adjuvant chemotherapy

The use of adjuvant chemotherapy is based on animal studies which have shown that chemotherapy is most effective when the tumour is small. It is thought that cytotoxic drugs eradicate a fixed proportion of cells at each cycle of chemotherapy

(Skipper, 1971; 1978). Other factors including the rate of growth, number of resting cells and drug delivery may be important. Animal tumours have been shown to exhibit Gompertzian growth characteristics, i.e. tumours grow more rapidly during the initial phases of growth, the rate of growth slowing as the tumour increases in size. It therefore follows that chemotherapy should be more effective against micrometastases than large bulky tumours.

Single agent

Several studies using single agents as adjuvant therapy were initiated in the 1960s, none of which showed significant benefit. Three studies, however, are of interest.

Oslo study   From 11 centres in Scandinavia 1188 patients were randomized to a 6-day postoperative course of cyclophosphamide (total dose 30 mg/kg) or no adjuvant therapy (Nissen-Meyer *et al.*, 1978; 1987). In 10 of the 11 centres cyclophosphamide was started on the day of surgery, but in 1 centre chemotherapy was not instituted for 3 weeks.

In the 10 centres giving chemotherapy immediately after surgery, 175 (34.5%) patients developed recurrence compared with 234 (45.1%) in the control group ($P<0.001$). There were 146 (28.8%) deaths in the treated group compared with 196 (37.8%) in the control group ($P<0.01$). The survival advantage started about 4 years and reached 10% after 10 years. Analysis of the data according to menopausal status and the presence or absence of axillary node metastases showed that the treatment advantage was maintained in each of these subgroups.

In contrast, in the single centre giving delayed chemotherapy there was no difference in recurrence rates or overall survival between the treated group and controls. This study was based on the premise that perioperative chemotherapy would eradicate the circulating tumour cells released at the time of surgery. This approach is at odds with the current concept that occult disseminated disease is already present at the time of presentation. Nevertheless, the advantage for treated patients has persisted (Houghton, Baum and Nissen-Meyer, 1988) and these results have rekindled interest in the use of perioperative systemic therapy.

NSABP (B-05) study   In this study 348 patients were randomized to receive either placebo or L-phenylalanine mustard (L-PAM) daily for 5 days every 6 weeks for 2 years. The initial analysis at 27 months reported that L-PAM had reduced the recurrence rate from 22% to 9%. As the data matured, however, this difference became less. The benefit was confined to premenopausal women, especially those less than 40 years of age with less than 3 nodes involved (Fisher *et al.*, 1977).

Guy's/Manchester study   In this study 370 patients were randomized to further treatment or L-PAM for two years. Although there was a trend towards an improvement in disease-free survival in treated patients, this failed to reach significance (Rubens *et al.*, 1983). There was no difference in survival between the groups. This study, therefore, failed to confirm the NSABP findings.

Combination chemotherapy

The first and most important study to use combination chemotherapy was initiated in Milan in 1973.

Milan study   In this study 386 patients were randomized to receive no further treatment or twelve cycles of CMF (cyclophosphamide 100 mg/m^2 orally days 1–14;

Table 6.10 Milan trial: 10-year results

		Control (%)	CMF (%)	P
Relapse-free survival	All patients	31.4	43.4	<0.001
	Premenopausal	31.4	48.3	<0.0005
	Postmenopausal	32.2	38.2	NS
Overall survival	All patients	47.3	55.1	NS
	Premenopausal	44.8	59.0	<0.02
	Postmenopausal	50.1	52.1	NS

methotrexate $40\,mg/m^2$ i.v. and 5-FU $600\,mg/m^2$ i.v. on days 1 and 8). At 10 years, 68.6% of the control group had relapsed compared with 56.6% of the CMF treated group (Table 6.10; $P<0.001$). Overall survival was also improved in the treated group; the advantage was confined to premenopausal patients (Bonadonna, Rossi and Valagussa, 1985). It has been suggested that the failure of postmenopausal patients to show benefit was due to the high proportion who received less than optimal doses of CMF (Bonadonna and Valagussa, 1981). Subsequent studies comparing 6 with 12 cycles of CMF showed no difference in disease-free and overall survival (Bonadonna *et al.*, 1983).

Manchester/Guy's study   In this study 327 patients were randomized to receive either no further treatment or adjuvant CMF. The CMF regimen used was similar to that reported by Bonadonna, except that the dose was reduced by 20%. At 3 years, relapse-free survival was significantly higher in patients receiving CMF; the benefit was confined to premenopausal women. There was no significant difference in overall survival (Howell *et al.*, 1984).

Whereas in the Milan study there was no difference in relapse-free or overall survival in premenopausal patients who did or did not develop amenorrhoea, in the Manchester/Guy's study premenopausal patients who developed amenorrhoea had a significantly greater relapse-free survival. Overall survival was also improved, although this did not reach significance.

West Midlands study   In this study 1083 women were randomized to chemotherapy or no further treatment. Node-positive patients received a 5-drug i.v. regimen every 3 weeks for 8 cycles. In these patients, adjuvant chemotherapy significantly prolonged relapse-free survival; there was no difference in overall survival between the groups. Node-negative patients received a 3-day oral regimen every 3 weeks for 8 cycles. In these patients, there was no difference in relapse-free or overall survival between the groups (Morrison *et al.*, 1987).

Glasgow study   In this study 214 women were allocated to receive adjuvant chemotherapy (CMF) or no further treatment; all received postoperative radiotherapy. There was an increase in disease-free interval in patients receiving chemotherapy irrespective of the number of nodes involved. There was a trend towards an improvement in disease-related survival in premenopausal patients with more than 3 nodes involved (McArdle *et al.*, 1986).

The results of these studies suggest:

1. The use of adjuvant chemotherapy (CMF) in premenopausal women with axillary node metastases significantly increases relapse-free survival. Overall survival may also be improved. The suggestion that the beneficial effects of adjuvant chemotherapy in premenopausal patients is due to ovarian suppression remains contentious (Padmanabhan, Howell and Rubens, 1986).
2. Overall survival in postmenopausal women is not influenced by the use of adjuvant chemotherapy. Failure to demonstrate benefit may be due to the use of suboptimal doses of chemotherapy.
3. Six-months' chemotherapy appears to be as effective as 12-months' therapy. It has, therefore, been suggested that courses of adjuvant chemotherapy should be limited to 6 months.

Meta-analysis

The role of adjuvant tamoxifen and chemotherapy has been clarified by a recent overview (Early Breast Cancer Trialists' Collaborative Group, 1988). Analysis of over 16 000 women randomized to receive tamoxifen or no further treatment showed that there was a 20% reduction in the odds of death in postmenopausal patients (Table 6.11), roughly equivalent to a 6% improvement in survival at 5 years. More prolonged use appeared to be more effective. No benefit was observed in premenopausal women.

Table 6.11 Survival following adjuvant tamoxifen or no systemic treatment

	Women aged < 50 (deaths/patients)			Women aged ⩾ 50 (deaths/patients)		
	Tamoxifen	Control	Improvement (%)	Tamoxifen	Control	Improvement (%)
Tamoxifen for ⩾ 2 years	282/1340	279/1326	1% ± 9	794/4408	968/4433	23% ± 4
Tamoxifen for ⩽ 1 year	116/497	108/489	−7% ± 15	570/1988	665/2032	15% ± 6
Total	398/1837	387/1815	−1 ± 8	1364/6396	1633/6465	20% ± 3

Analysis of over 9000 women randomized to receive chemotherapy or no further treatment showed that there was a 22% reduction in the odds of death in premenopausal patients (Table 6.12); no benefit was observed in postmenopausal women. If the analysis was confined to those women receiving combination chemotherapy, the beneficial effects were even greater; in premenopausal women the reduction in the odds of death was 26%, roughly equivalent to a 7% improvement in survival at 5 years.

This analysis shows that adjuvant tamoxifen in older women and chemotherapy in younger women can reduce short-term mortality. Tamoxifen is non-toxic and should therefore be given to all postmenopausal women with involved nodes regardless of oestrogen receptor status. Although patients with uninvolved nodes have an inherently better prognosis, the proportional reduction in mortality attributable to tamoxifen was similar in node-positive and node-negative patients.

Table 6.12 Survival following adjuvant chemotherapy or no systemic treatment

	Women aged < 50 (deaths/patients)			Women aged ≥ 50 (deaths/patients)		
	Treatment	Control	Improvement (%)	Treatment	Control	Improvement (%)
CMF	157/635	189/554	37% ± 9	277/1086	297/1105	9% ± 9
Polychemotherapy	352/1324	391/1202	26% ± 7	624/2315	663/2321	8% ± 6
Single agent	205/551	205/497	11% ± 10	296/627	265/282	4% ± 10
Total	557/1875	524/1497	22% ± 6	920/2942	871/2755	4% ± 5

Postmenopausal women with uninvolved nodes should probably also receive tamoxifen.

In contrast, chemotherapy should be considered for premenopausal women with involved lymph nodes regardless of oestrogen receptor status. Some node-negative women, for example those with oestrogen receptor-negative tumours, clearly have a poor prognosis and should also receive adjuvant chemotherapy.

Management of recurrent disease

Recurrence is greeted with dismay by the patient, and concern by the clinician. The likelihood of developing loco-regional recurrence depends on the type of surgery, the extent of axillary dissection and whether the patient received postoperative radiotherapy. Loco-regional recurrence may present as a small nodule or nodules in the skin flaps following mastectomy, axillary or supraclavicular node metastases or recurrence in the residual breast of patients treated by conservation. Further investigation at that time may reveal the presence of occult disseminated disease.

The initial aim of therapy should be to confirm the diagnosis by fine-needle aspiration, tru-cut or excision biopsy and to re-define the extent of disease. The incidence of occult disseminated disease in patients with a solitary nodule in a skin flap following mastectomy is relatively low; in contrast, in patients with supraclavicular node investment, further investigations may reveal the presence of asymptomatic metastases.

The management of local recurrence depends on the presence or absence of disseminated disease, extent of primary surgery and whether the patient received postoperative radiotherapy. In general, patients with loco-regional recurrence should, if they have not been previously irradiated and in the absence of disseminated disease, receive radiotherapy. Patients with recurrence in the residual breast following conservation surgery require mastectomy. Patients with loco-regional recurrence and disseminated disease should receive appropriate systemic therapy; they may also require radiotherapy to control the loco-regional disease.

Once a patient has developed metastatic disease her life expectancy is clearly limited, and any treatment must be regarded as palliative. Ideally, the aim of therapy should be to achieve the maximal and most enduring tumour response with minimal side-effects. In reality, however, in deciding appropriate treatment the clinician may have to balance the possibility of a response in a minority of patients against the likely side-effects which would be experienced by the majority.

Endocrine therapy

Endocrine therapy can be ablative or additive. Ablative techniques (oophorectomy, adrenalectomy and hypophysectomy) remove sources of endogenous oestrogen or oestrogen precursors thus depriving hormone-dependent tumours of the stimulus to continued growth. Additive therapy involves the systemic administration of naturally occurring or synthetic hormones, e.g. oestrogens, androgens, progestogens or corticosteroids. The precise mode of action of these substances is imperfectly understood, but it appears that they are capable of inducing regression of hormone-dependent tumours by altering the hormonal environment in which they are growing.

Until recently ovarian ablation has been the standard endocrine therapy for premenopausal women with advanced cancer. Patients most likely to respond include those with a long disease-free interval and metastases to bone; the mean duration of response is between 12 and 18 months.

Adrenalectomy and hypophysectomy are now seldom performed. The patients most likely to respond included those with a long disease-free interval, bone metastases and a prior response to endocrine therapy; the mean duration of remission is about 12–18 months. Adrenalectomy has been superseded by drugs such as aminoglutethimide; hypophysectomy has largely been abandoned because of the unacceptably high morbidity.

Oestrogens were once commonly used in postmenopausal women. Responses were commoner in soft tissue than elsewhere. Side-effects included anorexia, nausea and vomiting and fluid retention. Tumour flare was seen in about 10% of patients; hypercalcaemia could be induced by oestrogen administration. In approximately one-third of patients tumour regression occurred on stopping oestrogens.

Androgens and cortisone are now seldom used. Better responses to adrogens were obtained from patients with bony metastases. Virilization, however, was inevitable with prolonged use. Cortisone therapy did demonstrate subjective improvement in some patients with bone, brain or liver involvement; the duration of remission seldom exceeded 6 months. The use of these additive hormonal agents has now been largely superseded by the development of tamoxifen, aminoglutethimide and progestational agents.

Tamoxifen

Under physiological conditions oestrogens may enter all cells. However, only cells in hormone-sensitive organs (e.g. breast, uterus) possess soluble proteins in their cytoplasm (oestrogen receptors) which specifically bind these oestrogens. In tumours which are partially or wholly dependent on endogenous oestrogen for continuing growth, oestrogen binds to oestrogen receptors in the cytoplasm and the resulting oestrogen-receptor complex is translocated into the cell nucleus. Here it binds to specific acceptor sites in the chromatin initiating further cell replication.

Tamoxifen is a specific non-steroidal oestrogen antagonist. It has been shown to compete with oestrogen for the cytoplasmic oestrogen receptor. The resulting tamoxifen-oestrogen receptor complex is translocated into the nucleus, binds to the nuclear sites on the chromatin and inhibits further cell replication. Tamoxifen may also have a direct effect on breast cancer cells which does not involve the oestrogen receptor mechanism.

Tamoxifen has now been accepted as standard therapy for advanced disease in postmenopausal patients. Approximately 34% of patients achieve either a complete or partial response and a further 19% disease stabilization (Rose and Mouridsen, 1984). The mean duration of remission is 12–18 months, although many long-term survivors have been reported. The optimal dose would appear to be 20 mg daily; higher doses fail to produce further benefit. Women with predominantly soft-tissue disease are more likely to respond than those with visceral metastases. Side-effects are few, less than 3% are unable to tolerate the drug.

A similar response rate has now been reported in premenopausal women, although generally to a higher dose of tamoxifen. The results of a multicentre randomized study comparing oophorectomy with tamoxifen (20 mg b.d.) in premenopausal women showed no difference in overall response rate (21% v. 24%) or overall survival (Buchanan et al., 1986).

Tamoxifen is, therefore, generally accepted as the initial hormone treatment of choice for postmenopausal and some premenopausal women, not because the response rate is higher than other agents but because the incidence of side-effects is low.

Aminoglutethimide

Aminoglutethimide was originally thought to produce a 'medical adrenalectomy' by inhibiting steroid synthesis. It is now known to reduce adrenal cortical production of cortisol and androstenedione and aromatisation of androstenedione to oestrogens in peripheral tissues. The fall in serum cortisol stimulates ACTH release; patients should, therefore, be given corticosteroids.

Approximately 30% of postmenopausal women respond; good responses are obtained in bone and soft tissue (Powles, 1984). Comparison of surgical adrenalectomy with aminoglutethimide in postmenopausal women with advanced breast cancer has shown no difference in overall response rates (Santen et al., 1981). Approximately 50% of patients develop somnolence and lethargy during the first few weeks of therapy. Orthostatic hypotension and ataxia, blurred vision and a maculopapular rash may also occur. These symptoms may be minimized by increasing the dose incrementally. The possibility that low-dose aminoglutethimide with hydrocortisone may produce less toxicity while preserving the response rate is currently being investigated (Stuart-Harris et al., 1984).

Progestational agents

In the past, synthetic progestational agents were regarded as being ineffective; response rates were poor and the duration of response was less than other forms of endocrine therapy (Powles, 1984). Recently, however, interest has been revived in the use of high-dose medroxyprogesterone acetate (MPA) and megesterol acetate.

MPA is a synthetic progestational agent with anti-oestrogen, anti-androgen and anti-gonadotrophin effects. Although less than 20% of patients with advanced disease respond to low dose MPA, 43% respond to the equivalent of 500 mg/24h i.m. Side-effects include abscesses at the injection site; the use of high oral doses of MPA may circumvent this problem.

Megesterol acetate is an orally active synthetic progestational agent with a direct cytotoxic effect on breast cancer cells. Better responses are obtained with soft-tissue lesions, but some unexpected responses in patients with lung metastases occur. Approximately one-third of patients initially treated with tamoxifen will have a further response, the mean duration of response being about 6 months (Ross, Buzdar and Blumenschein, 1982). Toxic side-effects are mild and consist mainly of weight gain (Gregory *et al.*, 1985).

Combination therapy

The hypothesis that combinations of hormone therapies might prove more effective has also been tested. For instance, in the Marsden study postmenopausal patients were randomized to tamoxifen or a combination of tamoxifen, aminoglutethimide with hydrocortisone and danazol (TAD). Although the initial response rate for the combination (43%) was significantly better than tamoxifen alone (31%) there was no difference in overall survival (Powles *et al.*, 1984).

Cyclical combinations of tamoxifen and progestational agents have also been used in an attempt to improve the response rate. Tamoxifen reduces the oestrogen receptor content of tumour cells and increases the progesterone receptor content. Progestational agents reduce the concentration of both oestrogen and progesterone receptors. In theory, therefore, one hormone might be used to prime tumour cells in order to increase sensitivity to a second hormonal agent, and thereby achieve a higher response rate. Preliminary studies suggest that the response rate may be higher and the duration of response longer in patients receiving cyclical therapy, but there is no difference in overall survival (Garcia-Geralt *et al.*, 1986; Gunderson, Kvinnstand and Klepp, 1986).

In conclusion, therefore, randomized trials comparing tamoxifen with other hormonal agents and combination therapy showed no major differences in overall survival. The choice of treatment is, therefore, largely governed by the incidence of side-effects. Tamoxifen is widely used as first-line and megesterol acetate as second-line therapy.

Cytotoxic chemotherapy

The overall response rate for most commonly used single agents in advanced breast cancer lies between 19% and 35%, the median duration of response being 6 months or less. Adriamycin is probably the single most active agent with a response rate of 35–50% in previously untreated patients. Although higher response rates to single agents can be achieved by escalating the dose, at the present time it is conventional to treat patients with metastatic breast cancer with combination chemotherapy in an attempt to increase the response rate and minimize the extent of toxicity.

Overall, approximately 50% of patients will respond to combination chemotherapy, the median duration of response being 6–8 months. No one regimen of combination chemotherapy has been shown to be clearly more effective. Although studies have shown a higher response rate for combinations containing adriamycin, overall survival was similar in most studies. Currently, interest is focused on the use of alternating non-cross-resistant combinations which it is hoped may prolong the duration of response (Goldie, Coldman and Gudauskas, 1982).

Attempts to select appropriate therapy on the basis of '*in vitro*' sensitivity tests have failed to meet early expectations. The most commonly used technique is that of the human tumour clonogenic assay of Hamburger and Salmon (Jones *et al.*, 1985). Although the clonogenic assay correctly predicted that some patients would not respond to single agents it was unable to predict clinical response to combination chemotherapy. There is, therefore, at the present time no satisfactory 'in vitro' drug sensitivity assay system.

Because of the heterogeneity of most tumours, it has been suggested that combined endocrine and cytotoxic therapy might prove more effective than either alone. In general this has not proved to be so. Although the response rate of endocrine therapy alone may be less than to the combination, a proportion of women respond to chemotherapy on failure; overall survival is therefore no different (Forbes, 1986).

In summary, therefore, patients with metastatic breast cancer with oestrogen receptor-positive tumour, or in whom oestrogen receptor status was unknown, should receive tamoxifen as initial therapy. If the patient responds to tamoxifen she should have further endocrine treatment as second-line therapy on subsequent relapse. Patients who have failed to respond to tamoxifen should be considered for combination chemotherapy. Patients with oestrogen receptor-negative tumours with rapidly growing or visceral metastases should receive chemotherapy as first-line treatment.

The aim of therapy in patients with metastatic disease is to achieve good palliation and therefore the likely benefit obtained by some patients should always be balanced against the toxicity experienced by all. In some patients specific anti-cancer therapy, particularly chemotherapy, may be inappropriate and symptomatic measures only are indicated.

Symptomatic treatment

In addition to receiving anti-cancer therapy, or where anti-cancer therapy is inappropriate, many patients with advanced breast cancer may have specific problems which require symptomatic treatment.

Bone metastases

Bone is the commonest site for distant metastases in breast cancer, 85% of patients having osseous metastases at the time of death. Usually the pain becomes progressively more severe over several weeks; sudden pain, for instance in the back, may be due to vertebral collapse. Pathological fractures may occur in up to 30% of patients. The median survival from diagnosis to death is approximately 18 months (Coleman and Rubens, 1987).

It is not uncommon for patients to present with severe bone pain without radiological evidence of metastases, since 50% of the bony matrix has to be destroyed before the lesions can be detected radiologically. Isotope bone scan is a more sensitive method of detecting bone metastases, but specificity is poor (McNeil, 1984). In doubtful cases, bone biopsy or CT scan may be helpful. The assessment of response is particularly difficult since the changes associated with healing can be confused with tumour progression.

In isolated bone metastases radiotherapy is the treatment of choice. In patients with multiple bone metastases, only one of which is symptomatic, radiotherapy may be used in combination with systemic therapy to relieve pain. Radiotherapy will produce pain relief in approximately two-thirds of patients, the median duration of response being approximately 12 months (Tong, Gillick and Hendricson, 1982; Yarnold, 1985).

Patients with multiple bone metastases require systemic therapy. Approximately one-third will respond to endocrine therapy (Smith and Macauley, 1985); approximately one-quarter will demonstrate an objective tumour response to combination chemotherapy, although symptomatic improvement may occur in up to half the patients (Coleman and Rubens, 1987).

Surgical intervention may be required to stabilize a pathological fracture of long bone, usually proximal femur, and in some cases of spinal cord compression.

Hypercalcaemia

The true incidence of hypercalcaemia in breast cancer patients has not been clearly established. In one series, hypercalcaemia occurred in approximately one-third of patients with bone scan evidence of skeletal metastases (Ralston et al., 1982). There was, however, poor correlation between the degree of hypercalcaemia and extent of bony metastases. Although it is widely accepted that the major cause of hypercalcaemia in breast cancer is an increase in bone absorption due to an increase in osteoclast activity, other mechanisms may exist (Heath, 1989). It has been suggested that some tumour cells can elaborate hormonal agents with effects similar to PTH.

Patients with symptomatic hypercalcaemia require saline to correct dehydration, restore circulating fluid volume and improve urinary output. This may be sufficient in some patients with mild hypercalcaemia, but in most, further measures will be required.

Calcitonin inhibits bone resorption and renal tubular reabsorption; it produces a rapid fall in serum calcium and has relatively few side-effects (Hosking and Gilson, 1984). Unfortunately, responses are usually limited to a few days, although the concomitant use of glucocorticosteroids may prolong their effect.

Diphosphonates lower serum calcium by a direct action on osteoclast resorption of bone by rendering the phosphate molecule resistant to hydrolysis by phosphatases. Aminohydroxypropylidene diphosphonate (APD) has recently been compared with the combination of calcitonin and prednisolone (Ralston et al., 1985). Although the combination of calcitonin and prednisolone produced a more rapid fall in serum calcium, APD provided better long-term control. The combination of APD and calcitonin may be of particular value in patients with severe hypercalcaemia in whom a rapid but sustained reduction in serum calcium is desirable (Ralston et al., 1986). Oral dichloromethylene diphosphonate (clodronate) is poorly absorbed, but may be effective in controlling bone absorption (Stewart, 1983).

Hypercalcaemia is often a sign of a rapidly growing tumour. There is no evidence that control of the hypercalcaemia per se improves survival. It is, therefore, important that attempts to control the hypercalcaemia should be combined with effective anti-tumour therapy.

Pleural effusion

Pleural effusions are common in patients with breast cancer. Pleural tap and cytology will confirm the diagnosis in approximately 70% of cases; pleural biopsy may be useful in patients where cytology is unhelpful (Hausheer and Yarbro, 1985).

Paracentesis alone or tube drainage is seldom effective. Therefore, once the pleural effusion has been drained, tetracycline or bleomycin in 5 ml saline should be instilled into the pleural space in an attempt to control the effusion. Tetracycline will obliterate the pleural cavity in approximately 70% of patients with few side-effects apart from mild fever and pain. Similar results have been achieved with the use of bleomycin, although some drug-related deaths in the elderly due to hypotension have been reported. Talc is probably the most effective sclerosing agent, but its use should be reserved for patients who fail to benefit from tetracycline or bleomycin therapy. It produces an intense reaction with obliteration of the pleural cavity in over 90% of patients, but morbidity is high.

Malignant ascites

Ascites is a relatively uncommon complication. Traditional approaches such as fluid and salt restriction, diuretics, paracentesis and the intraperitoneal instillation of cytotoxic drugs are of little benefit. Techniques such as the instillation of cytotoxic drugs in large volumes of fluid to achieve uniform distribution of drugs, such as have been used in ovarian cancer, remain unproven.

A peritoneovenous shunt (Le Veen or Denver) may be appropriate in some patients. Such shunts are not without problems; these include shunt blockage, venous thrombosis and cardiac failure. However, most patients have at least temporary relief of ascites, and approximately one-half will not require further paracentesis (Souter et al., 1985). Tumour embolization through the catheter does occur, although it is unlikely to be of clinical relevance in patients with terminal cancer.

Malignant pericardial effusion

Secondary involvement of the heart and pericardium occurs rarely. If tamponade does occur, pericardiocentesis may be appropriate; usually, however, the fluid reaccumulates rapidly. Subxiphoid pericardial decompression may be performed under local anaesthesia (Osuch, Khandekar and Fry, 1985). If recurrent effusions occur in patients who otherwise have a reasonable prognosis a window may be created between the pericardial and peritoneal cavities.

Central nervous system

Approximately 30% of patients dying from breast cancer have central nervous system metastases at autopsy (Tsukada et al., 1983). In only one-third is the presence of metastases suspected before death. Isolated cerebral metastases are extemely rare; surgery is, therefore, rarely indicated. Most centres use a combination of dexamethasone and cerebral irradiation, although the combination has not been demonstrated to be superior to dexamethasone alone (Richter and Coia, 1985).

Spinal cord compression

If spinal cord compression occurs the outlook is very poor (Harrison et al., 1985). Patients with true paraplegia rarely, if ever, show evidence of neurological improvement. Surgical decompression may be indicated in patients with a solitary lesion in the spine; in the remaining patients there is no evidence to show that surgery is preferable to irradiation or vice versa.

Psychological morbidity

Anxiety and depression following mastectomy are common; Maguire and his colleagues (1978) found that 25% of women experience anxiety and depression 1 year after mastectomy. Not only does the patient have to cope with the suspicion that she may have incurable disease but she also has to face mutilating surgery, a threat to her femininity and consequent loss of self-esteem. Marital and sexual problems occur secondarily.

The incidence of morbidity may be further increased in women receiving postoperative radiotherapy or adjuvant chemotherapy (Hughson et al., 1986; 1987). Breast conservation, perhaps surprisingly, has not been shown to consistently reduce morbidity (Fallowfield, Baum and Maguire, 1986; Holmberg et al., 1989).

References

Andersson, I., Aspergren, K., Janzon, L. et al. (1988) Mammographic screening and mortality from breast cancer: the Malmo mammographic screening trial. British Medical Journal, 297, 943–948

Anon. (1987) Breast cancer screening. Lancet, i, 543–544

Armstrong, B. R. (1988) Oestrogen therapy after the menopause – boon or bane? Medical Journal of Australia, 148, 213–214

Atkins, H., Hayward, J. C., Klugman, D. J. and Wayte, A. B. (1972) Treatment of early breast cancer: a report after 10 years of a clinical trial. British Medical Journal, 2, 423–429

Baum, M., Brinckley, D. M., Dossett, J. A. et al. (1985) Controlled trial of tamoxifen as single adjuvant agent in management of early breast cancer: analysis of six years by Nolvadex Adjuvant Trial Organisation. Lancet, i, 836–840

Bergkvist, L., Adami, H. O., Persson, I. et al. (1989) The risk of breast cancer after estrogen and estrogen-progestin replacement. New England Journal of Medicine, 321, 293–297

Bloom, H. J. G. and Field, J. R. (1971) Impact of tumour grade and host resistance on survival of women with breast cancer. Cancer, 28, 1580–1589

Bonadonna, G., Rossi, A., Tancini, G. and Valagussa, P. (1983) Adjuvant chemotherapy in breast cancer. Lancet, i, 1157

Bonadonna, G., Rossi, A. and Valagussa, P. (1985) Adjuvant CMF chemotherapy in operable breast cancer: ten years later. World Journal of Surgery, 4, 707–713

Bonadonna, G. and Valagussa, P. (1981) Dose-response effect of adjuvant chemotherapy in breast cancer. New England Journal of Medicine, 304, 10–15

Brinkley, D. and Haybittle, J. L. (1971) Treatment of stage II carcinoma of the female breast. Lancet, ii, 1086–1087

Buchanan, R. B., Blamey, R. W., Durant, K. R. et al. (1986) A randomized comparison of tamoxifen with surgical oophorectomy in premenopausal patients with advanced breast cancer. Journal of Clinical Oncology, 4, 1326–1330

Cahill, C. J., Boulter, P. S., Gibbs, N. M. and Price, J. L. (1981) Features of mammographically negative breast tumours. British Journal of Surgery, 68, 882–884

Calle, R. (1985) Experience with breast conserving approaches at the Curie Institute. In Primary Management of Breast Cancer: Alternatives to Mastectomy (ed. J. S. Tobias and M. J. Peckham), Edward Arnold, London, pp. 59–79

Campbell, F. C., Blamey, R. W., Elston, C. W. et al. (1981) Oestrogen-receptor status and sites of metastasis in breast cancer. British Journal of Cancer, 44, 456–459

Cancer Research Campaign Working Party (1980) Cancer Research Campaign (King's/Cambridge) Trial for early breast cancer. A detailed update at the tenth year. Lancet, ii, 55–60

Clark, G. M., Osborn, C. K. and McGuire, W. L. (1984) Correlations between estrogen receptor, progesterone receptor and patient characteristics in human breast cancer. *Journal of Clinical Oncology*, **2**, 1102–1109

Cole, M. P. (1975) A clinical trial of an artificial menopause in carcinoma of the breast. In *Hormones and Breast Cancer* (ed. M. Namer and C. M. Lalann), Inserm, Paris, pp. 143–150

Coleman, R. E. and Rubens, R. D. (1987) The clinical course of bone metastases from breast cancer. *British Journal of Cancer*, **55**, 61–66

Collette, H. J., Rombach, J. J., Day, N. E. and De Ward, F. (1984) Evaluation of screening for breast cancer in a non-randomized study (The DOM Project) by means of a case-control study. *Lancet*, **i**, 1224–1226

Cooke, T., George, D., Shields, R. *et al.* (1979) Oestrogen receptors in early breast cancer. *Lancet*, **i**, 995–997

Coombes, R. C., Powles, T. J., Abbott, M. *et al.* (1980) Physical tests for distant metastases in patients with breast cancer. *Journal of the Royal Society of Medicine*, **73**, 617–623

Dixon, J. M., Anderson, T. J., Lamb, J. *et al.* (1984) Fine needle aspiration cytology, in relationships to clinical examinations and mammography in the diagnosis of a solid breast mass. *British Journal of Surgery*, **71**, 593–596

Dowle, C. S., Mitchell, A., Elston, C. W. *et al.* (1987) Preliminary results of the Nottingham breast self-examination education programme. *British Journal of Surgery*, **74**, 217–219

Early Breast Cancer Trialists' Collaborative Group (1988) Effects of adjuvant tamoxifen and of cytotoxic therapy on mortality in early breast cancer. An overview of 61 randomized trials among 28 896 women. *New England Journal of Medicine*, **319**, 1681–1692

Easson, E. C. (1968) Postoperative radiotherapy in breast cancer. In *Prognostic Factors in Breast Cancer* (ed. A. P. Forrest and P. B. Kunkler), Williams and Wilkins, Baltimore, pp. 118–135

Fallowfield, L. J., Baum, M. and Maguire, G. P. (1986) Effects of breast conservation and psychological mobidity associated with diagnosis and treatment of early breast cancer. *British Medical Journal*, **293**, 1331–1334

Fisher, B., Bauer, M., Margolese, R. *et al.* (1985a) Five-year results of a randomized clinical trial comparing total mastectomy and segmental mastectomy with or without irradiation in the treatment of breast cancer. *New England Journal of Medicine*, **312**, 665–673

Fisher, B., Glass, A., Redmond, C. *et al.* (1977) L-Phenylalanine mustard (L-PAM) in the management of primary breast cancer: an update of earlier findings and a comparison with those utilizing L-PAM plus 5-fluorouracil (5-FU). *Cancer*, **39**, 2883–2903

Fisher, E. R., Palekar, A. S., Gregorio, R. M. *et al.* (1978a) Pathological findings from the National Surgical Adjuvant Breast Project (Protocol No. 4). IV. Significance of tumour necrosis. *Human Pathology*, **9**, 523–530

Fisher, E. R., Redmond, C. and Fisher, B. (1980) Pathologic findings from the National Surgical Adjuvant Breast Project (Protocol No. 4). VI. Discriminants for 5-year treatment failure. *Cancer*, **46**, 908–918

Fisher, B., Redmond, C., Fisher, E. R. *et al.* (1985b) Ten-year results of a randomized clinical trial comparing radical mastectomy and total mastectomy with or without irradiation. *New England Journal of Medicine*, **312**, 674–681

Fisher, B., Redmond, C., Poisson, R. *et al.* (1989) Eight year results of a randomized clinical trial comparing total mastectomy and lumpectomy with or without irradiation in the treatment of breast cancer. *New England Journal of Medicine*, **320**, 822–828

Fisher, B., Slack, N. H. and Bross, D. J. (1969) Cancer of the breast: size of neoplasm and prognosis. *Cancer*, **24**, 1071–1080

Fisher, B., Slack, N. H., Cavanaugh, J. (1970) Postoperative radiotherapy in the treatment of breast cancer: results of the NSABP clinical trial. *Annals of Surgery*, **172**, 711–732

Fisher, E. R., Swamidoss, S., Lee, C. H. *et al.* (1978b) Detection and significance of occult axillary node metastases in patients with invasive breast cancer. *Cancer*, **42**, 2025–2031

Forbes, J. F. (1986) A randomized trial of sequential antioestrogen-cytotoxic chemotherapy, versus sequential cytotoxic chemotherapy – anti-oestrogen therapy, versus combined modality therapy in 339 patients with advanced breast cancer. *Reviews on Endocrine-related Cancer*, **18**, 43–50

Garcia-Giralt, E., Jouve, M., Panangi, T. *et al.* (1986) Disseminated breast cancer: sequential administration of tamoxifen and medroxyprogesterone acetate. Results of a controlled trial. *Reviews on Endocrine-related Cancer*, **18**, 27–32

Goldie, J. H., Coldman, A. J. and Gudauskas, G. A. (1982) Rationale for the use of alternating non-cross resistant chemotherapy. *Cancer Treatment Reports*, **3**, 439–449

Gregory, E. J., Cohen, S. C., Oines, D. W. and Mims, C. H. (1985) Megestrol acetate therapy for advanced breast cancer. *Journal of Clinical Oncology*, **3**, 155–160

Gundersen, S., Kvinnstand, S. and Klepp, O. (1986) Clinical use of tamoxifen and high-dose medroxyprogesterone acetate in advanced breast cancer. *Reviews on Endocrine-related Cancer*, **18**, 37–42

Harrison, K. M., Muss, H. B., Ball, M. R. *et al.* (1985) Spinal compression in breast cancer. *Cancer*, **55**, 2839–2844

Hausheer, F. H. and Yarbro, J. B. (1985) Diagnosis and treatment of malignant pleural effusion. *Seminars in Oncology*, **12**, 54–75

Hayward, J. C. (1977) The Guy's trial of treatments in early breast cancer. *World Journal of Surgery*, **1**, 314–316

Heath, D. A. (1989) Hypercalcaemia in malignancy. *British Medical Journal*, **298**, 1468–1469

Henderson, B. E., Pike, M. G. and Ross, R. K. (1984) Epidemiology and risk factors. In *Breast Cancer: Diagnosis and Mangement* (ed. G. Bonadonna), Wiley, Chichester, pp. 15–33

Holmberg, L., Omne-Pontén, M., Burns, T. *et al.* (1989) Psychological adjustment after mastectomy and breast-conserving treatment. *Cancer*, **64**, 969–974

Hosking, D. J. and Gilson, D. (1984) Comparison of the renal and skeletal actions of calcitonin in the treatment of severe hypercalcaemia of malignancy. *Quarterly Journal of Medicine*, **211**, 359–368

Host, H. and Brennhord, I. O. (1977) The effect of post-operative radiotherapy in breast cancer. *International Journal of Radiation Oncology, Biology and Physics*, **2**, 1061–1067

Houghton, J., Baum, M. and Nissen-Meyer, R. (1988) Is there a role for perioperative adjuvant therapy in the treatment of early breast cancer? *European Journal of Surgical Oncology*, **14**, 227–233

Howell, A., Bush, H., George, W. D. *et al.* (1984) Controlled trial of adjuvant chemotherapy with cyclophosphamide, methotrexate and fluorouracil for breast cancer. *Lancet*, **ii**, 307–311

Hughson, A. V. M., Cooper, A. F., McArdle, C. S. and Smith , D. C. (1986) Psychological impact of adjuvant chemotherapy in the first two years after mastectomy. *British Medical Journal*, **293**, 1268–1271

Hughson, A. V. M., Cooper, A. F., McArdle, C. S. and Smith, D. C. (1987) Psychosocial effects of radiotherapy after mastectomy. *British Medical Journal*, **294**, 1515–1518

Jones, D. R., Goldblatt, P. D. and Leon, D. A. (1984) Bereavement and cancer: some data on deaths of spouses from the longitudinal study of Office of Population Censuses and Surveys. *British Medical Journal*, **289**, 461–464

Jones, S. E., Dean, J. C., Young, L. A. and Salmon, S. E. (1985) The human tumour clonogenic assay in breast cancer. *Journal of Clinical Oncology*, **3**, 92–97

Kaae, S. and Johansen, H. (1977) Does simple mastectomy followed by irradiation offer survival comparable to radical procedures? *International Journal of Radiation Oncology, Biology and Physics*, **2**, 1163–1166

Kay, C. R. and Hannaford, P. C. (1988) Breast cancer and the pill – further report from the Royal College of General Practioners' Oral Contraceptive Study. *British Journal of Cancer*, **58**, 657–680

Lacour, J., Monique, L., Caceres, E. *et al.* (1983) Radical mastectomy versus radical mastectomy plus internal mammary dissection. Ten year results of an international cooperative trial in breast cancer. *Cancer*, **51**, 1941–1943

Leake, R. E., Laing, L., Calman, K. C. *et al.* (1981a) Oestrogen-receptor status and endocrine therapy of breast cancer: response rates and status stability. *British Journal of Cancer*, **43**, 59–66

Leake, R. E., Laing, L., McArdle, C. and Smith, D. C. (1981b) Soluble and nuclear oestrogen receptor status in human breast cancer in relation to prognosis. *British Journal of Cancer*, **43**, 67–71

Lythgoe, J. P. and Palmer, M. K. (1982) Manchester regional breast study: Five and ten-year results. *British Journal of Surgery*, **69**, 693–696

McArdle, C. S., Crawford, D., Dykes, E. H. *et al.* (1986) Adjuvant radiotherapy and chemotherapy in breast cancer. *British Journal of Surgery*, **73**, 264–266

McGuire, W. L., Horwitz, K. B., Pearson, O. H. and Segaloff, A. (1977) Current status of oestrogen and progesterone receptors in breast cancer. *Cancer*, **39**, 2934–2937

MacMahon, B., Cole, P., Lin, T. M. *et al.* (1970) Age at first birth and breast cancer risk. *Bulletin of the World Health Organisation*, **43**, 209–221

McPherson, K. M., Neil, A., Vessey, M. P. and Doll, R. (1983) Oral contraceptives and breast cancer. *Lancet*, **ii**, 1414–1415

McNeil, B. J. (1984) Value of bone scanning in neoplastic disease. *Seminars in Nuclear Medicine*, **14**, 277–286

McWhirter, R. (1964) Should more radical treatment be attempted in breast cancer? *American Journal of Roentgenology, Radium Therapy and Nuclear Medicine*, **92**, 3–13

Maguire, G. P., Lee, E. G., Bevington, D. J. *et al.* (1978) Psychiatric problems in the first year after mastectomy. *British Medical Journal*, **1**, 963–965

Mansi, J. L., Berger, U., Easton, D. *et al.* (1987) Micrometastases in bone marrow in patients with primary breast cancer: evaluation as an early predictor of bone metastases. *British Medical Journal*, **295**, 1093–1096

Meakin, J. W., Allt, W. E. C., Beale, F. A. *et al.* (1977) Ovarian irradiation and prednisolone following surgery for carcinomas of the breast. In *Adjuvant Therapy of Cancer* (ed. S. E. Salmon and S. E. Jones), Biomedical Press, Amsterdam, pp. 95–99

Meirik, O., Lund, E., Adami, H. O. *et al.* (1986) Oral contraceptive use and breast cancer in young women. A Joint National Case-control Study in Sweden and Norway. *Lancet*, **ii**, 650–653

Morris, J., Royle, G. T. and Taylor, I. (1989) Changes in the surgical management of early breast cancer in England. *Journal of the Royal Society of Medicine*, **82**, 12–14

Morrison, J. M., Howell, A., Grieve, R. J. *et al.* (1987) The West Midlands Oncology Association Trials of adjuvant chemotherapy for operable breast cancer. In *Adjuvant Therapy of Cancer V* (ed S. E. Salmon), Grune and Stratton, New York, pp. 311–318

Nissen-Meyer, R. (1975) Ovarian irradiation and its supplement by additive hormonal treatment. In *Hormones and Breast Cancer* (ed. M. Namer and C. M. Lalanne), Inserm, Paris, pp. 151–158

Nissen-Meyer, R., Host, M., Kjellgren, K. *et al.* (1987) Neoadjuvant chemotherapy in breast cancer: As single perioperative treatment and with supplementary long-term chemotherapy. In *Adjuvant Therapy of Cancer V* (ed. S. E. Salmon), Grune and Stratton, New York, pp. 253–261

Nissen-Meyer, R., Kjellgren, K., Malmio, K. *et al.* (1978) Surgical adjuvant therapy: results with one short course with cyclophosphamide after mastectomy for breast cancer. *Cancer*, **41**, 2088–2098

Osuch, J. R., Khandekar, J. D. and Fry, W. A. (1985) Emergency subxiphoid pericardial decompression for malignancy pleural effusion. *American Surgeon*, **51**, 298–300

Padmanabhan, N., Howell, A. and Rubens, R. D. (1986) Mechanism of action of adjuvant chemotherapy in early breast cancer. *Lancet*, **i**, 411–414

Paul, C., Skegg, D. C. G., Spears, G. F. S. and Kaldor, A. M. (1986) Oral contraceptives and breast cancer: a national study. *British Medical Journal*, **293**, 723–726

Peters, V. (1977) Wedge resection with or without radiation in early breast cancer. *International Journal of Radiation Oncology, Biology and Physics*, **2**, 1151–1156

Pike, M. C., Henderson, B. E., Krailo, M. D. *et al.* (1983) Breast cancer in young women and use of oral contraceptives: possible modifying effect of formulation and age at use. *Lancet*, **ii**, 926–929

Powles, T. J. (1984) Present role of hormonal therapy. In *Breast Cancer, Diagnosis and Management* (ed. G. Bonadonna), Wiley, Chichester, pp. 229–246

Powles, T. J., Ashley, S., Ford, H. T. *et al.* (1984) Treatment of disseminated breast cancer with tamoxifen, aminoglutethimide, hydrocortisone and danazol used in combination or sequentially. *Lancet*, **i**, 1369–1372

Ralston, S. H., Alzaid, A. A., Gardner, M. D. and Boyle, I. T. (1986) Treatment of cancer associated hypercalcaemia with combined aminohydroxypropylidene diphosphonate and calcitonin. *British Medical Journal*, **292**, 1549–1550

Ralston, S., Fogelman, J., Gardner, M. D. and Boyle, I. T. (1982) Hypercalcaemia of malignancy and metastatic bone disease: is there a causal link? *Lancet*, **ii**, 903–905

Ralston, S. J., Gardner, M. D., Dryburgh, F. J. *et al.* (1985) Comparison of aminohydroxypropylidene diphosphonate, mithramycin, and corticosteroids/calcitonin in treatment of cancer-associated hypercalcaemia. *Lancet*, **ii**, 907–910

Ravdin, R. G., Lewison, E. F., Slack, N. H. *et al.* (1970) Results of a clinical trial concerning the worth of prophylactic oophorectomy for breast carcinoma. *Surgery, Gynecology and Obstetrics*, **131**, 1055–1064

Reidy, J and Hoskins, O. (1988) Controversy over mammography screening. *British Medical Journal*, **297**, 932–933

Richter, M. P. and Coia, L. R. (1985) Palliative radiation therapy. *Seminars in Oncology*, **12**, 375–383

Rilke, F. (1984) Influence of pathologic factors on management. In *Breast Cancer: Diagnosis and Mangement* (ed. G. Bonadonna), Wiley, Chichester, pp. 35–62

Roberts, C. J., Farrow, S. C. and Charney, M. C. (1985) How much can the NHS afford to spend to save a life or avoid a severe disability? *Lancet*, **i**, 89–91

Roberts, M. M., Jones, V., Elton, R. *et al.* (1984) Risk of breast cancer in women with history of benign breast disease. *British Medical Journal*, **288**, 275–278

Rose, C. and Mouridsen, H. T. (1984) Treatment of advanced breast cancer with tamoxifen. *Recent Results in Cancer Research*, **91**, 230–242

Rose, C., Mouridsen, H. T., Thorpe, S. M. *et al.* (1985a) Anti-estrogen treatment of post-menopausal women with high risk of recurrence: 72 months of life-table analysis and steroid hormone receptor status. *World Journal of Surgery*, **9**, 765–774

Rose, C., Thorpe, S. M., Andersen, K. W. *et al.* (1985b) Beneficial effects of adjuvant tamoxifen therapy in primary breast cancer patients with high oestrogen receptor values. *Lancet*, **i**, 16–19

Ross, M. B., Buzdar, A. U. and Blumenschein, G. R. (1982) Treatment of advanced breast cancer with megestrol acetate after therapy with tamoxifen. *Cancer*, **49**, 413–417

Rubens, R. D., Hayward, J. L., Knight, R. K. *et al.* (1983) Controlled trial of adjuvant chemotherapy with melphalan for breast cancer. *Lancet*, **i**, 839–843

Sainsbury, J. R. C., Farndon, J. R., Needham, G. K. *et al.* (1987) Epidermal-growth-factor receptor status as predictor of early recurrence of and death from breast cancer. *Lancet*, **i**, 1398–1402

Santen, R. J., Worgul, T. J., Samojlik, E. *et al.* (1981) A randomized trial comparing surgical adrenalectomy with aminoglutethimide plus hydrocortisone in women with advanced breast cancer. *New England Journal of Medicine*, **305**, 545–551

Sattin, R. W., Rubin, G. L., Webster, L. A. *et al.* (1985) Family history and the risk of breast cancer. *Journal of the American Medical Association*, **253**, 1908–1913

Scottish Cancer Trials Office (MRC) Edinburgh (1987) Adjuvant tamoxifen in the management of operable breast cancer: The Scottish Trial. *Lancet*, **ii**, 171–175

Shapiro, S. (1989) Determining the efficacy of breast cancer screening. *Cancer*, **63**, 1873–1880

Skegg, D. C. G. (1987) Alcohol, coffee, fat and breast cancer. *British Medical Journal*, **295**, 1011–1012

Skipper, H. E. (1971) Kinetics of mammary tumour cell growth and implications for therapy. *Cancer*, **28**, 1479–1499

Skipper, H. E. (1978) Adjuvant chemotherapy. *Cancer*, **41**, 936–940

Skrabanek, P., (1985) False premises and false promises of breast cancer screening. *Lancet*, **ii**, 316–320

Skrabanek, P. (1988) The debate over mass mammography in Britain: The case against. *British Medical Journal*, **297**, 971–972

Smith, I. E. and Macauley, V. (1985) Comparison of different endocrine therapies in the management of bone metastasis from breast cancer. *Journal of the Royal Society of Medicine*, **9**, 15–17

Souter, R. G., Wells, C., Tarin, D. and Kettlewell, M. G. W. (1985) Surgical and pathological complications associated with peritoneovenous shunts in management of malignant ascites. *Cancer*, **55**, 1973–1978

Stadel, B. V., Rubin, G. L., Webster, L. A. *et al.* (1985) Oral contraceptives and breast cancer in young women. *Lancet*, **ii**, 970–973

Stewart, A. F. (1983) Therapy of malignancy-associated hypercalcemia. *American Journal of Medicine*, **74**, 475–480

Stewart, H. J. and Prescott, R. (1985) Adjuvant tamoxifen therapy and receptor levels. *Lancet*, **i**, 573

Stewart, H. J., Prescott, R. J. and Forrest, P. A. (1989) Conservation therapy of breast cancer. *Lancet*, **i**, 168–169

Stewart, J. F. and Rubens, R. D. (1984) General prognostic factors. In *Breast Cancer: Diagnosis and Management* (ed. G. Bonadonna), Wiley, Chichester, pp. 141–167

Stuart-Harris, R., Dowsett, M., Bozek, T. *et al.* (1984) Low-dose aminoglutethimide in treatment of advanced breast cancer. *Lancet*, **ii**, 604–606

Sutton, R., Campbell, M., Cooke, T. (1987) Predictive power of progesterone receptor status in early breast carcinoma. *British Journal of Surgery*, **74**, 223–226

Tabár, L., Fagerberg, C. J. G., Gad, A. *et al*. (1985) Reduction in mortaltiy from breast cancer after mass screening with mammography. *Lancet*, **i**, 829–832

Tong, D., Gillick, L. and Hendricson, E. (1982) Palliation of symptomatic osseous metastases: final results of the study by the Radiation Therapy Oncology Group. *Cancer*, **50**, 893–899

Tsukada, Y., Fonad, A., Pikren, J. W. and Lane, W. W. (1983) Central nervous system metastases from breast carcinoma: an autopsy study. *Cancer*, **52**, 2349–2354

Turner, L., Swindell, R., Bell, W. G. T. *et al*. (1981) Radical versus modified radical mastectomy for breast cancer. *Annals of the Royal College of Surgeons of England*, **63**, 239–243

UK National Case Control Study Group (1989) Oral contraceptive use and breast cancer risk in young women. *Lancet*, **i**, 973–982

UK Trial of Early Detection of Breast Cancer Group (1988) First results on mortality reduction in the UK trial of early detection of breast cancer. *Lancet*, **ii**, 411–416

Verbeek, A. L., Hendriks, J. H. C. L., Holland, R. *et al*. (1884) Reduction of breast cancer mortality through mass screening with modern mammography. *Lancet*, **i**, 1222–1226

Veronesi, U., Saccozzi, R., Del Vecchio, M. *et al*. (1981) Comparing radical mastectomy with quadrantectomy, axillary dissection, and radiotherapy in patients with small cancers of the breast. *New England Journal of Medicine*, **305**, 6–11

Veronesi, U. and Valagussa, P. (1981) Inefficiency of internal mammary nodes dissection in breast cancer surgery. *Cancer*, **47**, 170–175

Vessey, M., Baron, J., Doll, R. *et al*. (1983) Oral contraceptives and breast cancer: final report of an epidemiological study. *British Journal of Cancer*, **47**, 455–462

Wallgren, A., Arner, O., Bengström, J. *et al*. (1980) The value of preoperative radiotherapy in operable mammary carcinoma. *International Journal of Radiation Oncology, Biology and Physics*, **6**, 287–290

Wallgren, A., Baral, E., Carstensen, J. *et al*. (1986) Adjuvant Nolvadex treatment in postmenopausal women: the Stockholm experience. *Reviews on Endocrine-related Cancer*, Suppl. **17**, 35–38

Williams, M. R., Todd, J. H., Ellis, I. O. *et al*. (1987) Oestrogen receptors in primary and advanced breast cancer: an eight year review of 704 cases. *British Journal of Cancer*, **55**, 67–73

Yarnold, J. R. (1985) Role of radiotherapy in the management of bone metastases from breast cancer. *Journal of the Royal Society of Medicine*, **78**, 23–75

Chapter 7

Kidney

Alastair W. S. Ritchie

Introduction

Tumours of the kidney are much less common than those of the prostate or bladder
and account for only 2–3% of all adult malignancies. Tumours can be divided into
those arising from the parenchyma and those arising from the urothelium of the
collecting system. Diagnosis demands careful evaluation of all patients with
haematuria and the application of a well-developed imaging algorithm. Patients
with parenchymal tumours, presenting with systemic manifestations or with
symptoms related to metastases can tax the best clinician in making the diagnosis.
The management of localized and locally advanced disease is primarily surgical.
Metastatic disease has a variable clinical course and there are limited effective
treatment options. Recently, treatments with biological response modifiers have
resulted in some worthwhile responses in patients with renal carcinoma.

Tumours of the renal parenchyma

Incidence and diagnosis

The commonest malignant tumour of the kidney is the renal carcinoma, which is
also referred to as renal-cell carcinoma, renal adenocarcinoma and hypernephroma. The last name derives from the erroneous concept that such tumours
arose from the suprarenal gland. The term hypernephroma, although in common
usage, is therefore misleading and should be deleted from the medical vocabulary.
   Renal carcinoma has reported age-standardized incidence rates of 3.6–5.6 per
100 000 males and 1.7–3.4 per 100 000 females in the UK. The range indicates the
regional variation in UK incidence rates. There are also marked international
variations in incidence, being high in northern Europe and North America and low
in Africa, Asia and South America (Waterhouse *et al.*, 1976). There is some
evidence of increasing incidence in males (Kantor *et al.*, 1976; Ritchie, Kemp and
Chisholm, 1984). The disease affects males more often than females (approximately 2:1) and can occur at any age, although it is most common in the 6th and 7th
decades. Careful post-mortem studies on hospital inpatients have shown that a
large number of cases are not diagnosed during life (Hajdu and Thomas, 1967;
Hellsten, Berge and Wehlin, 1981). For example, a series of 16 294 autopsies
performed in Malmo, Sweden, revealed 350 cases of renal carcinoma, 235 of which
were unrecognized during life (Hellsten, Berge and Wehlin, 1981). In Los Angeles

County, the proportion of incidentally diagnosed cases was unchanged in two 4-year periods: 16% in 1976–1979 and 14% in 1980–1983 (Ritchie and deKernion, 1988) but in a small series, Konnak and Grossman (1985) reported that 7 of 56 (13%) of their tumours were discovered incidentally during the period 1961 to 1973, whereas 22 of 46 (48%) were incidental findings during the 4 years from 1980. A greater proportion of asymptomatic tumours are confined to the kidney (Ritchie and deKernion, 1988) and available data suggest better survival than in patients with symptomatic tumours. It is likely that increasing use of diagnostic ultrasound, CT and magnetic resonance imaging will result in diagnosis of more asymptomatic tumours in the future.

The clinical presentation of renal carcinoma is varied and there may be delay in making the diagnosis if the patient has non-specific symptoms or presents with symptoms related to a para-neoplastic syndrome. A number of such syndromes have been described and these allow the disease to mimic many other conditions (Laski and Vugrin, 1987). The commonest presentation, however, is with haematuria and investigation then leads to the finding of a renal mass. The evalution of such a renal mass requires adherence to now well-defined diagnostic pathways to differentiate tumour from cystic and other non-malignant conditions (Bosniak, 1986). A normal intravenous urogram does not exclude the diagnosis of renal carcinoma. Of 9 small neoplasms less than 3 cm in diameter when first imaged, 3 were not visible on the IVU, even in retrospect and a further 3 were overlooked (Curry, Schabel and Betsill, 1986).

Classification and pathology

Tumours of the kidney can be benign or malignant and primary or secondary (metastatic). There is considerable debate surrounding the term adenoma as some pathologists do not believe in the existence of this lesion considering all such tumours as small renal carcinomas.

The gross appearance of renal carcinoma is variable but the typical appearance is of a yellow tumour with areas of haemorrhage and necrosis. The tumour may produce a pseudocapsule, caused by compression of surrounding healthy kidney by mechanical expansion. Areas of tumour infiltration may be obvious and evidence of penetration of the capsule and Gerota's fascia should be sought. Intrarenal veins may show invasion and extension of tumour may reach the main renal vein(s) and vena cava.

Renal carcinoma has a number of cell types but any one tumour is rarely homogeneous. Papillary, granular, alveolar, spindle-cell and mixed-cell types are described. Nuclear pleomorphism and mitotic activity are usually prominent. There is no clear relationship between the predominant cell type and prognosis, although the presence of spindle cells in conjunction with poor grade has been reported to imply a poor outcome.

Oncocytoma

Oncocytomas have a characteristic appearance, being usually well circumscribed with a uniform tan colour and in some cases a central scar, with radiations into the surrounding tumour. The lesions may be multicentric and bilateral. Renal oncocytomas comprise about 4% of all parenchymal tumours previously grouped as renal carcinoma. Oncocytes are altered epithelial cells that have an abundant homogeneous eosinophilic cytoplasm and usually a small round nucleus. The cells contain abundant mitochondria with a paucity of other cytoplasmic organelles. Oncocytes have been described in other tissues and apparently increase in numbers with advancing age. The origin of renal oncocytes is controversial (Klein and Valensi, 1976; Eble and Hull, 1984). Oncocytomas are incidental findings in approximately 70% of cases and have a low but not absent potential for local penetration and metastases. Many renal carcinomas have oncocytic features in certain areas but may have aggressive clinical behaviour. Thus the term oncocytoma has to be reserved for a tumour composed solely of oncocytes (Lieber and Tsukamoto, 1986).

Juxtaglomerular tumour

The rare juxtaglomerular tumour is associated with the clinical syndrome of hypertension and hypokalaemia. This tumour is thought to arise from the renin-secreting juxtaglomerular cells. The tumours are usually small (3–5 cm in diameter) situated in the cortex and appear well circumscribed. Neither local recurrence nor metastases have been described with this tumour.

Prognosis

Survival after nephrectomy for renal carcinoma is related to the anatomical extent of the disease, the grade, the DNA content of the tumour, the cell type and the size. The presence or absence of metastases is the most important determinant of survival. Patients with no evidence of metastases have a 90% 2-year survival compared with 20% for those with metastases (Selli et al., 1983).

For patients without distant metastases, survival is also related to the local anatomical extent of the disease with involved lymph nodes having a significant adverse effect on survival (Table 7.1). Five-year survival rates of up to 93% have been reported for tumours confined by the renal capsule (Selli et al., 1983). For all other stages, there is a significant decline in survival, suggesting the presence of clinically undetected metastatic disease at the time of nephrectomy. Patients at

Table 7.1 Relationship of anatomical extent of tumour to survival (Based on data from Skinner et al. (1971))

Anatomical extent of tumour	% Survival	
	5 Year	10 Year
Confined by renal capsule	65	56
Renal vein alone	66	49
Renal vein + perinephric fat	50	33
Renal vein + regional nodes	0	0
Perinephric fat alone	47	20
Regional nodes alone	33	17
Direct extension to nearby structures	0	0

particular risk of recurrent/metastatic disease are those with obvious tumour extension to nearby structures, those with positive regional lymph nodes and those with evidence of tumour penetration into the perinephric fat. Such patients are therefore potential candidates for adjuvant therapy after nephrectomy.

Metastatic renal carcinoma is not always a rapidly progressive disease. A study of 181 patients with metastases has shown that improved survival in a subgroup of patients was associated with long disease-free interval between nephrectomy and appearance of metastases, good performance status, metastases limited to the lungs and removal of the primary tumour. The subgroup of patients with favourable characteristics had a mean survival of 24 months and 50% were alive at 5 years. This compared with a 5-year survival for the whole group, of 9% (Maldazys and deKernion, 1986).

The prognostic significance of the DNA content of renal tumour cells has been reported in recent studies (Otto *et al.*, 1984; Ljunberg, Stenling and Roos, 1986; Ljunberg *et al.*, 1986; Rainwater *et al.*, 1987). Better prognosis, in terms of tumour recurrence and survival, has been noted for patients with diploid/near diploid DNA content when compared to patients with an aneuploid pattern. In a further study, the DNA content of primary renal carcinoma, measured by flow cytometry in 32 patients, was correlated with tumour recurrence and survival. Three subgroups of patients were studied: patients without metastases at the time of nephrectomy and two groups of patients who had metastases at the time of nephrectomy (those who survived for more than 2 years, or less than 2 years). Comparison of ploidy with staging and standard histological parameters was performed. None of the patients who presented without metastases died from their disease during the period of follow-up. Eleven patients out of 13 in this group had diploid/near diploid pattern and only 1 patient has developed metastases. Patients with metastatic disease and a diploid/near diploid DNA content had a significantly better survival than those with aneuploid primary tumours. Statistical analysis revealed that grade and ploidy contributed significant but independent prognostic information. It was concluded that DNA content is a useful prognostic indicator (deKernion *et al.*, 1989). The implications of such findings are that DNA content may be useful in a prospective fashion in helping to select patients for adjunctive nephrectomy and in stratifying patients entering clinical trials.

Management of the primary tumour

The standard treatment of localized renal carcinoma is radical nephrectomy. This implies removal of the kidney within its fascial envelope, the ipsilateral adrenal and the upper two-thirds of the ureter. The term does not imply a radical lymph node dissection although this has been advocated as an integral part of the surgery by Robson, Churchill and Anderson, (1969). Early ligation of the renal vessels is desirable and is most easily achieved be an anterior, transperitoneal approach or a thoraco-abdominal approach. The latter approach gives particularly good exposure, especially for large upper pole tumours on the left side. Local tumour extension may necessitate resection of nearby structures such as portions of mesentery, colon, pancreas and diaphragm. Such extended nephrectomies may result in long-term disease control and are therefore worthwhile in the absence of metastases.

The encouraging results of parenchymal preserving surgery in those with single kidneys or with bilateral tumours have stimulated a reappraisal of the need for radical nephrectomy in every patient. An appraisal of available data suggests that enucleation is an inadequate procedure, likely to leave behind tumour which has penetrated the pseudocapsule around the tumour. Partial nephrectomy with a wide margin of normal kidney may be a reasonable alternative for small, peripheral, incidental tumours (Ritchie and deKernion, 1988). There seems little to recommend simple as opposed to radical nephrectomy as the latter procedure may fail to render tumour free those with microscopic penetration of the capsule and is technically no easier a procedure. In the absence of a controlled comparison of the alternatives, radical nephrectomy seems likely to remain the standard treatment if the opposite kidney is normal.

Lymphadenectomy

The role of lymphadenectomy at the time of removal of the primary tumour continues to cause debate and is currently the subject of a prospective trial. A review of surgical reports has shown that regional node metastases are present in 5–10% of tumours confined by the renal capsule, approximately 30% of tumours extending beyond the capsule and 50% of those with distant metastases (Pizzocaro, 1986). Post-mortem studies have shown that the presence of regional lymph node metastases in the retroperitoneum correlate significantly with node metastases above the diaphragm (Hellsten, Berge and Linell, 1983). In addition, distant nodes such as those in the axilla and inguinal regions may contain tumour when the regional nodes are clear (Hulten et al., 1969). The benefit of formal lymphadenectomy is therefore unlikely to be considerable and although some authors have claimed a 3–10% improvement in survival following lymphadenectomy (Marshall, 1986), close analysis of such calculations reveals that the data are retrospective and incomplete. Biopsy of regional nodes can be useful for prognosis if positive, and involves no extra morbidity. Long-term survival in patients with nodal metastases has been reported to be as high as 35% at 5 years after extensive lymphadenectomy but cumulative data from other series reveals a much lower figure of 17% (Marshall, 1986).

Adjunctive nephrectomy

If the patient has distant metastases or obvious bulky lymph node involvement removal of the primary may seem illogical. Certainly there is no overall demonstrable survival benefit (Johnson, Kaesler and Samuels, 1975). Some argue that removal of the primary may induce 'spontaneous' regression of metastases but the incidence of postoperative 'spontaneous' regression is very small (<1%) and when it does occur is usually only a partial regression with subsequent disease progression. Furthermore, nephrectomy in a patient with metastatic disease has a measurable mortality and variable morbidity. A survey of British urologists showed, however, that 89% did not consider the presence of metastases a contraindication to nephrectomy (Ritchie and Chisholm, 1983) and there are circumstances in which nephrectomy should be performed. Patients with symptoms related to the primary and patients with knowledge of the existence of the primary may benefit symptomatically and psychologically from surgery. Retrospective analyses of data from clinical trials of immunotherapy, have suggested some survival advantages in those in whom the primary was completely removed, especially those with small pulmonary metastases and nephrectomy may therefore be justified in the context of a clinical trial.

As noted above DNA content may help in predicting those patients likely to have useful survival after nephrectomy.

Tumour extension to the vena cava

Tumour extension to the vena cava occurs in up to 10% of patients. This fact implies that all patients should have imaging studies of the renal vein and cava before surgery in order to establish the presence of and extent of any tumour extension. Ultrasound offers a non-invasive method of imaging but the vessels may be obscured by bowel gas. If there is doubt or difficulty with ultrasound imaging, then alternative methods such as computed tomography or inferior vena cavography (via a femoral vein puncture) may be required to provide this essential information.

The presence of tumour in the vena cava used to be considered as implying a poor prognosis and many such patients were deemed inoperable. Studies by Skinner, Pfister and Colvin (1972) and Cherrie et al. (1982) have shown that venous extension alone does not impart a poor prognosis, if it is completely removed. Positive lymph nodes in association with the venous extension are, however, linked to diminished survival (vide supra). Successful surgery involves accurate assessment of the upper level of the caval extension. This may involve imaging via the superior vena cava. Extension above the level of the hepatic veins usually necessitates a combined cardiac and urological approach to avoid the risks of large blood loss and fragmentation of the tumour thrombus. Direct invasion of the wall of the vena cava may require resection of the cava.

Radiotherapy

Radiotherapy may be of value in the management of painful bony metastases. The tumour is relatively radioresistant however. Early, uncontrolled studies suggested that preoperative adjuvant radiotherapy improved survival but a randomized study performed by Van der Werf-Messing (1973) showed no difference in survival at 5 years if 3000 rad or no therapy was given before surgery. Similar results are available for postoperative radiotherapy, with uncontrolled reports suggesting improved survival but a controlled study by Finney (1973), comparing surgery alone with surgery and postoperative radiotherapy, showed that the survival of those treated with postoperative radiotherapy was worse. Although still a controversial topic, there seems little objective evidence to support the use of radiotherapy in the management of local disease.

Management of metastatic disease

Approximately 25% of patients have metastases at the time of presentation and, as noted above, a significant proportion of those presenting with clinically localized disease will develop metastases during follow-up. Options for treatment of metastatic disease include surgery, hormonal therapy, radiotherapy, cytotoxic chemotherapy, immunotherapy and combination therapy. Palliative therapy is also important.

Surgery

Surgical excision of solitary metastases has produced long-term disease-free survival. In 1939 Barney and Churchill reported excision of a primary renal tumour and a solitary pulmonary metastasis, the patient surviving for 23 years before dying of ischaemic heart disease. Solitary metastases have been reported to occur in 1.6–3.2% of patients at diagnosis but such reports come from referral centres and may therefore be an overestimate of the true incidence. In reality, solitary metastases are an unusual clinical problem and a diligent search will reveal other evidence of widespread disease. The benefit claimed for surgical treatment may therefore relate more to tumour biology than to the surgical procedure (Golimbu *et al.*, 1986).

Hormonal therapy

Medroxyprogesterone acetate (MPA) has been popular in the management of metastatic disease following the work of Bloom (1973). Recent work has, however, raised doubt about the hormone-dependent status of human renal carcinoma. When MPA was administered as adjuvant therapy in a randomized study of 136 patients with non-metastatic disease, no benefit was noted in treated patients and side-effects were evident in 50% (Pizzocaro *et al.*, 1986). Actuarial 5-year survival was 73% for the untreated group and 67% for the treated group. Sex steroid receptor hormones were studied in 10 of these tumours and the autologous normal kidney. Oestradiol and progesterone binding sites were found more frequently in the healthy kidney than in the tumour. No correlation could be found between steroid receptors in the tumour and later response to hormonal therapy at relapse.

Patients with metastatic disease may report symptomatic benefit from treatment with MPA but the objective response rate of approximately 4% (see Table 7.3), has reduced enthusiasm for this form of systemic management.

Cytotoxic chemotherapy

There are no consistently effective single agents or combinations active against renal carcinoma (deKernion, 1983). In view of the toxicity of such agents, it is therefore not logical to 'try out' chemotherapy unless this is being done within the confines of a phase I/II study.

Immunotherapy

The rationale for immunotherapy in renal carcinoma is based on an accumulation of indirect evidence that there is a host–tumour interaction mediated through the immune system. Traditional approaches to solid tumour immunotherapy have been adequately reviewed elsewhere and have largely consisted of attempts to actively stimulate host immunity using a variety of tumour 'vaccines' with or without adjuvants (Ritchie and deKernion, 1989). Table 7.2 lists some of the agents used in conventional immunotherapy. Use of such agents has been largely unsuccessful. The advent of recombinant DNA technology and refined understanding of cellular immunology has enabled production of biological response modifiers (interferons and interleukins) on a scale that has permitted their clinical use.

Table 7.2 Immunotherapy for metastatic renal carcinoma

Conventional immunotherapy
BCG
Transfer factor
Polymerized tumour cells
Tumour cells + *C. parvum*
Immune RNA
Tumour necrosis factor
Thymosin fraction 5

Contemporary immunotherapy
Interferons (single agent and combination)
Interferons + chemotherapy
Monoclonal antibodies/conjugates
Interleukin 2 (IL-2)
IL-2 + LAK cells
IL-2 + TIL

Interferons

Although interferons are included under the banner of immunotherapy, their mode of action in renal carcinoma is not defined. There are a number of possibilities as interferons have a number of biological effects, including a direct anti-proliferative effect, anti-oncogene effects and effects on immune modulation, antigen expression and phenotypic reversion. It is clear that interferons bind to cell surface receptors to form a complex which is then internalized and induces transcription of a number of genes. The presence of such receptors in the various cellular subtypes of renal carcinoma merits further investigation. Furthermore, the relationship between the presence of such receptors and response to interferon has not been investigated.

Alpha interferons appear to have response rates in excess of those for gamma and beta interferons. The overall response rate (complete and partial response) in a total of 754 patients in 15 different studies of alpha interferon was 16% (Selby, 1990). Intramuscular and intravenous injections seem to have no benefit over subcutaneous injection and the latter is easier for the patient to do himself. Side-effects are universal, reversible and dose dependent. A 'flu-like' illness is the common side-effect, which can be ameliorated by the use of non-steroidal anti-inflammatory agents and bed-time administration. The median time to response with alpha interferon is 2–4 months and the treatment should therefore be continued for at least 2 months before response can be judged. There are no clear data indicating prolongation of survival following treatment.

Based on results of animal studies and the encouraging results of maintenance therapy in malignant melanoma, interferons may have a place as adjuvant therapy for those at risk of the development of metastases after nephrectomy. Adjuvant studies are in progress in Europe but no data are yet available.

Interferons have been used in combination (e.g. alpha and gamma) and in association with chemotherapy (e.g. vinblastine). Whilst there is some evidence of synergism (Table 7.3), the toxicity of such combinations may be worse than that of interferon alone.

At the time of writing, only one company (F. Hoffmann-La Roche & Co. Ltd) has a UK product licence for alpha interferon (Roferon) in renal carcinoma.

Table 7.3 Accumulated results of interferon alpha 2a studies (Based on data from Holdener, E. E. (F. Hoffman–La Roche & Co. Ld)

Treatment	No. of patients	% showing response
Interferon alpha 2a	557	12
Interferon alpha 2a + Vinblastine	370	24
Medroxyprogesterone acetate	30	4

Adoptive immunotherapy

Adoptive immunotherapy can be defined as transfer to the tumour-bearing host of active immunologic reagents such as immunocytes, antibodies or other modulators of the immune response. In humans, lymphokine activated killer (LAK) cells have no effect when used alone on solid tumours *in vivo*. Interleukin-2 (IL-2) alone has some effects, in terms of tumour response, when given in high bolus dosage and is the subject of intense investigation at present. It has been shown that LAK cells are generated *in vivo* after 3–4 weeks of high dose IL-2 therapy (Ellis *et al.*, 1987). The cells, isolated from peripheral blood of patients being treated with IL-2, can be shown to lyse the NK-resistant cell line Daudi and fresh tumour cells in 4-hour ^{51}Cr release assays. High-dose IL-2 therapy, however, is not without side-effects due to a capillary leak syndrome, which is reversible and directly attributable to the IL-2. To investigate the possibility that continuous infusion may circumvent the side-effects related to large pulses of IL-2, West *et al.* (1987) reported modest response and lowered side-effects with such a regimen. The best results in solid tumours in both animals and man, have been associated with treatment with LAK cells and IL-2 given together. Responses have been reported in a variety of solid tumours (Rosenberg *et al.*, 1985; 1987; West *et al.*, 1987; Rosenberg, 1988). It is noteworthy that of all the patients with advanced cancer treated by LAK cells plus IL-2, the most responsive non-lymphomatous tumour has been renal carcinoma with a 31% response rate (CR + PR) compared with an 18% response rate for melanoma and 11% for colorectal cancer (Rosenberg, 1988).

An alternative to the use of LAK cells generated from peripheral blood lymphocytes, is to use the lymphocytes which infiltrate the tumour. The attraction of this approach being that the tumour-infiltrating lymphocytes (TIL) may be biologically more relevant having been exposed to the tumour associated antigens. Belldegrun, Muul and Rosenberg (1988) have recently described a method for generation of activated tumour-infiltrating lymphocytes (aTIL) from fresh renal carcinomas. The technique involves enzymatic disaggregation and culture of the resultant cell suspension in medium containing IL-2. Active expansion (5–15 fold) of the aTIL was shown to occur over 10–14 days. Subsequent reculture in fresh medium with IL-2 resulted in further expansion over a period of approximately 34 days, resulting in a 50 000 fold increase in the total number of lymphocytes. The scientific study of the immunology of this LAK/TIL phenomenon is not just an academic exercise. This new adoptive immunotherapy has been criticized (Moertel, 1986), mainly on account of the toxicity and expense. Thus if the most effective cells can be identified and selectively expanded *in vitro*, it may be possible to reduce the dose of IL-2 required in addition to the transferred cells and lead to diminished toxicity in the future.

Palliative therapy

Palliation with a variety of methods of pain control, radiotherapy and early internal fixation of bone metastases in weight-bearing areas all have a place in selected patients. Arterial embolization may be of value in selected patients who are not considered fit for nephrectomy but have troublesome symptoms related to the primary. In a series of 29 patients with metastatic or inoperable renal tumour 19 (65%) were considered to have obtained useful palliation with control of haematuria and relief of pain being most prominent. Four patients, 3 with bilateral tumours had successful highly selective embolization. The technique is not without hazard however and 5 patients had complications including renal failure, pulmonary embolus and large bowel infarction (Ritchie *et al.*, unpublished).

Summary

In summary, surgery remains the most effective treatment available for renal carcinoma. Survival after surgery is a function of the anatomical extent of the disease and the majority of patients presenting with renal carcinoma could benefit from systemic adjuvant therapy. Recent studies have clarified the prognostic factors in metastatic disease and these must be taken into account in future clinical trials. Interferons and adoptive immunotherapy with LAK cells and interleukin-2 appear to offer the best hope of response in metastatic renal carcinoma. Treatment toxicity remains a problem. Complete responses, notably rare in earlier attempts at immunotherapy, are an important feature of these treatments, which hopefully will be the basis for improved disease control in the future.

Urothelial tumours of the kidney

Incidence and diagnosis

Tumours arising from the transitional epithelium of the collecting system account for up to 10% of all renal tumours. Over 90% are transitional-cell carcinomas with true benign transitional tumours (papilloma) being very rare. Squamous-cell carcinomas account for 7–9% of renal urothelial tumours and are associated with chronic inflammation usually caused by calculi. It was only with the revised classification of disease sponsored by WHO in 1967 that ICD 189 was subdivided into 189.0 (parenchymal tumours) and 189.1,2 (tumours of the pelvis and ureter). Accurate data on the relative incidence of such tumours has therefore only been available for a short time. Available data suggest that the number of registered cases of upper tract urothelial tumours is increasing in both sexes (Figure 7.1) but it is not clear whether this represents a genuine increase in incidence or reflects better diagnostic methods. For example, the recent availability of good quality urine cytology may have stimulated a more thorough search for upper tract tumours in patients with negative cystoscopy and positive urine cytology.

Urothelial tumours of the kidney occur most commonly in the 6th and 7th decades and the data shown in Figure 7.1 indicate that they occur more commonly in males (M:F = 2.1:1).

The tumours show international variation in incidence and are classically associated with residence in the Balkan countries and excessive analgesic ingestion (especially phenacetin). The latter two associations are also related to a higher

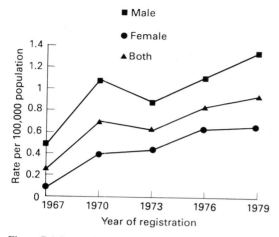

Figure 7.1 Age standardized incidence rates for ICD 189.1 (Based on Scottish Cancer Registration data 1967–1979)

incidence of bilateral tumours. Others aetiological factors are similar to those of bladder urothelial cancer (Wallace, 1988). Upper tract tumours may occur in association with bladder tumours and vice versa. The implication of this observation is that the patient who has had a urothelial tumour requires follow-up and supervision of the entire urinary tract, or at least those parts left behind by the surgeon.

Presentation

The commonest presentation is with haematuria, be this frank or microscopic. Up to 15% of patients are asymptomatic and the diagnosis may be made by chance during investigation for other suspected pathology. Loin pain may be described as a dull ache or be more acute if caused by clots of blood and/or tumour passing down the ureter. The patient may present with systemic symptoms related to advanced local or metastatic disease. Renal failure may occur if the tumours or resulting blood clots produce obstruction to the outflow tract. There are rarely any physical signs. A renal mass is palpable in less than 10% of patients.

The diagnosis depends heavily on good quality intravenous urography in a suitably prepared patient. This investigation should be done in all patients with haematuria and periodically in those being followed after a previous diagnosis of urothelial cancer at other sites. The presence of a filling defect, distortion of the calyces and the finding of a poorly or non-functioning kidney all raise the possibility of a urothelial tumour. Filling defects may require better definition with retrograde ureteropyelography which is best done with a combination of screening under image intensification and single shot radiographs. Oblique views and post drainage images may be helpful in the identification of small lesions.

Urine cytology by an experienced cytopathologist is most helpful when unequivocally positive but may be negative in the presence of well-differentiated tumours. The combination of a typical filling defect on IVU and positive voided urine cytology can establish the diagnosis. If the voided urine cytology is negative or equivocal then urine samples can be obtained from the upper tract at the time of retrograde studies. The acquisition of the sample can be assisted by lavage of the renal pelvis with saline or by brushing the lesion. This is best performed before injection of contrast as this may distort the cytological appearances producing a false positive result. False positive cytology may also result from coincidental inflammatory lesions of the urinary tract such as calculi and infection. Sarnacki *et al.* (1971) have reported a 6% false positive rate and a false negative rate of up to 38% in a study of 2400 urine specimens from 1400 patients. The diagnosis of urothelial malignancy can not therefore be made by cytological studies in isolation.

Diagnostic ureteroscopy can be performed if the foregoing studies fail to establish a diagnosis. Ureteroscopy using rigid instruments is more likely to produce valuable additional information for ureteric lesions than calyceal lesions as the view above the pelvi-ureteric junction is limited. Flexible ureteroscopes are not widely available but may give a better view of the pelvis and calyces.

In the presence of ureteric obstruction, antegrade pyelography using percutaneous needle puncture may occasionally be necessary. This technique should be used with caution, however, as there is a small but definite risk of tumour implantation after puncture of the collecting system. This caveat should be extended to the risk of perforation of the ureter at the time of ureteroscopy.

Ultrasound is less useful for urothelial lesions than in the diagnosis of parenchymal renal tumours but may be performed in the evaluation of a non-functioning kidney. Similarly, computed tomography is less sensitive in the diagnosis of small collecting system tumours and is not usually necessary in making the diagnosis. Tumours of the collecting system may invade the renal parenchyma and vice versa. When it is not clear from the IVU whether a lesion arises from the parenchyma or the collecting system, then CT with and without contrast may be of considerable value (Gatewood *et al.*, 1982). The distinction of parenchymal from urothelial tumours is of practical importance as the necessity for complete removal of the ureter depends upon the nature of the tumour.

Preoperative biopsy or fine aspiration cytology is not usually necessary or desirable on account of the risks of malignant cellular extravasation. The procedures recommended by the UICC for assessment are physical examination, imaging and endoscopy.

Staging

Preoperative staging should include a chest X-ray. Bone scintiscan and abdominal CT may be added if the symptoms or imaging studies raise the possibility of local invasion and if cytology suggests a high grade lesion. The TNM clinical and pathological classification is similar to that used in bladder cancer. Assessment of function in the opposite kidney is necessary before planning definitive management.

Management

Definitive management is by surgical removal of the kidney, ureter and a cuff of bladder mucosa around the ureter. Subtotal removal of the upper urinary tract on the side of the lesion is associated with a significant risk (up to 84%) of recurrent malignancy in the ureteric stump (Droller, 1986).

Traditionally the nephro-ureterectomy has been performed by a retroperitoneal approach through two incisions. The kidney and upper ureter are mobilized through a standard loin approach to the kidney. Maintaining continuity of the ureter, the kidney is placed in a pouch in the retroperitoneum and the superior incision closed. Using a separate incision, the distal ureter is then dissected from within and outside the bladder to allow *en bloc* removal.

A modification of the two incision approach has been suggested by Abercrombie (1972). This modified nephro-ureterectomy involves transurethral resection of the intramural ureter using a resectoscope. The resection is carried through the full thickness of the bladder until the ureter is seen lying free in the perivesical fat. The bladder is drained with a catheter and the patient turned for a standard loin approach to the kidney. A ligature is placed around the ureter early in the dissection. The ureter can be removed from above by careful finger dissection. This approach has the obvious advantage of avoiding the lower incision and ensures complete removal of the ureter. The defect in the bladder wall heals readily with catheter drainage for 8 days. Concern expressed about a higher incidence of local tumour recurrence at the site of the distal resection (Hetherington, Ewing and Philp, 1986) has not been confirmed (Abercrombie *et al.*, 1988). Both the modified approach and conventional nephro-ureterectomy are associated with a 30% probability of subsequent bladder tumours. The modified approach should be confined to renal tumours however – ureteric tumours are not considered suitable.

Endoscopic management

Patients with bilateral tumours or compromised renal function in the opposite kidney may not be suitable for definitive management by nephro-ureterectomy. In such patients, local management may be effected by segmental resection or endoscopic techniques either using the ureteroscope or by percutaneous access to the collecting system. Percutaneous approaches have the advantage of a better view and the ability to insert larger instruments for resection or coagulation of the tumour. The disadvantage of this approach, however, is the difficulty of assessment of the depth of tumour penetration and the need to irradiate the percutaneous tract to prevent tumour implantation. Long-term follow-up of patients treated by endoscopic surgery is not available and, as yet, these techniques cannot be recommended for patients with a normal contralateral kidney and ureter.

Chemotherapy and biological therapy

Where surgical resection is not possible chemotherapy may be used by both systemic and topical application. Infusion of agents with proven efficacy against urothelial lesions of the bladder (e.g. mitomycin C and Bacille Calmette-Guérin) can be performed via a nephrostomy tube and responses have been reported. Systemic chemotherapy with cisplatin-based combination regimens is in the early stages of assessment.

Prognosis

Evaluation of the results of nephro-ureterectomy for transitional-cell tumours of the kidney is complicated by the variety of staging systems reported in the literature. Furthermore, factors which may influence the outcome such as tumour grade and the association with urothelial tumours, or carcinoma-in-situ at other sites, are not consistently reported. Within these limitations it appears that the prognosis for patients having low-grade tumours with no evidence of muscle invasion is excellent (5-year survival > 90%). Penetration of tumour into the peripelvic or perirenal area, in association with high tumour grade, carries a poor prognosis (5-year survival 5–10%) (Mufti *et al.*, 1989).

Summary

The diagnosis of upper tract urothelial tumours requires constant vigilance and methodical assessment of all patients with haematuria. The results of surgical treatment for confined tumours are excellent. The challenge for the future is to explore new treatment methods, such as percutaneous resection and topical chemotherapy, which preserve functioning renal tissue and establish their place in the overall management and follow-up of these patients.

Secondary tumours

Metastases to the kidney are usually silent. The factors favouring the diagnosis of renal metastases are small, multifocal avascular renal masses in association with widespread metastases elsewhere in the body. Renal metastases do not usually involve the renal venous system (Pagani, 1983). When both kidneys are involved the commonest primary is a lymphoma, whereas if one kidney is involved the commonest primary is the lung (Klinger, 1951). Other primary sources are the breast and uterus.

References

Abercrombie, G. F. (1972) Nephro-ureterectomy. *Proceedings of the Royal Society of Medicine*, **65**, 1021–1022

Abercrombie, G. F., Eardley, I., Payne, S. R. *et al.* (1988) Modified nephro-ureterectomy. Long term follow-up with particular reference to subsequent bladder tumours. *British Journal of Urology*, **61**, 198–200

Barney, J. D. and Churchill, E. J. (1939) Adenocarcinoma of the kidney with metastasis to the lung: Cured by nephrectomy and lobectomy. *Journal of Urology*, **42**, 269–276

Belldegrun, A., Muul, M. and Rosenberg, S. A. (1988) Interleukin-2 expanded tumor-infiltrating lymphocytes in human renal cell cancer: isolation, characterization and antitumor activity. *Cancer Research*, **48**, 206–214

Bloom, H. J. G. (1973) Hormone-induced and spontaneous regression of metastatic renal cancer. *Cancer*, **32**, 1066–1071

Bosniak, M. A. (1986) The current radiological approach to renal cysts. *Radiology*, **158**, 1–10

Cherrie, R. J., Goldman, D. G., Lindner, A. and deKernion, J. B. (1982) Prognostic implications of vena caval extension of renal cell carcinoma. *Journal of Urology*, **128**, 910–912

Curry, N. S., Schabel, S. I. and Betsill, W. L. (1986) Small renal neoplasms: diagnostic imaging, pathologic features and clinical course. *Radiology*, **158**, 113–117

deKernion, J. B. (1983) Treatment of advanced renal cell carcinoma – traditional methods and innovative approaches. *Journal of Urology*, **130**, 2–7

deKernion, J. B., Mukamel, E., Ritchie, A. W. S. *et al.* (1989) The prognostic significance of the DNA content of renal carcinoma. *Cancer*, **64**, 1669–1673

Droller, M. J. (1986) Transitional cell cancer: upper tracts and bladder. In *Campbell's Urology* (eds. P. C. Walsh, R. F. Gittes, A. D. Perlmutter, *et al.*) Philadelphia, Saunders, pp. 1343–1440

Eble, J. N. and Hull, M. T. (1984) Morphological features of renal oncocytoma: a light and electron microscopic study. *Human Pathology*, **15**, 1054–1059

Ellis, T. M., Braun, D. P., Creekmore, S. P. *et al.* (1987) Appearance and phenotypic characterization of circulating Leu 19⁺ cells in patients receiving recombinant IL-2. *Proceedings of the American Association of Cancer Research*, **28**, 373

Finney, R. (1973) The value of radiotherapy in the treatment of hypernephroma – a clinical trial. *British Journal of Urology*, **45**, 258–269

Gatewood, O. M. B., Goldman, S. M., Marshall, F. F. and Siegelman, S. S. (1982) Computerized tomography in the diagnosis of transitional cell carcinoma of the kidney. *Journal of Urology*, **127**, 876–887

Golimbu, M., Al-askari, S., Tessler, A. and Morales, P. (1986) Aggressive treatment of metastatic renal cancer. *Journal of Urology*, **136**, 805–807

Hajdu, S. I. and Thomas, A. G.(1967) Renal cell carcinoma at autopsy. *Journal of Urology*, **97**, 978–982

Hellsten, B., Berge, T. and Linell, F. (1983) Clinically unrecognized renal carcinoma: Aspects of tumour morphology, lymphatic and haematogenous metastatic spread. *British Journal of Urology*, **55**, 166–170

Hellsten, S., Berge, T. and Wehlin, L. (1981) Unrecognized renal cell carcinoma. Clinical and diagnostic aspects. *Scandinavian Journal of Urology and Nephrology*, **8**, 269–272

Hetherington, J. W., Ewing, R. and Philp, N. H. (1986) Modified nephro-ureterectomy: a risk of tumour implantation. *British Journal of Urology*, **58**, 368–370

Hulten, L., Rosencrantz, T., Seeman, T. *et al.* (1969) Occurrence and localization of lymph node metastases in renal carcinoma. *Scandinavian Journal of Urology and Nephrology*, **3**, 129–133

Johnson, D. E., Kaesler, K. E. and Samuels, M. L. (1975) Is nephrectomy justified in patients with metastatic renal carcinoma? *Journal of Urology*, **114**, 27–29

Kantor, A. L. F., Meigs, J. W., Heston, J. F. and Flannery, J. T. (1976) Epidemiology of renal cell carcinoma in Connecticut, 1935–1973. *Journal of the National Cancer Institute*, **57**, 495–500

Klein, M. J. and Valensi, Q. J. (1976) Proximal tubular adenomas of kidney with so-called oncocytic features; a clinico-pathologic study of 13 cases of a rarely reported neoplasm. *Cancer*, **38**, 906–909

Klinger, M. E. (1951) Secondary tumours of the genitourinary tract. *Journal of Urology*, **65**, 144–153

Konnak, J. W. and Grossman, H. B. (1985) Renal cell carcinoma as an incidental finding. *Journal of Urology*, **134**, 1094–1096

Laski, M. E. and Vugrin, D. (1987) Paraneoplastic syndromes in hypernephroma. *Seminars in Nephrology*, **7**, 123–130

Lieber, M. M. and Tsukamoto, T. (1986) Renal oncocytoma. In *Tumours of the Kidney* (eds. J. B. deKernion and M. Pavone-Macaluso). International Perspectives in Urology, Vol. 13. Williams & Wilkins, Baltimore, pp. 306–319

Ljunberg, B., Forsslund, G., Stenling, R. and Zetterberg, A. (1986) Prognostic significance of the DNA content in renal cell carcinoma. *Journal of Urology*, **135**, 422–426

Ljunberg, B., Stenling, R. and Roos, G. (1986) Prognostic value of deoxyribonucleic acid content in metastatic renal cell carcinoma. *Journal of Urology*, **136**, 801–804

Maldazys, J. D. and deKernion, J. B. (1986) Prognostic factors in metastatic renal carcinoma. *Journal of Urology*, **136**, 376–379

Marshall, F. F. (1986) Lymphadenectomy for renal cell carcinoma. In *Tumours of the Kidney* (eds. J. B. deKernion and M. Pavone-Macaluso). International Perspectives in Urology, Vol. 13. Williams & Wilkins, Baltimore, pp. 87–97

Moertel, C. G. (1986) Editorial. On lymphokines, cytokines and breakthroughs. *Journal of the American Medical Association*, **256**, 3141

Mufti, G. R., Gove, J. R. W., Badenoch, D. F. *et al.* (1989) Transitional cell carcinoma of the renal pelvis and ureter. *British Journal of Urology*, **63**, 135–140

Otto, U., Baisch, H., Huland, H. and Kloppel, G. (1984) Tumour cell deoxyribonucleic acid content and prognosis in human renal cell carcinoma. *Journal of Urology*, **132**, 237–239

Pagani, J. J. (1983) Solid renal mass in the cancer patient: second primary renal cell carcinoma versus renal metastasis. *Journal of Computer Assisted Tomography*, **7**, 444–448

Pizzocaro, G. (1986) Lymphadenectomy in renal adenocarcinoma. In *Tumours of the Kidney* (eds. J. B. deKernion and M. Pavone-Macaluso). International Perspectives in Urology, Vol. 13. Williams &

Wilkins, Baltimore, pp. 75–86

Pizzocaro, G., Piva, L., Salvioni, R. *et al.* (1986) Adjuvant medroxyprogesterone acetate and steroid receptor hormones in category M0 renal cell carcinoma. An interim report of a prospective randomized study. *Journal of Urology*, **135**, 18–21

Rainwater, L. M., Hosaka, Y., Farrow, G. M. and Lieber, M. M. (1987) Well differentiated clear cell renal carcinoma: significance of nuclear deoxyribonucleic acid patterns studied by flow cytometry. *Journal of Urology*, **137**, 15–20

Ritchie, A. W. S. and Chisholm, G. D. (1983) The management of renal carcinoma: A questionnaire survey. *British Journal of Urology*, **5**, 591–594

Ritchie, A. W. S. and deKernion, J. B. (1988) Incidental renal neoplasms: incidence in Los Angeles County, treatment and prognosis. *Progress in Clinical and Biological Research*, **269**, 347–356. EORTC Genitourinary Group Monograph 5. *Progress and Controversies in Oncological Urology II*, (ed. F. H. Schroder), Alan Liss, Inc., New York. 1988

Ritchie, A. W. S. and deKernion, J. B. (1989) Immunobiology of renal carcinoma. In: *Scientific Foundations in Urology*, 3rd edn (eds. G. D. Chisholm and W. R. Fair) Heinemann, London, pp. 540–548

Ritchie, A. W. S., Kemp, I. W. and Chisholm, G. D. (1984) Is the incidence of renal carcinoma increasing? *British Journal of Urology*, **56**, 571–573

Robson, C. J., Churchill, B. M. and Anderson, W. (1969) The results of radical nephrectomy for renal cell carcinoma. *Journal of Urology*, **101**, 297–301

Rosenberg, S. A., Lotze, M. T., Muul, L. M. *et al.* (1985) Observations on the systemic administration of autologous lymphokine-activated killer cells and recombinant interleukin-2 to patients with metastatic cancer. *New England Journal of Medicine*, **313**, 1485–1492

Rosenberg, S. A., Lotze, M. T., Muul, L. M. *et al.* (1987) A progress report on the treatment of 157 patients with advanced cancer using lymphokine-activated killer cells and interleukin-2 or high dose interleukin-2 alone. *New England Journal of Medicine*, **316**, 889–897

Rosenberg, S. A. (1988) Immunotherapy of cancer using interleukin-2: current status and future prospects. *Immunology Today*, **9**, 58–62

Sarnacki, C. T., McCormack, L. J., Kiser, W. S. *et al.* (1971) Urinary cytology and the clinical diagnosis of urinary tract malignancy: a clinicopathologic study of 1400 patients. *Journal of Urology*, **106**, 761–764

Selby, P. (1990) Progress in the treatment of renal cell carcinoma. Conference Proceedings (in press)

Selli, C., Hinshaw, W., Woodard, B. H. and Paulson, D. F. (1983) Stratification of risk factors in renal cell carcinoma. *Cancer*, **52**, 899–903

Skinner, D. G., Covin, R. B., Vermillion, C. D. *et al.* (1971) Diagnosis and mangement of renal cell carcinoma: a clinical and pathologic study of 309 cases. *Cancer*, **28**, 1165–1177

Skinner, D. G., Pfister, F. G. and Colvin, R. (1972) Extension of renal cell carcinoma into the vena cava: the rationale for aggressive surgical management. *Journal of Urology*, **107**, 711–716

van der Werf-Messing, B. (1973) Carcinoma of the kidney. *Cancer*, **32**, 1056–1061

Wallace, D. M. A. (1988) Occupational urothelial cancer. *British Journal of Urology*, **61**, 175–182

Waterhouse, J., Muir, C., Cornea, P and Powell, J. (eds.) (1976) *Cancer Incidence in Five Continents*, Vol. II IARC Scientific Publication No. 15, Lyon

West, W. H., Tauer, K. W., Yannelli, J. R. *et al.* (1987) Constant-infusion recombinant interleukin-2 in adoptive immunotherapy of advanced cancer. *New England Journal of Medicine*, **316**, 898–905

Chapter 8

Bladder cancer

G. D. Chisholm

Introduction

Carcinoma of the bladder is the fifth most common cancer in the UK, after lung, colorectal, breast and stomach cancers. The lifetime risk of developing bladder cancer is 1 in 53, compared to 1 in 11 for lung, 1 in 20 for prostate and 1 in 42 for stomach. In 1983 there were 7693 registrations of bladder cancer for men and 2877 for women in the UK. The deaths from 1984 data are 3625 men and 1619 women. The 5-year survival from 1980 data was 50%. These collective data from the Office of Population Censuses and Surveys, Scottish and Northern Ireland Offices and ICFR indicate the size of the problem but because of the nature of the disease these figures do not emphasize the large work load that the regular follow-up of these patients produces on any health care system.

The male to female ratio in most western countries is 3:1 and the incidence begins to rise sharply after the 5th decade of life. The clinical impression that there is an increasing incidence of carcinomas is supported by epidemiological data (Devesa and Silverman, 1978).

Carcinoma of the bladder is one of the most carefully studied tumours in respect of aetiological factors and especially the hazards to workers in a variety of industries. The chemicals that have been identified as carcinogens in man are aromatic amines that are used in a variety of industries under a variety of names (Table 8.1).

Table 8.1 Human bladder carcinogens (Rübben, Lutzeyer and Wallace, 1985)

2-Naphthylamine	Orthotoluidine
Benzidine	Phenacetin
4-Aminobiphenyl	Chlornaphazine
Dichlorobenzidine	Cyclophosphamide
Orthodianisidines	

An important characteristic of industrial carcinogenesis is the long lag period between exposure to the carcinogen and development of the tumour: the time may range from 20 years to 40 years. It may therefore be difficult to determine, from a routine clinical history, the relevance of past occupations in the genesis of the cancer (Table 8.2) but guidelines have been published and information is available

Table 8.2 Occupations where workers are known to have been exposed to bladder carcinogens (A) and occupations where there is an increased risk but exposure to carcinogens has not been proved (B) (Rübben, Lutzeyer and Wallace, 1985)

A. Chemical dye manufacture and other chemicals	B. Leather work
Manufacture of rubber articles (tyres, cables)	Aluminium
Gas works producing coal gas	refining
Rodent operator	Hairdressing
Laboratory work	Tailoring
Sewage work	Textiles
Manufacture of firelighters	Printing in general
Textile printing	
Kimono painting	

on the procedures for industrial compensation (BAUS Subcommittee on Industrial Bladder Cancer, 1988; Wallace, 1988).

Other aetiological factors in bladder cancer include cigarette smoking, chronic urinary infection, bilharzia and bladder exstrophy, the latter two being associated with squamous-cell carcinomas. The debate about the risk from saccharine and cyclamate sweeteners and excessive coffee drinking indicates that if there is an association, it is very weak (Weinberg et al., 1983).

Experimental bladder carcinogenesis has attracted much interest (Hicks, 1982). The main clinical interest lies in whether or not urothelial injury increases the risk of bladder carcinogenesis and whether or not some form of prophylactic treatment should be used to reduce the incidence of recurrences and the theoretical risk of implantation tumours (Wallace et al., 1984). This problem is still the subject of debate and has now been studied in clinical trials (see superficial bladder cancer).

The relevance of oncogenes in the development of bladder cancer has attracted much recent interest (Malone et al., 1985). The most frequently detected oncogene that transforms cells (from non-tumour to one with a tumour-developing capability) in human solid tumours belongs to the ras family of cellular oncogenes. There is some evidence that ras oncogenes may exert transforming activity by over-expression of gene productes. Evidence for this has come from immunohistochemical studies when an increased expression of ras p21 was demonstrated in cases of carcinoma-in-situ and dysplasia with normal urothelium (Viola et al., 1985). Low-grade lesions showed essentially similar light staining to normal urothelium whereas high-grade lesions showed intense staining. This increase in protein product expression has been confined in other malignancies and another product of H-ras, p55, has been found in the urine of bladder cancer patients at levels which roughly correlate with grade and stage and are especially elevated in patients who have had multiple recurrences (Stock et al., 1987). Regardless of whether oncogenes actually cause cancer or are merely secondary events in the disease, their products are very important in following cell behaviour; it may be that in the future, oncogene analysis will have a role in the assessment of the bladder cancer patient.

Presentation

Most patients with bladder cancer are diagnosed as the result of signs or symptoms. Less than 10% are diagnosed incidentally or as a result of routine screening methods. The principal presentation is haematuria which may be either macroscopic or microscopic and these require separate discussion.

Macroscopic haematuria

Haematuria may be uniformly mixed throughout the urine i.e. total haematuria or may be seen mainly at the end of micturition, i.e. terminal haematuria. The latter is generally associated with disease of the bladder neck and urethra while the former indicates a cause at a higher level in the urinary tract; however, this common distinction is not absolute. Haematuria that causes both patient and doctors to react quickly will be gross painless haematuria but the degree of haematuria may have little relationship to the seriousness of the cause and painful haematuria requires just as urgent an assessment as painless haematuria. The colour of the urine may range from bright red to tea-coloured and colours other than red may be misinterpreted by a patient to indicate strong or concentrated urine. There are a number of pigments and dyes that can cause confusion in interpreting the appearance of the urine, but on microscopy there are no red cells and tests for haemoglobin are negative. A number of drugs have the potential to cause haematuria either by affecting the coagulation system or by causing glomerular damage but the clinical history should establish the likelihood of such a cause.

The proportion of patients with bladder cancer that present with haematuria varies from 70% to 95% (Hendry et al., 1981). Malignant disease of the urothelium is diagnosed in up to 22% of patients with haematuria (Turner et al., 1977). Wallace and Harris (1965) emphasized that the earlier this sign was investigated, then the chances of cure were more likely to be increased.

Because the main delay appeared to be in hospital appointments and investigations, a haematuria diagnostic service was evaluated in two major London hospitals (Turner et al., 1977; Hendry et al., 1981) and in a district general hospital (Talbot, Bannister and Hills, 1984). The studies showed that between 57% and 85% of patients had their symptoms for less than a month whereas in a study in the US, Hopkins, Ford and Soloway (1983) found 46% had symptoms for less than a month before diagnosis. The claimed advantage of a haematuria service was the greater proportion of operable invasive tumours; this advantage was mainly in category T2 tumours though differences compared with routine cases were not as impressive as might have been expected and it thus remains to be demonstrated that a haematuria clinic is economically justifiable.

Microscopic haematuria

Asymptomatic microscopic haematuria is a relatively common clinical problem which is often incompletely investigated or accepted as within 'normal' range. Earlier counting chamber techniques led to a number of studies defining the number of red cells in the urine in the normal population. The full investigation of every person with any red cells is clearly impractical and an arbitrary level can be interpreted from the sensitivity of the dipstick method of testing: this method detects at least 20 000 rbc/ml, equivalent to 8 rbc/hpf but even this can lead to a number of people referred for investigation solely on the basis of a positive 'stix' test. Dipstick methods have virtually replaced other classic methods for urine screening and because of the ease of the test it is advisable to refer for urological assessment all asymptomatic patients who have at least two positive tests. An evaluation of dipstick reliability has been reported by Arm, Peile and Rainford (1986) and Arm *et al.* (1986). In a group of 100 patients in whom there was either known or suspected haematuria, the dipstick results were compared with cell counts on unspun urine under phase contrast microscopy. The patients were divided into three groups: (i) Dipstick consistently negative, (ii) Dipstick trace only, (iii) Dipstick more than a trace. In the second group, i.e. those where there is most doubt as to the significance of the finding, 22 of 27 patients had an identifiable source of bleeding, 3 were negative on routine tests (but no renal biopsy), 1 had exercise related haematuria and 1 had an inflamed ureteric orifice that remained unexplained. This study endorsed the view that a persistent trace dipstick reading merits further investigation.

In an attempt to distinguish upper from lower urinary tract bleeding, Birch and Fairley (1979) advocated the use of phase contrast microscopy to examine the urine. Red cells that arise via glomerular lesions are dysmorphic and this finding should lead to a renal biopsy. When the red cells are not dysmorphic, further radiological and urological screening is indicated.

In practical terms, up to 10% of cases with microscopic red cells in the urine will prove to have a bladder cancer (Carson, Segura and Greene, 1979; Golin and Howard, 1980; Gillat and O'Reilly, 1987).

Other presentations

Bladder cancers may mimic almost any symptom of a urinary tract disorder. Thus 'cystitis', especially in a male over the age of 50, is highly suspicious. Infection is a common association with bladder cancer (approximately 40%) and causes symptoms of bladder irritation. A patient with outflow urinary tract symptoms thought to be due to prostatic enlargement may have an associated tumour, either an entirely chance finding or an aggressive tumour already involving the prostate. The tumour may have infiltrated to the extent of reducing bladder capacity or may be so proliferative as to fill the bladder. A bladder tumour overlying or infiltrating a ureteric orifice may present with renal and/or ureteric pain. Rarely, the disease may be so advanced and present with anaemia and weight loss.

Pain might be thought to be a feature of advanced invasive cancer and this may occasionally be true. It is, however, also a common association with carcinoma-in-situ. Riddle *et al.* (1976) reported that patients with flat carcinoma-in-situ commonly had a dull but persistent ill-defined pain that could be either suprapubic, penile or perineal.

Dipstick urinalysis by a general practitioner has been discussed, but patient screening either because of a known industrial risk or as a routine health check may prove positive. Other patients with a known risk, such as bilharziasis or analgesic (phenacetin) abuse, may have positive urine test for blood. The use of dipstick screening is easy and highly cost effective; the use of exfoliative cytology should be limited to the known high-risk group, i.e. those exposed to a known bladder carcinogen.

Diagnostic and staging procedures

Imaging techniques

Intravenous urography
Sherwood in 1983 wrote that 'the adult patient with haematuria needs a cystoscopy to find his bladder tumour, not an IVU (which will probably miss it)'. This

comment emphasizes the limitations of the procedure and reminds the clinician that it is the information about the upper urinary tract that is the main value of an IVU. Thus an IVU is essential to exclude a second, upper tract transitional-cell carcinoma and will give information about the presence or absence of obstruction. Dilatation of the ureter usually indicates that the tumour in the bladder is invading muscle in the region of the ureteric orifice. If the kidney is non-functioning, a tumour of the renal pelvis or ureter cannot be excluded and further investigation by ultrasound CT and possibly an antegrade pyelogram may be needed. Any problem relating to the state of the upper urinary tract must be resolved before the management of a bladder lesion can be planned. It is for this reason that an IVU precedes cystoscopy in the sequence of investigations.

The bladder film of the IVU may show a filling defect and give an indication of the size of the tumour but any information on tumour infiltration can only be an inspired guess.

Calcification over the tumour usually indicates an invasive high-grade lesion. A large 'prostate' shadow may hide a lesion though these are sometimes seen retrospectively on the post-micturition films.

Special techniques of double contrast cystography using sterile barium are rarely indicated unless there is suspicion about the contents of a diverticulum, and even this has largely been superseded by CT.

Ultrasound

Ultrasound is increasingly used as an alternative to an IVU in screening the urinary tract of a patient with prostatism (Fidas *et al.*, 1987). This may detect a bladder tumour incidentally but transabdominal ultrasound as a method of diagnosing and staging bladder tumours is of little practical value. Perurethral ultrasound provides better anatomical detail and can be used in staging (Braeckman *et al.*, 1987); it does not replace standard methods.

Computed tomography

It had been hoped that CT would provide the precision to preoperative assessment of a bladder tumour that is lacking from the time honoured bimanual examination. Localized thickening or flattening of the bladder wall, irregularity of the line between the wall and perivesical fat are described as features of invasion but the extent of the invasion is imprecise and cannot separate a T2 from T3a tumour. Invasion to the extent of a T4 tumour is usually reliable though even this should not be used as a decision for non-operability since CT tends to overstage the tumour.

Thus CT at best is only useful as an estimate of tumour size and stage. CT to assess pelvic lymphadenopathy may be more accurate than lymphography and it has the advantage of identifying internal iliac and obturator nodes. However, CT, as with any other imaging technique can only show distortion or overall enlargement of the nodes and cannot evaluate microscopic metastases.

Magnetic resonance imaging

Advances in the technology of MRI are such that its use in staging of bladder and other pelvic tumours may soon offer advantages over conventional techniques.

Cytology

Examination of the urine as a diagnostic procedure was described by Papanicolaou and Marshall in 1945. The value of this procedure depends on the degree of cellular dysplasia of the tumour: low-grade tumours are often accompanied by negative urinary cytology and cannot therefore be used as a substitute for regular cystoscopy in the follow-up of a patient who has an established tumour. By contrast, the high-grade tumour and especially the patient with carcinoma-in-situ will readily shed tumour cells but it is the group of patients in whom conventional follow-up will be close and early radical treatment considered.

One of the most important groups to benefit from screening by urinary cytology is those who have been exposed to an industrial carcinogen (Glashan, Wijesinghe and Rileym, 1981).

The technique of flow cytometry has been developed in an effort to quantify the cellular abnormality in terms of grade and prognosis. The method provides information about the rate of cell division by measuring abnormal levels of DNA per cell and so gives an accurate profile of a tumour (Hadjissotiriou et al., 1987). Flow cytometry analysis is being used in a variety of tumour studies and as the technique becomes more readily available so it is expected that it will prove to be useful both in screening and for histopathological grading because of the speed, objectivity and reproducibility of the method.

Cystoscopy, biopsy and bimanual examination under anaesthetic

The most important diagnostic procedure in bladder cancer remains a cystoscopy and biopsy of the tumour. Current endoscopic equipment gives a perfect view of the bladder mucosa though bleeding or infection may restrict the clarity. The tumour is assessed in size and gross appearance; the depth of penetration is assessed from a bimanual examination with the patient fully relaxed under anaesthesia.

The biopsy is usually obtained with the resectoscope with the intention of obtaining tissue from the tumour base to determine the depth of muscle penetration. A superficial papillary tumour may be so small that it is completely removed by cup-biopsy forceps: the base is then diathermized.

Random biopsy and prognostic factors

At the time of the first assessment it is essential to look closely at the apparently normal bladder mucosa and any area that looks red, or raised, or velvety should be biopsied and examined separately. Schade and Swinney (1973) noted a wide range of urothelial atypia in random biopsies taken from bladders taken with established invasive tumours. Others have studied the extent of urothelial changes in the form of bladder maps (Koss, Nakanishi and Freed, 1977). In a study of 154 patients with bladder cancer, Wallace et al. (1979) detected carcinoma-in-situ in 4.5% of biopsies from normal-looking mucosa, in 14% of those where the biopsy was from flat red mucosa and in 42% where the mucosa was granular or velvety. In a prospective study of new patients with superficial bladder cancer the following prognostic factors were monitored: tumour size, number of tumours, grade and histology from random biopsies of normal urothelium (Smith et al., 1983). The strongest predictor of recurrence was any pathological change in the random biopsy (i.e. any degree of either dysplasia or carcinoma-in-situ). Poor histological grade was a strong predictor of subsequent muscle invasion. Others have confirmed this predictive role for random bladder biopsies (Wolfe, Olsen and Hojgaard, 1985) but it must be emphasized that there are considerable differences amongst pathologists as to the definition of dysplasia and even carcinoma-in-situ.

Summary

Essential requirements in the diagnosis and assessment of a patient with bladder cancer are intravenous urogram, cystoscopy, biopsy and examination under anaesthesia. Added precision to the grade and stage and prognosis can be obtained from random biopsies and from flow cytometry but these investigations require both the facilities and the expertise. None of the other imaging techniques has established a place in routine practice and there is no substitute for good histopathology, good biopsy sampling in determining the stage of the tumour (Chisholm et al., 1980).

Management

Bladder cancer has been staged according to two systems – the Jewett–Strong–Marshall system and the TNM system. Both have endeavoured to identify factors, mainly depth of penetration of the tumour, that warrant separate description because of the significant difference in prognosis.

The Jewett and Strong (1946) and Marshall (1952) classification was based on studies of autopsy and cystectomy specimens: thus Stage O involved epithelium only, Stage A – lamina propria, Stage B1 – superficial bladder muscle, B2 – penetration to deep layer of bladder muscle and C involved perivesical fat. The distinction between B1 and B2 was due to the remarkable prognostic advantage for cystectomy patients when tumour invasion was confined to the inner half of the muscle wall.

The TNM system, developed in 1950, described not only the primary tumour (T) but lymph nodes (N) and metastases (M) (Wallace, Chisholm and Hendry, 1975). Criticized as unnecessarily complex, the TNM does give a better indication of size and extent of the disease but as with all classifications there is debate about the validity of some of the definitions (Chisholm et al., 1980). Nevertheless, Stages O and A are comparable to Ta, T1, Stages B1 and B2, comparable to T2 and T3a and Stage C with T3b.

In 1952, Melicow and Hollowell introduced the term carcinoma-in-situ for epithelial malignancy and this led to important changes in the understanding of the natural history of bladder cancer. The relevance of in situ change not only in apparently normal looking urothelium but in the prostatic ducts and urethra has led to a sharper awareness of the influence of this form of the disease on prognosis. Also, because of its unpredictable and often aggressive nature, it is suggested that this form of bladder cancer be given separate status in any discussion.

Thus, from a management point of view there are three main treatment groups:

1. Superficial bladder cancer: Ta, T1 (or O, A)
2. Carcinoma-in-situ: TIS or CIS
3. Invasive (into bladder muscle): T2, T3a, T3b (or B1, B2, C)

Superficial bladder cancer (Ta, T1)

Standard treatment
The majority of bladder cancers are Ta, T1 and while most of these are easy to treat, the development of further tumours occurs in about 70% and a significant proportion of these new tumours, or recurrences, have a higher grade of malignancy than the original lesion (Heney et al., 1982; Pocock et al., 1982).

The reported mortality from bladder cancer presenting with superficial tumours is 4–12% at 5 years; the overall survival rate following transurethral resection is about 70% (Williams, Hammonds and Saunders, 1977). Thus superficial bladder cancer must be regarded as a potentially dangerous tumour and a programme of regular follow-up is essential. Great efforts have been made to identify some characteristic of the initial tumour that might indicate the risk of recurrence (Heney *et al.*, 1982; Pocock *et al.*, 1982); grade of the tumour is undoubtedly the most important but size and multiplicity are also relevant risk factors. It is also of note that if the first follow-up cystoscopy at 3 months is clear then this is also a very favourable prognostic factor.

Transurethral resection is the basis of treatment for all apparently superficial bladder tumours. The resection achieves not only removal of the exophytic tumour but provides adequate tissue, including some superficial muscle, for the pathologist to describe accurately the level of tumour penetration. Review of the material with the pathologist is essential and if it is confirmed that the tumour is either pTa or pTl then a regular programme of follow-up is all that is required.

If there are multiple tumours or a very large but apparently superficial tumour, this is best removed using the continuous flow resectoscope so that continuous vision of the area is sustained and the risk of perforating the bladder wall is minimized.

If the resection is to be anything more than two to three cuts, it is recommended that the irrigation solution is isotonic, e.g. 1.5% glycine.

It is the opinion of this author that the initial management of a superficial lesion is incomplete unless random biopsies from apparently normal mucosa are taken; it is probable that two biopsies are adequate, one within 2 cm of the primary lesion and the other more distant. Any visible mucosal abnormality should also be biopsied. These biopsies are also reviewed with the pathologist and if severe dysplasia or CIS is diagnosed this raises the index of suspicion of risk of recurrence and further biopsies should be taken at the first 3-month review; should these also prove to be abnormal then some form of intravesical treatment is recommended.

The question of how long should a patient be followed with check cystoscopies is often asked but there is no simple answer. Five tumour-free years is the minimum; exceptions are made for the frail and those with other medical problems. All patients who smoke must be advised that they are only adding to their recurrence risk.

Prophylaxis with intravesical chemotherapy
The idea that the intravesical instillation of a chemotherapeutic agent might reduce the recurrence rate was first explored by Jones and Swinney (1961) who used thiotepa. Though there was some beneficial effect there were also reports of myelosuppression from thiotepa absorption. Since then, many intravesical agents have been studied in an attempt to find the optimum drug. Although a number of studies confirm that thiotepa, after resection of the tumour, reduced recurrence rates, the dose, its frequency of use and the overall cost effectiveness remained in doubt. A Medical Research Council study compared the effect of a single instillation of thiotepa at the time of primary treatment, with five instillations at 3-month intervals, with a control of no instillation and found no benefit from thiotepa to justify its use in either regime (MRC Working Party on Urological Cancer, 1985).

Mitomycin C (MMC) was first used for superficial bladder cancer in Japan and the US. Most of the early data showed that it was an effective drug against existing superficial tumours but it was also expensive and there was initial reluctance to use it for tumour prophylaxis. In 1983 both Huland and Otto and Devonec *et al.* reported an impressive advantage for prophylactic MMC, compared to a non-treatment group after transurethral resection of the tumour. Tumour progression rates following MMC have shown wide variations but Smith *et al.* (1986) showed that the progression rate after MMC was similar to that with Epodyl and Methotrexate.

In 1984, the Medical Research Council undertook a randomized trial of prophylactic MMC using the same protocol as for the thiotepa study; no results have been published but an interim analysis indicates a prophylactic value for MMC.

Other chemotherapeutic agents have been studied. Fitzpatrick *et al.* (1979) showed that Epodyl does have long-term prophylactic value but once a recurrence develops then an alternative treatment is required. Zincke *et al.* (1983) showed that prophylactic Adriamycin reduced tumour recurrence from 81% in the placebo group to 38% in the treated group. Results with a range of other chemotherapeutic agents have been less impressive and show little or no advantages between MMC, thiotepa, and Epodyl and Adriamycin in prophylaxis.

Recently, BCG has been shown to be highly effective both in prophylaxis and in treatment and this therapeutic approach is discussed in the next section.

Two aspects of intravesical therapy require comment. The first is the economic aspect of the treatment. At least 30% of patients with superficial transitional-cell carcinoma never have any further recurrence and if these could be identified then much unnecessary treatment could be saved. With this in mind, the Medical Research Council have begun a comparison of Epodyl and MMC given only to those at the time of their first recurrence. The second aspect of intravesical therapy concerns the large amount of data that is uncontrolled. Few studies allow reasonable comparison and many are uninterpretable. The need for properly controlled clinical trials remains as important as ever.

Treatment with either intravesical chemotherapy or BCG
In a small proportion of patients with superficial bladder cancer either their extent or their rate and number of recurrences defy even the expert resectionist. It is in this highly selected group that the previously described chemotherapeutic agents have also been studied and shown to be effective. For example, MacFarlane and Tolley (1985) used MMC for superficial tumours no longer readily controlled endoscopically and reported a complete response rate of 40%. There is, however, no suggestion that these agents should replace proper endoscopic methods as primary treatment. Since there are no adequate comparative data, it is not possible to rank these agents in an order of efficacy; indeed, most reviews comment that the results are suprisingly uniform (Messing and deKernion, 1985) but it is also evident that case selection has a major influence on results and their interpretation.

In recent years intravesical BCG has been introduced as an alternative to intravesical chemotherapy (Morales, Eidinger and Bruce, 1976).

Initial results were varied but with increasing experience it appears that BCG may well give the best results of any intravesical treatment and it also appears that it is especially effective in treating urothelial dysplasia and/or CIS (Droller, 1986). In a randomized prospective study comparing TUR alone with TUR plus BCG for recurrent superficial tumours, the addition of BCG significantly reduced the number of recurrent tumours and increased the mean time to recurrence from 3 months to 18 months (Herr *et al.*, 1985). BCG is effective both in treatment and prophylaxis of Ta, Tl tumours and CIS. Complete responses to treatment of Ta, Tl tumours has been reported in 40 to 60%, and to treatment of CIS in 42 to 71% and complete prophylaxis in 48 to 100% (Morales, 1984; Droller, 1986). Haaff *et al.*, 1986 reported a 46% response rate for superficial papillary tumours from a single course but if they added a second course for the treatment failures, the cumulative rate was 69%. There is now evidence to suggest that if a patient fails to respond to two courses then the response to any further BCG is low and alternative therapy should be considered (Catalona *et al.*, 1987). The optimal regime for BCG prophylaxis has yet to be determined but there is no evidence so far to suggest that 3-months prophylaxis is better than the standard 6-week course of instillation.

It is important to be aware that a wide range of complications has now been reported – most commonly cystitis and haematuria; it is even more important to be aware that a fever may be an early warning of progressive systemic BCG infection which will require hospitalization and anti-tuberculosis therapy (Lamm *et al.*, 1989).

Urologists are in the best position to carry out intravesical treatment and especially if the treatments are linked with a check cystoscopy. However, close monitoring of response to early recognition of tumour progression make these treatments full of risks for those not fully familiar with this rapidly developing subject.

Carcinoma-in-situ (CIS)

The clinical presentation of CIS and the diagnostic problems including interpretation of pathological and cytological material, show considerable differences from other tumours of the bladder (Melicow 1952; Koss, Nakanishi and Freed, 1977; Utz *et al.*, 1980). The increasing use of endoscopic mucosal biopsy from both apparently normal and suspicious areas of bladder epithelium has produced a dilemma in treatment when the abnormalities of CIS are found. There is also a genuine dilemma for the pathologists many of whom disagree over the diagnosis of CIS and the varying degrees of epithelial dysplasia (Webb, 1985).

From a practical point of view CIS will be discussed under four headings.

Primary CIS

This lesion has been called flat intra-epithelial neoplasia (Barlebo, Sorensen and Ohlson, 1972) or flat carcinoma-in-situ (Riddle *et al.*, 1976) and refers to CIS that occurs in a bladder where there is no associated exophytic tumour and no previous history of urothelial tumour. The presentation of these patients is commonly associated with outflow tract obstructive symptoms and often with haematuria. Many of these patients have an ill-defined pain either suprapubic, penile or perineal (Riddle *et al.*, 1976). Urinary cytology is an important test in the detection of these patients. Endoscopically, the epithelium may be inflamed and oedematous, so-called 'malignant cystitis', but the diagnosis has been made in some with entirely normal appearing mucosa. Multiple mucosal biopsies are essential to establish the diagnosis.

The management dilemma has arisen from the fact that CIS, in a high proportion of patients, progresses to invasive disease. It is also evident that it is not radiosensitive and Riddle *et al.* (1976) concluded that where there is widespread disease, cystectomy is the best choice; for lesions that are localized, the combination of diathermy with or without intravesical chemotherapy is recommended. Recently, experience with BCG has shown that this may be the best initial treatment for CIS (Droller, 1986).

CIS associated with invasive bladder cancer
In 1968 Schade and Swinney reported their findings in mucosal biopsies taken from 100 cases of invasive bladder cancer: the mucosa was normal in only 5, CIS occurred in 30, and cellular atypia in 42 and the remainder had varying degrees of metaplasia, inflammation and cystitis glandularis. This high incidence of associated urothelial abnormalities emphasized the field change in bladder cancer and hastened the demise of partial cystectomy for invasive tumours.

CIS associated with superficial bladder cancer
Multiple mucosal biopsies have also been responsible for the increased awareness of urothelial abnormalities even in patients with a superficial Ta, Tl lesion (Wallace *et al.*, 1979; Smith *et al.*, 1983).

The practical significance of a positive random biopsy is that not only must the follow-up be meticulous but the patient should be considered for some form of intravesical treatment. The decision will depend upon the extent of the field change and also the pathological description. It is probable that there are no real differences between severe dysplasia and CIS so that if the changes are extensive, the patient would be of high risk and a course of intravesical BCG would be the treatment of choice. Lesser degrees of cellular atypia and limited focal change constitute a lower risk and such a patient would be suitable for either MMC or Epodyl given after the check cystoscopy.

CIS can be a sinister finding in these patients and both patient and urologist may be unwilling to adopt aggressive treatment for a condition which is difficult to see and may cause few symptoms. A conservative approach is justifiable only if there is regular 3-monthly follow-up. If there is any evidence of progression and invasion despite intravesical therapy then cystectomy remains the treatment of choice (Stanisic *et al.*, 1987).

CIS in prostatic ducts (and prostatic urethra)
Prostatic involvement by transitional-cell carcinoma is not a single entity and can only be described in histological detail on the basis of an adequate TUR biopsy.

The finding of CIS of the prostatic ducts and prostatic urethra when there is similar involvement in the bladder was reported by Melicow and Hollowell (1952). The importance of this observation is twofold: the first is that intravesical therapy for CIS will be inappropriate and the second is that a cystectomy for invasive bladder cancer must take account of the presence of CIS both in the bladder and in the urethra (Seemayer *et al.*, 1975). There is thus a good case to be made for the routine biopsy of the prostatic urethra and suburethral prostatic tissue as a staging procedure in patients with bladder CIS as well as high-grade bladder tumour (Mahadevia, Koss and Tar, 1986).

It has also been observed that CIS and invasive transitional-cell cancer originating from the periurethral prostatic ducts can occur without associated bladder tumours (Kopelson *et al.*, 1978; Sawczuk *et al.*, 1985).

The existence of a third variant, the penetration of the prostate by an infiltrating bladder cancer (pT4a), indicates that a clear distinction should be made between these different forms of transitional-cell carcinoma involving the prostate since their management and prognosis are different (Chibber *et al.*, 1981; Wolfe and Lloyd-Davies, 1981).

Invasive transitional-cell carcinoma (T2, T3a, T3b)

It would be an understatement to say that there was uncertainty as to the best form of treatment for bladder cancer, once it has invaded bladder muscle, i.e. T2, T3a, T3b. The reason for this uncertainty lies in the fact that most of the so-called standard treatments (radical cystectomy, radiotherapy or combination of these two) all give approximately the same 5-year survival data (20–40%). However, with selection, it is possible to give a bias towards one or the other treatment. It is also true that better staging and surgical technique make it impossible to compare reports of current surgical series with earlier results. Even where clinical trials have been carried out, the problems of selection and the interpretation of data prevent any convincing conclusion from being made.

Primary radical cystectomy
The feasibility of radical cystectomy for bladder cancer began in about 1950 when the ileal conduit became an acceptable form of urinary diversion. Prior to this, the operative mortality had been anything from 15% to 40% and the hazards of urinary diversion into the sigmoid colon created a high incidence of morbidity. In 1962, Whitmore and Marshall recommended the inclusion of regional node dissection in an attempt to improve local control.

Whitmore (1980) has reviewed the experience of the Memorial Sloan–Kettering Cancer Centre experience throughout this period. Between 1949 and 1959, primary cystectomy alone was carried out on 137 patients. At 5 years 33% were alive with no evidence of disease, 48% died of tumour and 18% died without recurrence. It was also evident from this experience and from others, that even microscopic lymph node disease indicated a very poor prognosis. Thus, Smith and Whitmore (1981) reported that only 7% of 134 patients treated by radical cystectomy and node dissection with positive lymph nodes survived 5 years. The actuarial survival ranged from 7 months when nodes above the common iliac bifurcation were involved to 22 months for a single node metastasis. This gloomy experience led urologists to explore the possibilities of surgery combined with radiotherapy, see later.

However, the role of radiotherapy in the management of bladder cancer has been sharply questioned in recent years (Radwin, 1980) and some urologists have continued to prefer radical cystectomy alone as the treatment of choice for invasive bladder cancer. In a review of 197 consecutive patients treated between 1971 and 1982, both with and without preoperative radiotherapy, Skinner and Lieskovsky (1984) found no advantages for the radiotherapy-treated group; their overall results were 75% 5-year survival rate, free of tumour for pT2 and pT3a disease, and 44% pT3a and pT3b disease. Montie, Straffon and Stewart (1984) also reviewed their cystectomy alone results and found 40% 5-year survival rate for T3a, T3b, T4a patients and claimed these to be comparable to other series that combined surgery with radiotherapy.

The major disadvantage of cystectomy – the need for a urinary diversion – has led to a surge in the use of continent ileostomy (e.g. Kock pouch) and other recontructive techniques. The reader is referred elsewhere for update reviews and descriptions of these procedures (Lilien and Camey 1984; Ashken, 1987; Skinner, Boyd and Lieskovsky, 1988) as well as the techniques for radical cystectomy (Montie, 1983).

The combination of radiotherapy with surgery was developed in the hope that this would lead to improved results by, at least, controlling local recurrence. Whitmore (1980) in his review of different treatments was able to show an improvement in the 5-year survival rate from 33% to 42% with combination treatment; he claimed that because the data were from the same institution many of the selection variables were minimized. However, there remains a danger in comparing historical data especially when there are evident improvements in operative technique.

Different preoperative radiotherapy regimes have been tried, e.g. 6000 cGy in 30 fractions over 6 weeks, 4000 cGy in 20 fractions over 4 weeks, 2000 cGy in 5 fractions over 1 week.

The highest dose must be considered a definitive radical course with surgery reserved for treatment failure (see later). The debate as to whether any of these preoperative regimes has been beneficial has not been resolved in the few clinical trials that have attempted a comparison (Prout, Slack and Bross, 1971; Miller, 1977; Anderstrom et al., 1983). A general conclusion by Montie, Straffon and Stewart (1984) was that there appears to be no major differences between cystectomy with or without radiotherapy. By contrast Plowman (1985) reviewed similar large Dutch, British and American studies and concluded that all of the 5-year survival figures showed an improved survival with invasive bladder cancer after combined treatment when compared with the historical treatment data base.

Primary radical radiotherapy

The proponents of radical radiotherapy as primary treatment for invasive bladder cancer maintain that since there are no major differences between the results of surgery or preoperative radiotherapy plus surgery or radiotherapy alone, then at least the latter offers the chance for the patient to retain the bladder and avoid the problem of urinary diversion. Comparison of the results of these three main lines of treatment is almost impossible because no such comparative study has been made.

Reference has been made to comparisons between preoperative radiotherapy plus cystectomy with cystectomy alone. The main clinical trial of these treatments in the UK was undertaken by the Institute of Urology and the Royal Marsden Hospital (Bloom et al., 1982). This study took 10 years to accrue 199 patients from 8 centres. The corrected 5-year survivals were 38% for the combined treatment and 29% for radiotherapy alone ($P = 0.2$). This trend towards an advantage for combined treatment was greater in the under 65 age group so that the combined treatment for this group has become a popular approach. Nevertheless, similar survival rates after radical radiotherapy have been reported from the London Hospital (Blandy et al., 1980) and Edinburgh (Duncan and Quilty, 1986) so that for many urologists there is no convincing evidence that makes one form of treatment better than the other. Comparisons of mortality, morbidity, local recurrence and distant recurrence are approximately similar.

The term 'salvage cystectomy' has come to mean cystectomy either for persistent or recurrent tumour or for bladder symptoms after a full course of radiotherapy. Once again, selection features strongly in determining when and who should have a salvage cystectomy. Indeed, Smith et al. (1985) showed that by no means all patients whose tumour failed to respond to radiotherapy would require a cystectomy and many were managed well by more conservative endoscopic methods. The claim that salvage cystectomy is associated with unnecessarily high morbidity has not been borne out in recent reports (Hope-Stone *et al.*, 1981; Freiha and Faysal, 1983; Quilty *et al.*, 1986).

Neo-adjuvant chemotherapy

As with many other solid tumours, disappointment in the various forms of conventional treatment has led to the study of a range of systemic chemotherapeutic agents. Also, part of this disappointment has arisen from the inescapable fact that apparently localized tumours have often spread beyond the limits of surgical excision or field of radiotherapy at the time of primary treatment.

Among the most active drugs are cisplatin, methotrexate, cyclophosphamide, Adriamycin and 5-fluorouracil (Loening, 1984). In single agent studies, these agents give objective response rates of 20–40%. Unfortunately, complete responses are few (0–10%) and often only of short duration. Combination chemotherapy regimens have generally produced response rates higher than for single agents alone. Regimens containing Adriamycin without cisplatin are no more effective than Adriamycin alone (Yagoda, 1983). There is some evidence that cisplatin and Adriamycin, with or without cyclophosphamide may be more active than cisplatin alone. The combination of cisplatin and methotrexate achieved a 68% objective response rate and 21% complete remission in patients with recurrent or metastatic transitional-cell carcinoma (Carmichael *et al.*, 1985).

Using the formidable combination of methotrexate, vincristine, Adriamycin and cisplatin (M-VAC) Sternberg *et al.* (1985) reported a complete clinical remission in 18 of 45 patients (40%) with an overall response rate of 67%. The side-effects from these drugs are considerable and despite these promising results, it remains uncertain whether chemotherapy offers an acceptable palliation or useful long-term benefits in patients with metastatic carcinoma of the bladder.

The fact that there is such a measurable response rate has led to a number of studies using chemotherapy prior to either radical radiotherapy or radical cystectomy, usually with cisplatin and methotrexate. Pearson and Raghavan (1985) using cisplatin only, recorded a 76% symptomatic improvement with a 60% objective response; the further experience and a full review of neo-adjuvant chemotherapy has recently been reported by Raghavan (1988). An alternative approach giving concurrent cisplatin and radiotherapy for high stage and high-grade cancers (T3b, T4a) achieved a 75% downstaging and 76% overall survival at 3-year median follow-up; these results of a pilot study have now been followed by a collaborative randomized trial that is in progress in Canada.

To date, no prospective randomized trial of systemic neo-adjuvant chemotherapy has been completed. There remains considerable controversy over the merits of different protocols and different combinations and it must be emphasized that until such studies are completed these new approaches can only be regarded as experimental.

Palliative treatment

Perhaps the most difficult surgical decisions in bladder cancer arise either in those who present with advanced incurable disease or whose disease progresses after primary definitive treatment. At one extreme is the patient whose bladder tumour is so extensive as to cause obstructive uraemia; at the other is the patient whose definitive radiotherapy has removed all evidence of cancer yet he/she has intolerable urinary frequency and haematuria as a result of bladder contraction and radiotherapy telangiectasia. For the former, relief of the obstruction may not be the best decision if the patient is then left to face untreatable bladder symptoms or painful metastases. For the latter, a cystectomy and urinary diversion may be the only way to ensure a tolerable quality of life. The risks of such palliative surgery need to be weighed against that quality of life.

The choice of palliation for these and similar clinical problems requires the expertise of a specialist centre for only experience can tell the relative merits of a group of not very satisfactory options. This subject has been well reviewed by Kurth (1985) and is strongly recommended to the reader seeking a detailed analysis of the various forms of palliative treatment.

References

Anderstrom, C., Johansson, S., Nilsson, S. *et al.* (1983) A prospective randomized study of pre-operative irradiation with cystectomy or cystectomy alone for invasive bladder carcinoma. *European Urology*, **9**, 142–147

Arm, J. P., Peile, E. B. and Rainford, D. J. (1986) Significance of dipstick haematuria 2. Correlation with pathology. *British Journal of Urology*, **58**, 218–223

Arm, J. P., Peile, E. B., Rainford, D. J. *et al*, (1986) Significance of dipstick haematuria 1. Correlation with microscopy of the urine. *British Journal of Urology*, **58**, 211–217

Ashken, M. H. (1987) Stomas continent and incontinent. *British Journal of Urology*, **59**, 203–207

Barlebo, H., Sorensen, B. L and Ohlsen, A. S. (1972) Carcinoma-in-situ of the urinary bladder: flat intra-epithelial neoplasia. *Scandinavian Journal of Urology and Nephrology*, **6**, 213–223

BAUS Subcommittee on Industrial Bladder Cancer (1988) Occupational bladder cancer: A guide for clinicians. *British Journal of Urology*, **61**, 183–191

Birch, D. E. and Fairley, K. F. (1979) Haematuria – glomerular or non-glomerular? *Lancet*, **ii**, 845–846

Blandy, J. P., England, H. R., Evans, S. J. W. *et al.* (1980) T3 Bladder cancer – the case for salvage cystectomy. *British Journal of Urology*, **52**, 506–510

Bloom, H. J. G., Hendry, W. F., Wallace, D. M. and Skeet, R. G. (1982) Treatment of T3 bladder cancer, controlled trial of preoperative radiotherapy and radical cystectomy versus radical radiotherapy. *British Journal of Urology*, **54**, 136–151

Braeckman, J., Keuppens, F., Chaban, M. and Denis, L. (1987) Ultrasound in urological oncology. *European Journal of Surgical Oncology*, **13**, 475–483

Carmichael, J., Cornbleet, M. A., MacDougall, R. H. *et al.* (1985) Cis-platin and methotrexate in the treatment of transitional cell carcinoma of the urinary tract. *British Journal of Urology*, **57**, 299–302

Carson, C. C., Segura, J. W. and Greene, L. F. (1979) Clinical importance of microhematuria. *Journal of American Medical Association*, **241**, 149–150

Catalona, W. J., Hudson, M. A., Gillen, D. P. *et al.* (1987) Risks and benefits of repeated courses of intravesical Bacillus Calmette-Guérin therapy for superficial bladder cancer. *Journal of Urology*, **137**, 220–224

Chibber, P. J., McIntyre, M. A., Hindmarsh, J. R. *et al.* (1981) Transitional cell carcinoma involving the prostate. *British Journal of Urology*, **53**, 605–609

Chisholm, G. D., Hindmarsh, J. R., Howatson, A. G. *et al.* (1980) TNM (1987) in bladder cancer: use and abuse. *British Journal of Urology*, **52**, 500–505

Devesa, S. S. and Silverman, D. T. (1978) Cancer incidence and mortality trends in United States. *Journal of National Cancer Institute*, **60**, 545–571

Devonec, M., Bouvier, R., Sarkissian, J. *et al.* (1983) Intravesical instillation of mitomycin C in the prophylactic treatment of recurring superficial transitional cell carcinoma of the bladder. *British Journal of Urology*, **55**, 382–385

Droller, M. J. (1986) Bacillus Calmette-Guérin in the management of bladder cancer. *Journal of Urology*, **135**, 331–333

Duncan, W. and Quilty, P. M. (1986) The results of a series of 963 patients with transitional cell carcinoma of the urinary bladder previously treated by radical megavoltage X-ray therapy. *Radiotherapy and Oncology*, **7**, 299–310

Fidas, A., Mackinlay, J. Y., Wild, S. R. and Chisholm, G. D. (1987) Ultrasound as an alternative to intravenous urography in prostatism. *Clinical Radiology*, **38**, 479–482

Fitzpatrick, J. K., Khan, O., Oliver. R. T. D. and Riddle, P. R. (1979) Long-term follow-up in patients with superficial bladder tumours treated with intravesical Epodyl. *British Journal of Urology*, **51**, 545–548

Freiha, F. S and Faysal, M. H. (1983) Salvage cystectomy. *Urology*, **22**, 496–498

Gillat, D. A. and O'Reilly, P. H. (1987) Haematuria analysed – a prospective study. *Journal of the Royal Society of Medicine*, **80**, 559–560

Glashan, R. W., Wijesinghe, D. P. and Rileym, A. (1981) The early changes in the development of bladder cancers in patients exposed to known industrial carcinogens. *British Journal of Urology*, **53**, 571–577

Golin, A. L. and Howard, R. S. (1980) Asymptomatic microscopic hematuria. *Journal of Urology*, **124**, 389–391

Haaff, E. O., Dresner, S. M., Ratliff, T. L. and Catalona, W. J. (1986) Two courses of intravesical Bacillus Calmette-Guérin for transitional cell carcinoma of the bladder. *Journal of Urology*, **136**, 820–824

Hadjissotiriou, G. G., Green, D. K., Smith, G. *et al.* (1987) Bladder cancer flow cytometry profiles in relation to histological grade and stage. *British Journal of Urology*, **60**, 239–247

Hendry, W. F., Manning, N., Perry, N. M. *et al.* (1981) The effects of a haematuria service on early diagnosis of bladder cancer. In *Bladder Cancer, Principles of Combination Therapy* (eds. R. T. D. Oliver, W. F. Hendry and H. J. G. Bloom), Butterworths, London, pp. 19–25

Heney, N. M., Nocks, B. N., Daly, J. J. *et al.* (1982) Ta and Tl bladder cancer: location, recurrence and progression. *Journal of Urology*, **54**, 152–157

Herr, H. W., Pinsky, C. M., Whitmore, W. F. *et al.* (1985) Experience with intravesical Bacillus Calmette-Guérin therapy of superficial bladder tumours. *Urology*, **25**, 119–123

Hicks, R. M. (1982) The development of bladder cancer. In *Scientific Foundations of Urology* 2nd edn, (eds. G. D. Chisholm and D. I. Williams), Heinemann Medical, London, pp. 711–722

Hope-Stone, H. F., Blandy, J. P., Oliver, R. T.D. and England, H. (1981) Radical radiotherapy and salvage cystectomy in the treatment of invasive carcinoma of the bladder. In *Bladder Cancer: Principles of Combination Therapy* (eds. R. T. D. Oliver, W. F. Hendry and H. J. B. Bloom), Butterworths, London, pp. 127–138

Hopkins, S. C., Ford, K. S. and Soloway, M. S. (1983) Invasive bladder cancer: support for screening. *Journal of Urology*, **130**, 61–63

Huland, H. and Otto, U. (1983) Mitomycin instillation to prevent recurrence of superficial bladder carcinoma. *European Urology*, **9**, 84–86

Jewett, H. J. and Strong, G. H. (1946) Infiltrating carcinoma of the bladder: Relation of depth of penetration of the bladder wall to incidence of local extension and metastases. *Journal of Urology*, **55**, 366–372

Jones, H. C. and Swinney, J. (1961) Thiotepa in the treatment of tumours of the bladder. *Lancet*, **ii**, 615–618

Kopelson, G., Harisiadis, I., Romas, N. A. *et al.* (1978) Periurethral prostatic duct carcinoma. *Cancer*, **42**, 2894–2902

Koss, L. G., Nakanishi, I and Freed, S. Z. (1977) Nonpapillary carcinoma in situ and atypical hyperplasia in cancerous bladders. Further studies of surgically removed bladders by mapping. *Urology*, **9**, 422–455

Kurth, K. H. (1985) Palliative treatment. In *Bladder Cancer* (eds. E. J. Zingg and D. M. A. Wallace), Springer-Verlag, Heidelberg, pp. 263–297

Lamm, D. L., Steg, A., Bocon-Gibod, L. *et al.* (1989) Complications of Bacillus Calmette-Guérin immunotherapy: review of 2603 patients and comparison of chemotherapy complications. In *BCG in Superficial Bladder Cancer. Progress in Clinical and Biological Research*, Vol.310. Liss, New York, pp. 335–355

Lilien, O. M. and Camey, M. (1984) Twenty-five years experience with replacement of the human bladder (Camey procedure). *Journal of Urology*, **132**, 886–891

Loening, S. (1984) Chemotherapy as an adjuvant to cystectomy for advanced urothelial cancer. *Urological Clinics of North America*, **11**, 699–708

MacFarlane, J. R. and Tolley, D. A. (1985) Intravesical mitomycin C therapy for superficial bladder cancer. Report of a multicentre phase II study. *British Journal of Urology*, **57**, 172–174

Mahadevia, P. S., Koss, L. G. and Tar, I. J. (1986) Prostatic involvement in bladder cancer. *Cancer*, **58**, 2096–2102

Malone, P. R., Visvanathan, K. V., Ponder, B. A. *et al.* (1985) Oncogenes and bladder cancer. *British Journal of Urology*, **57**, 664–667

Marshall, V. F. (1952) The relation of the preoperative estimate to pathological demonstration of the extent of vesical neoplasms. *Journal of Urology*, **68**, 714–723

Melicow, M. M. (1952) Histological study of vesical urothelium intervening between gross neoplasms in total cystectomy. *British Journal of Urology*, **68**, 261–279

Melicow, M. M. and Hollowell, J. W. (1952) Intraurothelial cancer: carcinoma-in-situ. Bowen's disease of the urinary system. *Journal of Urology*, **68**, 763–772

Messing, E. and deKernion, J. B. (1985) Chemotherapy of bladder cancer. In *Bladder Cancer* (eds. E. J. Zingg and D. M. A. Wallace), Springer-Verlag, Heidelberg, pp. 235–262

Miller, L. S. (1977) Bladder cancer: superiority of preoperative irradiation and cystectomy in clinical stages B2 and C. *Cancer*, **39**, (Suppl.) 973–980

Montie, J. E. (1983) Technique of radical cystectomy. *Seminars in Urology*, **1**, 53–59

Montie, J. E., Straffon, R. A. and Stewart, B. H. (1984) Radical cystectomy without radiation therapy for carcinoma of the bladder. *Journal of Urology*, **131**, 477–482

Morales, A. (1984) Long-term results and complications of intracavitary Bacillus Calmette-Guérin therapy for bladder cancer. *Journal of Urology*, **132**, 457–459

Morales, A., Eidinger, D. and Bruce, A. W. (1976) Intracavitary Bacillus Calmette-Guérin in the treatment of superficial bladder tumours. *Journal of Urology*, **116**, 180–183

MRC Working Party on Urological Cancer (1985) The effect of intravesical thiotepa on the recurrence rate of newly diagnosed superficial bladder cancer. *British Journal of Urology*, **57**, 680–685

Papanicolaou, G. N. and Marshall, W. F. (1945) Urine sediment smears as a diagnostic procedure in cancers of the urinary tract. *Science*, **101**, 519

Pearson, B. S. and Raghavan, D. (1985) First-line intravenous cisplatin for deeply invasive bladder cancer: update on 70 cases. *British Journal of Urology*, **57**, 690–693

Plowman, P. N. (1985) Radiotherapy. In *Bladder Cancer* (eds. E. J. Zingg, and D. M. A. Wallace), Springer-Verlag, Heidelberg, pp. 207–221

Pocock, R. D., Ponder, B. A. J., O'Sullivan, J. P. *et al.* (1982) Prognostic factors in non-infiltrating carcinoma of the bladder: a preliminary report. *British Journal of Urology*, **54**, 711–715

Prout, G. R. Jr, Slack, N. H. and Bross, I. D. (1971) Preoperative irradiation as an adjuvant in the surgical management of invasive bladder carcinoma. *Journal of Urology*, **105**, 223–321

Quilty, P. M., Duncan, W., Chisholm, G. D. *et al.* (1986) Results of surgery following radical radiotherapy for invasive bladder cancer. *British Journal of Urology*, **58**, 396–405

Radwin, H. M. (1980) Radiotherapy and bladder cancer: a critical review. *Journal of Urology*, **124**, 43–46

Raghavan, D. (1988) Pre-emptive (neo-adjuvant) intravenous chemotherapy for invasive bladder cancer. *British Journal of Urology*, **61**, 1–8

Riddle, P. R., Chisholm, G. D., Trott, P. A. and Pugh, R. C. B. (1976) Flat carcinoma-in-situ of bladder. *British Journal of Urology*, **47**, 829–833

Rübben, H., Lutzeyer, W. and Wallace, D. M. A. (1985) The epidemiology and aetiology of bladder cancer. In *Bladder Cancer* (eds. E. J. Zingg and D. M. A. Wallace), Springer-Verlag, Heidelberg, pp. 1–21

Sawczuk, I., Tannenbaum, M., Olsson, C. A. and White, R. de V. (1985) Primary transitional cell carcinoma of prostate periurethral ducts. *Urology*, **25**, 339–343

Schade, R. O. K. and Swinney, J. (1968) Pre-cancerous changes in bladder epithelium. *Lancet*, **ii**, 943–946

Schade, P. O. and Swinney, J. (1973) The association of urothelial atypism with neoplasia: its importance in treatment and prognosis. *Journal of Urology*, **109**, 619–622

Seemayer, T. A., Knaack, J., Thelmo, W. L. *et al.* (1975) Further observations on carcinoma-in-situ of the urinary bladder: silent but extensive intraprostatic involvement. *Cancer*, **36**, 514–520

Sherwood, T. (1983) The abdomen. In *Roads to Radiology* (eds. T. Sherwood, A. K. Dixon, D. Hawkins and M. L. J. Abercrombie), Springer-Verlag, Heidelberg, pp. 59–72

Skinner, D. G., Boyd, S. D. and Lieskovsky, G. (1988) Creation of the continent Kock ileal reservior as an alternative to cutaneous urinary diversion. In *Diagnosis and Management of Genitourinary Cancer* (eds. D. G. Skinner and G. Leiskovsky), Saunders, Philadelphia, pp. 653–674

Skinner, D. G. and Lieskovsky, G. (1984) Contemporary cystectomy with pelvic node dissection compared to pre-operative radiation therapy plus cystectomy in management of invasive bladder cancer. *Journal of Urology*, **132**, 1069–1072

Smith, G., Elton, R. A., Beynon, L. L. *et al.* (1983) Prognostic significance of biopsy results of normal looking mucosa in cases of superficial bladder cancer. *British Journal of Urology*, **55**, 559–665

Smith, G., Elton, R. A., Chisholm, G. D. *et al.* (1986) Superficial bladder cancer. Intravesical chemotherapy and tumour progression to muscle invasion or metastases. *British Journal of Urology*, **58**, 659–663

Smith, G., Quilty, P. M., Duncan, W. *et al.* (1985) The role of endoscopic treatment after radical radiotherapy for invasive bladder cancer. *British Journal of Urology*, **57**, 694–699

Smith, J. A. and Whitmore, W. F. (1981) Salvage cystectomy for bladder cancer after failure of definitive irradiation. *Journal of Urology*, **125**, 643–645

Stanisic, T. H., Donovan, J. M., Lebouton, J. and Graham, A. R. (1987) Five-year experience with intravesical therapy of carcinoma-in-situ: an inquiry into the risks of 'conservative' management. *Journal of Urology*, **138**, 1158–1161

Sternberg, C. N., Yagoda, A., Scher, H. I. *et al.* (1985) Preliminary results of M-Vac for transitional cell carcinoma of the urothelium. *Journal of Urology*, **133**, 403–307

Stock, L. M., Brosman, S. A., Fahey, J. L. and Liu, B. C. (1987) Ras related oncogene protein as a tumor marker in transitional cell carcinoma of the bladder. *Journal of Urology*, **137**, 789–792

Talbot, R. W., Bannister, J. J. and Hills, N. H. (1984) A haematuria diagnostic service in a district general hospital. *Annals of Royal College of Surgeons England*, **66**, 348–350

Turner, A. G., Hendry, W. F., Williams, G. B. and Wallace, D. M. (1977) A haematuria diagnostic service. *British Medical Journal*, **2**, 29–31

Utz, D. C., Farrow, G. M., Rife, C. C. *et al.* (1980) Carcinoma in situ of the bladder. *Cancer*, **45**, 1842–1848

Viola, M. V., Fromowitz, F., Oraves, S. *et al.* (1985) Ras oncogene p21 expression is increased in pre-malignant lesions and high grade bladder carcinoma. *Journal of Experimental Medicine*, **161**, 1213–1218

Wallace, D. M. and Harris, D. C. (1965) Delay in treating bladder tumours. *Lancet*, ii, 332–334

Wallace, D. M., Chisholm, G. D. and Hendry, W. F. (1975) TNM classification for urological tumours (UICC) – 1974. *British Journal of Urology*, **47**, 1–12

Wallace, D. M. A. (1988) Occupational urothelial cancer. *British Journal of Urology*, **61**, 175–182

Wallace, D. M. A., Hindmarsh, J. R., Webb, J. N. *et al.* (1979) The role of multiple mucosal biopsies in the management of patients with bladder cancer. *British Journal of Urology*, **51**, 535–540

Wallace, D. M. A., Smith, J. H. F., Billington, S. *et al.* (1984) The promotion of bladder tumours by endoscopic procedures in an animal model. *British Journal of Urology*, **56**, 658–662

Webb, J. N. (1985) Histopathology of bladder cancer. In *Bladder Cancer* (eds. E. J. Zingg and D. M. A. Wallace), Springer-Verlag, Heidelberg, pp. 23–51

Weinberg, D. M., Ross, R. K., Mack, T. M. *et al.* (1983) Bladder cancer etiology. A different perspective. *Cancer*, **51**, 675–680

Whitmore, W. F. Jr (1980) Integrated irradiation and cystectomy for bladder cancer. *British Journal of Urology*, **52**, 1–9

Whitmore, W. F. Jr and Marshall, V. F. (1962) Radical total cystectomy for cancer of the urinary bladder: 230 consecutive cases five years later. *Journal of Urology*, **87**, 857–868

Williams, J. L., Hammonds, J. C. and Saunders, N. (1977) T1 bladder tumours. *British Journal of Urology*, **49**, 663–668

Wolf, H., Olsen, P. R. and Hojgaard, K. (1985) Urothelial dysplasia concomitant with bladder tumours. A determinant for future new occurrences in patients treated by full-course radiotherapy. *Lancet*, **i**, 1005–1008

Wolfe, J. H. N. and Lloyd-Davies, R. W. (1981) The management of transitional cell carcinoma in the prostate. *British Journal of Urology*, **53**, 253–257

Yagoda, A. (1983) Chemotherapy for advanced urothelial cancer. *Seminars in Urology*, **1**, 60–72

Zincke, H., Utz, D. C., Taylor, W. F. *et al.* (1983) Influence of thiotepa and doxorubicin instillation at the time of transurethral surgical treatment of bladder cancer or tumor recurrence: a prospective, randomized, double-blind controlled trial. *Journal of Urology*, **129**, 505–509

Chapter 9

Prostate

David Kirk

Adenocarcinoma of the prostate, one of the commonest malignancies in the male, shares with carcinoma of the breast the important therapeutic implications of hormonal sensitivity. However, public perception of these two diseases is very different. Carcinoma of the prostate is a disease of old men, and concern rightly is concentrated on the young women with family responsibilities who too often are the victims of breast cancer. While the old age of typical prostatic cancer sufferers is an important factor in their management, all urologists will testify to the size of the problem caused by this disease, a problem arising as much from the morbidity and the resulting social problems it causes as from its mortality statistics.

Prostatic cancer – the problems

The first radical prostatectomy was performed at the dawn of the twentieth century (Young, 1905) yet the merits of so treating early tumours still is debated (Stamey, 1982). Hormonal treatment has been practised for nearly 50 years (Huggins and Hodges, 1941). Its correct timing is still uncertain and despite recent developments, there is little evidence that any of the treatments now available gives a man with prostatic cancer a better outlook than he had in Huggins' day (Smith, 1987). The following questions still cannot be answered with confidence:

- Does radical prostatectomy cure a significant number of men with prostatic carcinoma?
- Are alternatives such as radiotherapy as effective for local treatment of early disease?
- When should patients receive hormonal treatment?
- What is the correct choice of hormonal treatment?
- Is combination therapy – 'Total Androgen Ablation' – more effective than standard hormonal treatment?
- How should the patient be managed when he relapses after hormonal treatment?
- Is it possible to reduce the mortality from prostatic cancer?

The natural history of prostatic carcinoma

Histological evidence of carcinoma can be found in the prostates of 30% of men over 50 years old and 100% of those over 90 (Franks, 1954). Progression from these incidental foci to frank carcinoma (McNeal, 1969), occurs so slowly that the majority of men with such lesions will reach the end of their lives before clinically significant disease occurs. As the tumour in the prostate develops, its histological grade, its invasive potential and its ability to metastasize may increase in proportion to its volume; a tumour of less than 1 ml volume seems unlikely to metastasize but metastases may be inevitable with a tumour volume over 4 ml (McNeal *et al.*, 1986).

The prostate can be divided on the basis of structure, function and pathology into a number of zones (McNeal, 1981). Benign hypertrophy affects its inner portion while carcinomas arise in the peripheral, posterior and apical part of the gland.

The age of the prostatic cancer patient

Prostatic carcinoma predominantly affects elderly men, whose life expectation is short and who are likely to be afflicted by other potentially fatal conditions. Indeed, of the deaths occurring during the Veterans Administration Cooperative Urological Research Group (VACURG) studies (Byar, 1973) only half were ascribed to prostatic cancer (Table 9.1). This has a number of implications.

Table 9.1 Veterans Administration Prostate Study 1. Deaths in placebo treated patients (data from Byar, 1973)

	Stage III (T3 M0)	Stage IV (TX M1)
Patients	262	223
Deaths	177	189
Cause of death:		
Ca prostate	26%	56%
Cardiovascular	50%	29%
Other causes	24%	15%

1. For those patients destined to die from other causes, treatment of their prostatic cancer cannot increase their life span.
2. Many patients with asymptomatic disease may die from other causes before they need treatment on symptomatic grounds.
3. Any advantage to the remainder from early treatment will be at the expense of subjecting those who will not live to benefit from it to the same treatment and its potential side effects.

Clearly the age of many men with prostatic cancer will produce additional social and medical problems which will bear on its management. A young woman with family responsibilities suffering from advanced breast cancer would probably welcome the chance of an extra few months life at whatever price in side-effects from her treatment. The typical elderly man with prostatic cancer might be a frail widower living a lonely life in a high rise flat and for him the balance sheet might be different.

Staging and grading of prostatic cancer

Staging (Table 9.2)

In the UK the UICC (Union Internationale Contre Cancer) TNM system is favoured. Although a recent revision has been proposed, it is subject to some controversy, and its more familiar predecessor (Wallace, Chisholm and Hendry, 1975) will be used in this chapter. In America the stage is described by a single letter category, A–D, covering both primary and metastatic disease. Originally the stages were numbered 1–4 (Whitmore, 1956), and were so categorized in the important VACURG trials. The lettered designations have been subdivided by Jewett (1975) and others, e.g. A1 (occult nodule) and A2 (diffuse occult disease), such modifications often varying from centre to centre.

Table 9.2 Staging conventions for carcinoma of prostate

UICC		USA
T0	Occult; clinically undetected disease	A
(T0a)	Focal	(A1)
(T0b)	Diffuse	(A2)
T1	Nodule not distorting gland	B (B1)
T2	Nodule distorting gland, but not invading capsule	B (B2)
T3	Tumour invading capsule but not fixed or invading other organs	C
T4	Fixed tumour; tumour invading other organs	C
	Any tumour with metastases	D
N1–4	Lymph node metastases	(D1)
M1–4	Distant metastases	(D2)

Histological grade

In the Gleason scoring system (Gleason, Mellinger and the Veterans Administration Cooperative Urological Research Group, 1974), five patterns of the tumour are given numbers from 1 to 5 (Figure 9.1). To accommodate the variations seen in most tumours the two commonest patterns in the tumour are so numbered, the two numbers being added to give a 'Gleason score' from 2 to 10. It takes no account of cytological changes but despite alternative systems (e.g. Gaeta, 1981) a high Gleason score does correlate with a poor prognosis at least at a statistical level (Gleason *et al.*, 1974) and it has become the most widely accepted system.

Assessment of prostatic cancer

Diagnosis and assessment of primary tumour

In the majority of patients, the diagnosis will be made from TUR chippings. Where a TUR is not indicated therapeutically, a needle biopsy may be a better method of sampling a small tumour in the periphery of the gland. Transperineal biopsy avoids the septic problems associated with the transrectal route (Hillyard, 1987). However, sepsis is not a problem with transrectal *fine-needle* aspiration with a

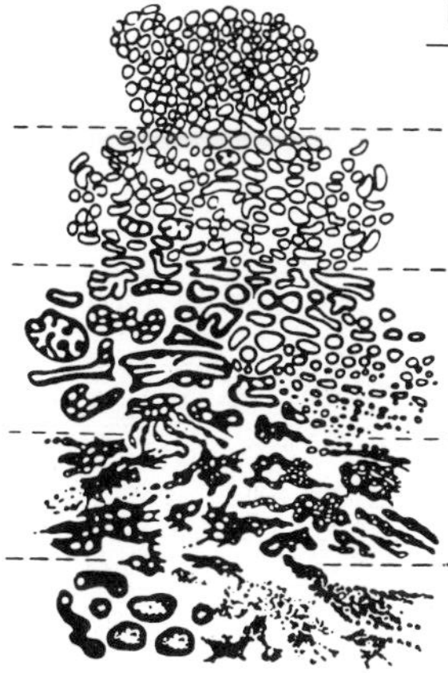

Pattern	Margins of tumour areas	Gland pattern	Gland size	Gland distribution
1	Well defined	Single, separate, round	Medium	Closely packed
2	Less defined	Single, separate, rounded, but more variable	Medium	Spaced up to one gland diameter apart, on average
3 or	Poorly defined	Single, separate, more irregular	Small, medium, or large	Spaced more than one gland diameter apart, rarely packed
3	Poorly defined	Rounded masses of cribri-form or papillary epithelium	Medium or large	Rounded masses with smooth sharp edges
4	Ragged infiltrating	Fused glandular masses or 'hypernephroid'	Small	Fused in ragged masses
5 or	Ragged infiltrating	Almost absent, few tiny glands or signet ring cells	Small	Ragged anaplastic masses of epithelium
5	Poorly defined	Few small lumina in rounded masses of solid epithelium central necrosis?	Small	Rounded masses and cords with smooth, sharp edges

Prostatic adenocarcinoma (histological patterns)

Figure 9.1 Grading of prostatic carcinoma: principles of Gleason's scoring system. (Courtesy of Schering.)

Franzen needle (Kaufman *et al.*, 1982) which is useful where an adequate cytology service is available.

Histochemical techniques for demonstrating PAP (prostatic acid phosphatase) (Jobsis *et al.*, 1978) and PSA (prostate-specific antigen) (Ford *et al.*, 1985) in biopsy material can be useful in difficult situations, for example, patients who present with metastases at unusual sites.

Transrectal ultrasonography
Rectal examination, even with the practised finger of the experienced urologist, is inaccurate both in diagnosing and in staging prostatic cancer (Grayhack and Bockrath, 1981). Ultrasonography has proved a considerable advance in assessing the prostate (Resnick, 1985). A probe in the rectum can display the size of the prostate, variations in its consistency, areas of calcification and breaches of its capsule. With this information tumours can be diagnosed and staged with considerable accuracy (Lee *et al.*, 1985). Ultrasonography can be used to assess progression in the absence of treatment and response following treatment. It can detect tumours too small to be felt on digital rectal examination. Modern portable machines can be used in clinic and operating theatre, enabling needle biopsies to be taken under vision (Hastak, Gammelsaard and Holm, 1982) and radioactive seeds for treating localized disease to be inserted as a closed procedure (Holm *et al.*, 1983).

Diagnosis of metastases

Most urologists base their management on an assessment of the stage of the tumour and would consider at least measurement of serum prostatic acid phosphatase (PAP), bone scintigraphy and radiology essential before deciding on treatment.

Acid phosphatase
Although PAP levels have long been recognized as an indicator of treatment response (Huggins and Hodges, 1941), elevations of PAP in serum occur only in advanced disease, and probably are a reflection of tumour bulk. Indeed a significant elevation often is taken to indicate metastatic disease (Pontes *et al.*, 1981). On the other hand, Stamey and his colleagues found no correlation between elevated PAP (using a sensitive radioimmunoassay) and the presence of extracapsular tumour spread (Stamey *et al.*, 1989a), and patients with elevated PAP alone have a better prognosis than patients with metastatic disease defined by a positive bone scan (Goodman *et al.*, 1989). PAP is not a tumour marker in the sense that αFP and βHCG are in testicular tumours, neither is it a productive screening test. Once carcinoma has been confirmed histologically, changes in PAP can be useful in indicating response to treatment and in detecting progression in patients who are managed conservatively, or in those who have responded to treatment. However, changes in levels of *alkaline* phosphatase may be a more sensitive indicator of response and of disease progression than PAP (Bishop *et al.*, 1985), and the whole role of PAP measurement must now be reconsidered following the development of the serum PSA assay.

Prostate-specific antigen
Besides being a useful histochemical marker of prostatic tissue (Ford *et al.*, 1984), prostate-specific antigen (PSA) is found in increased levels in the serum of patients

with prostatic carcinoma (Ferro *et al.*, 1987). PSA is a more sensitive indicator of prostatic carcinoma than PAP, although mild elevations occurring in benign prostatic hypertrophy reduce its specificity. It rises in proportion to clinical stage, and with increasing Gleason score (Stamey and Kabalin, 1989).

Prostate-specific antigen falls not only in response to successful hormonal therapy (Stamey *et al.* 1989a), but also after local treatment (Stamey, Kabalin and Ferrari, 1989; Stamey *et al.*, 1989b). It appears to be the first marker to rise as an indication of relapse after hormonal treatment (Killian *et al.*, 1985), although the current lack of effective treatment for such relapsed patients reduces the value of this observation at present. PSA undoubtedly is a significant advance in the management of the disease but its final role perhaps has yet to be determined. One unresolved problem is that results from the different assays currently available are not interchangeable, and until a universal standard is achieved, comparison of data and hence agreement on the value of this new tumour marker will remain problematic (Stamey and Kabalin, 1989).

Bone scintigraphy
Radioisotope bone scanning with technetium-99m is the standard method of demonstrating bony metastases (McKillop, 1986), and when there is extensive disease of typical distribution (Figure 9.2) the appearance is diagnostic.

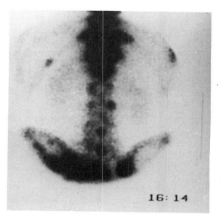

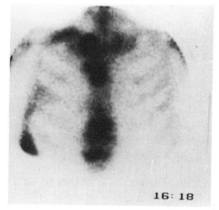

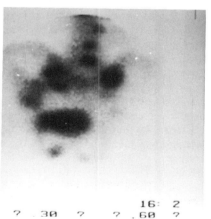

Figure 9.2 Metastatic prostatic carcinoma: bone scan showing typical distribution of increased technetium-99 uptake in axial skeleton

Confirmatory X-rays to demonstrate radiologically visible metastases coinciding with the hot spots or to exclude benign lesions (e.g. old fractures, arthritis) which also increase isotope uptake may be necessary in equivocal cases. Radiology is less sensitive than bone scanning, and a skeletal survey alone would miss metastases in many patients.

There is a significant difference in survival between patients with negative and those with positive scans (Lund *et al.*, 1984). A normal scan is an essential prerequisite to 'curative' local treatment such as radical prostatectomy (Walsh and Lepor, 1987). An improvement in a positive scan is a useful indicator of response to treatment, certainly one more reliable than X-rays (Pollen, 1981), although changes sometimes are difficult to interpret. A scan 3–6 months after treatment is useful, as is one if relapse is suspected, although changes in serum alkaline phosphatase (Bishop *et al.*, 1985) or PSA (Killian *et al.*, 1985) might be a more sensitive indicator of response or relapse.

Lymph node staging
In much of routine practice, especially in the UK, the lymph node component of the TNM is neglected. A staging pelvic lymphadenectomy is considered desirable before radical prostatectomy (Walsh and Lepor, 1987). When the seed implantation for interstitial radiotherapy was done by the retropubic route, lymphadenectomy likewise was performed as part of the procedure (Herr, 1980). With ultrasound-guided insertion of radio-iodine seeds, with external beam irradiation, and other closed treatments, much of the advantage to the patient would be obviated by the burden of lymphadenectomy. Fine-needle aspiration of suspicious nodes demonstrated by lymphangiography (Gothlin, 1976) or CT scanning, or sampling nodes under vision by pelvioscopy (Hald and Rasmussen, 1980) are less invasive alternatives. However, the presence of node involvement can be predicted to a great extent from the stage of the tumour (Wajsman, 1981), and assessment of the lymph node stage, while important in clinical research, is much less significant in the routine practice of most urologists, especially when local curative treatment is not a consideration.

Criteria of response to treatment in prostatic cancer

Assessing the benefits of treatment in prostatic cancer, especially in clinical trials, poses a number of problems. In localized disease, a long period of follow-up, during which deaths from other causes will occur, is necessary to obtain survival data. Disease control in terms of local or distant progression can be shorter-term aims, and indeed in an elderly population may be more relevant.

Advanced prostatic cancer also presents difficulties. In the absence of transrectal ultrasonography, assessment of changes in the primary tumour is difficult and subjective. Metastatic disease rarely occurs in easily measurable forms such as lung or liver metastases. While bone scan appearances frequently improve after successful treatment their interpretation can be difficult. Lytic radiological lesions, recalcification of which is a reliable indicator of response, are less common than sclerotic lesions which often do not change or may even intensify (Pollen, 1981). PSA may become a useful indicator of response (Killian *et al.*, 1985) but alterations in PAP levels are less precise.

A number of research organizations, e.g. the National Prostatic Cancer Project

(NPCP), (Loening *et al.*, 1983), have established response criteria in an attempt to overcome these difficulties. They define complete and partial regression, and tumour progression, but 'stabilization' of previously progressing disease also has been defined as an objective response. This concept has been criticized (Beynon and Chisholm, 1984). Certainly in practical terms it leaves the patients no better off, and its inclusion creates 'objective response rates' which tend to over-value the treatment in question, especially in hormone-relapsed patients.

Management of carcinoma of the prostate

Treatment of occult (TO, stage A) disease

A proportion of TURs performed on clinically benign glands will reveal malignant tissue. Having ensured by checking PAP levels and a bone scan that the tumour truly is localized to the prostate what should be done? Occult disease occurs in two forms (Sheldon, Williams and Fraley, 1980), which are designated in America as stages A1 and A2, and can be described as TOa and TOb under the TNM system.

The TOa focus
This consists of a small localized focus too small to produce a palpable nodule usually with a low grade as indicated by the Gleason score (Beynon *et al.*, 1983). Patients with such tumours have a good prognosis and their survival approaches their natural life expectation. While there is some consensus that its good prognosis makes active treatment inappropriate for most patients with TOa disease, some patients do slowly progress (Walsh and Lepor, 1987) and there is always the worry that both the grade and extent of the tumour elsewhere in the gland might be greater than in the TUR chips.

TOb occult disease
Here the tumour occupies a large proportion of the tissue and has a poor Gleason grade. Patients with this type of tumour have a poor prognosis and it is argued that they should be treated actively. It is likely that many men with TOb tumours have lymph node metastases (Catalona and Scott, 1986), and these clearly must contribute to the poor prognosis of this group of patients as a whole. The prognosis of similarly affected patients without lymph node involvement is less clear. Either they share with TOa tumours a good prognosis or they could represent a group where therapeutic zeal is justified.

Since prostatic carcinoma arises in the peripheral portion of the gland, a small focus of tumour among some TUR chippings might indicate a tumour truly of stage TOa or might be due to the TUR just encroaching into a peripheral TOb tumour. Advocates of a 'second look' TUR have shown that occasionally the stage will be altered by re-resecting the prostate (Ford *et al.*, 1984). The author would combine this with needle biopsies of the periphery of the gland. Active treatment of such upstaged tumours has only been reported anecdotally and the value of this procedure is debatable (Walsh and Lepor, 1987).

The treatment of confined localized disease

The palpable (T1) nodule confined without distortion to the gland is considered the classical indication for radical prostatectomy (Jewett, 1970). Stage T1 is equivalent to the lower spectrum of stage B in the USA and was subclassified by Jewett (1975) as stage B1.

The British view of radical prostatectomy has been that it is applicable to so few cases that the side-effects, universal impotence and frequent incontinence, and dubious benefits severely question its value. This raises wrath from across the Atlantic (Moon, 1985). What evidence can we call on to resolve what is seen as a major dichotomy between British and American Urology (Fraser, 1985)?

Men suitable for this treatment have tumours of favourable prognosis. Therefore it is a procedure appropriate only for the younger patient (certainly under 70 years) and its success has to be measured in terms of *15*-year survival figures. In reported series one-third of patients are alive at the end of this time, with perhaps one-half of deaths being from other causes (Stamey, 1982). Similar 15-year survival figures can be produced by radiotherapy (Bagshaw, Ray and Cox, 1985), and by those who adopt a conservative approach (Barnes, 1969).

Anecdotal series, however carefully followed and however well reported, fail to resolve the issue. Unfortunately there have been only *two* controlled trials. The VACURG trial randomly compared patients treated by radical prostatectomy with an untreated group (Byar and Corle, 1981). No survival benefit emerged, although disease progression has occurred in more patients in the untreated group. The number of patients was small, stage A1 (TOa) patients were included and the methods used to exclude metastatic disease would now be considered inadequate, so that the current relevance of the trial is questioned (Catalona and Scott, 1986).

Paulson compared treatment by radiotherapy with radical prostatectomy (Paulson *et al.*, 1982). Because survival data take many years to gather, the end-point chosen was distant progression. On this criterion, a statistically significant difference in favour of radical prostatectomy emerged. It has been suggested (Gittes, personal communication) that a less than optimal radiotherapy regime was adopted and that this rather than a superiority of surgical treatment accounted for the difference. However, if radical prostatectomy is better than radiotherapy (whether adequate or not), it will also be better than no treatment. This presupposes that the adopted end-point is reasonable, and in prostatic cancer with its unusual history, and with the availability of hormonal therapy, earlier progression does not always mirror poorer survival.

Stamey (personal communication) has commented that if Hugh Hampton Young had performed radical prostatectomy on only half his patients this question would have been answered long ago. As it is, not far from the centenary of the first such operation, arguments about its value demand a good controlled trial for their resolution.

The other issue is the question of side-effects. The perineal operation of Young and Jewett almost invariably produced impotence (Schmidt, 1981) and incontinence was a frequent complication. Using Walsh's nerve sparing technique, retropubic radical prostatectomy can be performed without interfering with potency (Walsh, Lepor and Eggleston, 1983). As damage to the distal bladder sphincter mechanism now is more readily avoided, these two major complications no longer have to be weighed against the possible benefits of radical prostatectomy (Walsh, 1986). In the UK most individual urologists see too few suitable cases to enable them to develop and retain the expertise to perform such surgery. If this *is* the correct way to treat early prostatic tumours, we may have to overcome our British reluctance to refer patients to others with the necessary skills. Indeed interest in radical prostatectomy is increasing in the UK (McNicholas *et al.*, 1989) and if a more critical attitude develops in America (Stamey, 1982), transatlantic agreement on this issue may yet occur.

Alternatives to radical surgery

External beam radiotherapy
Irradiation has been accepted as effective treatment for localized disease (Bagshaw, Ray and Cox, 1985), and is the method of local treatment most widely practised in the UK (Tolley and Robinson, 1984). Its merits compared to radical surgery hinge largely on whether the regime shown by Paulson to be less effective in terms of preventing tumour progression was therapeutically adequate. Other than this study, most published data are from uncontrolled series which are difficult to compare directly with other modalities.

While surgical treatment of T3 tumours is possible (Zincke *et al.*, 1984), radiotherapy more often is chosen by those who favour active treatment of the more advanced localized tumour (Walsh and Lepor, 1987).

External beam irradiation has a significant complication rate (Lindholt and Hansen, 1986). Most published series contain patients with complications of a catastrophic nature – for example fistulae requiring bowel and urinary diversion. The prognosis depends on the tumour grade (Ritchie *et al.*, 1985), indicating that the biology of the patient's disease may have as great a bearing on the outcome as how he is treated.

Perhaps too much has been made of possible benefits from radiotherapy in terms of survival. Many reported series contain men with locally advanced tumours which must be past cure if only because of unsuspected lymph node metastases (Prout *et al.*, 1981). The true value of radiotherapy probably is local control of the primary tumour – not an insignificant benefit as many men, particularly in the later stages of their disease, are made miserable by recurring outflow obstruction. The author has found radiotherapy a useful palliation, avoiding repeat TURs, and for this purpose can be equally appropriate for those with metastatic disease.

Interstitial radiotherapy
Implantation of radioisotope seeds originally was an open retropubic operation (Herr, 1980). It now can be done as a semi-closed procedure, ^{125}I seeds being introduced through needles inserted via the perineum, under guidance of a rectal ultrasound probe (Holm *et al.*, 1983). Long-term results are available for the open technique (Grossman *et al.*, 1982) but those for whom the technique is recommended have in any case a good prognosis.

'Radical' TUR and laser treatment
In this new approach to local treatment, after an aggressive TUR using a rectal ultrasound probe to ensure adequate clearance, the residual prostatic tissue is then destroyed with a YAG laser, the apical region of the gland being dealt with from above by passing the probe through a suprapubic cystotomy (McNicholas *et al.*, 1988). These authors now appear to have abandoned the technique in favour of radical prostatectomy (McNicholas *et al.*, 1989).

Should TUR be avoided in early prostatic cancer?

There has been much concern that a TUR may disseminate the tumour (Hanks, Leibel and Kramer, 1983), and adversely affect progression and survival. However, comparing patients in uncontrolled series could be misleading, since those needing TUR may have more aggressive tumours (Meacham *et al.*, 1989). The controversy is yet to be resolved. One recent analysis of data on men receiving radiotherapy suggested TUR caused a two-fold increase in risk of disease progression (Forman *et al.*, 1986), while Paulson and Cox (1987) could detect no effect in men undergoing radical prostatectomy. Although the question really demands a prospective trial, where a patient has severe local symptoms, or is in retention, current evidence is not sufficient to deny him the prompt and reliable relief possible from TUR.

Treatment of advanced localized disease

Attempts at *curing* prostatic carcinoma are directed largely at stage T1 tumours. Many patients with more advanced tumours will have no evidence of metastatic disease. It is attractive to consider that such men still are curable if their local disease is eradicated, or at least that disease progression can be delayed, and that this will improve survival. Even if these objectives are not realized, treatment might prevent local progression which can cause recurrent urinary symptoms, retention, or ureteric obstruction.

There is little general agreement on how these patients should be managed. Radical prostatectomy is not impossible for some T3 tumours (Zincke *et al.*, 1984) although adequate excision of tumour will preclude the nerve sparing technique and continence must be at greater risk. While radiotherapy is perhaps more appropriate for localized disease (Walsh and Lepor, 1987) many British urologists employ hormonal treatment for patients with T3 MO tumours (Tolley and Robinson, 1984). Since the prognosis of men with negative bone scans, as far as death from prostatic cancer is concerned, is relatively good (Lund *et al.*, 1984), a case can be made for deferring any treatment. Patients so managed may require a further TUR if local symptoms recur (Handley *et al.*, 1988) which might then become an indication either for radiotherapy, or hormonal treatment.

It is impossible to adjudicate between these options. However, the relatively good prognosis of T3 MO disease and the old age of most patients, does make good sense of an expectant approach, provided that the urologist is alert to the needs of the occasional patient whose disease progresses rapidly.

Hormonal therapy

The discovery of the hormonal sensitivity of prostatic cancer (Huggins and Hodges, 1941) provided one of the earliest opportunities to treat effectively a tumour which had spread beyond the scope of surgical cure. Hormonal therapy came rapidly into use and in 1950 Nesbit and Baum reported 1818 patients treated in a number of centres in the USA. Compared with previous experience, dramatically better survival curves were obtained for patients treated with hormones, and the conclusion was drawn that this was a life-prolonging therapy.

Nesbit and Baum (1950) used the term 'control group' to describe patients from a report on pre-hormonal prostatic cancer (Nesbit and Plumb, 1946), with whom hormonal treated patients were compared. The dangers of historical controls were particularly acute at that time, a period of dramatic medical advance. The introduction of antibiotics alone must have improved considerably the life expectancy of the elderly men who are the typical victims of advanced prostatic cancer. However, hormonal treatment was considered so effective that treatment, usually with oestrogens, was started immediately in any man in whom the diagnosis was even suspected.

In this environment it was a courageous step for the Veterans Administration Cooperative Urological Research Group (VACURG) to introduce into their trials a control arm of patients initially treated with placebo only (Byar, 1973). They found that the survival of those patients initially in the placebo groups was similar to that of those treated with DES or undergoing orchiectomy from the start. Hormonal treatment did affect tumour growth, because those patients with tumours initially confined to the prostate progressed to develop metastases more slowly if receiving hormonal therapy. Why did they not live longer? When the placebo-treated patients' disease progressed, they could be 'withdrawn' and commenced on hormonal therapy. Since placebo-treated patients started on hormonal treatment on progression seemed to live as long as patients treated with hormones from the time of diagnosis of their disease it was suggested that hormonal treatment could safely be deferred until symptoms from metastases or other demanding indications occurred.

The VACURG studies caused a reappraisal of the need to treat all patients with prostatic cancer as soon as the diagnosis was made. Increasingly, in the absence of bone pain or other symptoms, treatment has been deferred until a specific indication occurs. In addition, with the realization that the benefits in terms of survival from hormonal therapy are at best questionable few would now consider treatment in the absence of histological proof of the diagnosis except in the most extreme circumstances.

Although the case for deferring treatment has been said to have been resolved by the VACURG trials (Fraser, 1985), a survey conducted in 1982 showed that two-thirds of British urologists still favoured early treatment (Tolley and Robinson, 1984). Two recently reported retrospective studies give somewhat conflicting views. One could show no obvious detriment from such a practice (Parker *et al.*, 1985) but there has to be concern that another group practising deferred treatment found that a number of their patients died from prostatic cancer before treatment could be instituted (Handley *et al.*, 1988).

Clinical trials can only satisfactorily answer the question for which they were designed. The VACURG studies only revealed the *possibility* of deferring treatment on retrospective analysis of the results. In answering the question 'immediate or deferred therapy?' these studies were deficient in a number of respects (Kirk, 1987a). While their vital role in *suggesting* the option of deferring treatment is undisputed, the general applicability of this principle has yet to be determined, and perhaps awaits the result of a study currently being performed in the UK by the Medical Research Council (Kirk, 1985).

Management of advanced but asymptomatic disease

This then is the problem. A man presents with a T3 or T4 tumour causing outflow obstruction (even retention), readily manageable by TUR of the prostate. Bone scan etc. shows either no metastases or any metastases are asymptomatic. The patient delighted with the results of his TUR and considering himself 'cured' may not thank the urologist for any side-effects of hormonal treatment prescribed while he is asymptomatic, but he *is* suffering from cancer for which there is an effective form of treatment. Arguments can be advanced either for starting treatment immediately or for deferring it until unquestionable need arises (Kirk, 1987b).

It has not definitely been shown that early treatment produces *no* survival benefit although a few months extra life may not be a great advantage to an elderly man. Some reported data seems to show that patients with metastases have a poorer response rate to treatment. Does this mean that prostatic tumours lose their hormone sensitivity as they advance, which would favour earlier treatment, or is it simply that non-sensitive tumours are more aggressive and present at a more advanced stage?

Leaving aside the question of response and survival, other advantages are suggested for early treatment. Recurrent outflow obstruction is a common reason for abandoning deferred treatment (Handley *et al.*, 1988). Patients may not have specific symptoms, such as back pain but still feel unwell if their tumour is uncontrolled. A catastrophe such as sudden paraplegia could occur unheralded in an untreated patient. Many urologists are happier treating their patients immediately in the hope of preventing these problems.

While there may be some justification for this concern (Handley *et al.*, 1988) increasing numbers of urologists are deferring hormone treatment in suitable patients without regretting this choice (Parker *et al.*, 1985). The problems may be avoidable by careful follow-up and attention to all aspects of the patient's disease. Deferred treatment is not neglect. As in stage 1 testicular teratoma, surveillance is not the easy option, and should only be considered where the urologist has the time and facilities, there is good communication with the patient and his general practitioner, and prompt action can be taken about any problem as it arises.

Advanced disease with symptomatic metastases or complications

Prostatic cancer may present with pain from metastatic disease, pathological fracture, spinal cord compression, or with uraemia due to ureteric obstruction. Here the need for treatment requires no discussion. Fortunately, this situation in *prostatic* cancer is far from hopeless and the availability of hormonal treatment justifies aggressive management which might not be appropriate if the same problem occurred in, for example, bladder or bronchial cancer. If the problem is one of bone pain only, the institution of hormonal therapy alone may be necessary. More complicated situations will require additional measures, for example internal fixation of fractures or spinal decompression.

Uraemia in a patient with prostatic cancer might be due to bladder outflow obstruction. If there is no encroachment onto the ureters, a TUR alone might solve the problem, and the need for hormonal therapy becomes debatable along the lines discussed in the previous section. Alternatively, the ureters may be obstructed by invading tumour. The priority then is to establish drainage of the upper tracts, usually by percutaneous nephrostomy, in the hope that the obstructing tumour will respond to subsequent hormonal therapy.

The general requirement for histological proof before starting treatment can with justification sometimes be relaxed in those presenting with very advanced disease. An elderly man with proven skeletal metastatic disease could be given hormonal therapy without subjecting him to biopsy, on the grounds that the only primary tumour likely to be amenable to effective treatment is one in the prostate.

The choice of hormonal therapy

The hormonal treatment of prostatic cancer depends on the tumour retaining the androgen sensitivity of the normal prostate. In considering the regulation of androgen levels (Figure 9.3) it is important to note the control of luteinizing hormone (LH) by luteinizing hormone releasing hormone (LHRH), the negative feedback of testosterone on the pituitary and the LH independent secretion of androgens by the adrenal gland. Both testosterone and the adrenal androgens are converted in the prostate by the enzyme 5α-reductase to dihydrotestosterone (Figure 9.4).

Of the methods of hormonal manipulation available until recently, diethyl stilboesterol (DES) had fallen into disrepute due to its cardiovascular toxicity, although this problem is dose related and treatment with 1 mg daily may have a minimal risk of such complications (Smith, 1987). The steroidal anti-androgen cyproterone acetate (Tunn, Graff and Senge, 1983) is a satisfactory drug whose main disadvantage is its high cost, a major problem where treatment may be necessary for months or years. Thus, although it is irreversible, and involves albeit a minor surgical operation, orchiectomy remained popular. It appears to have no long-term complications, and does not depend on the patient's compliance (Stamey, 1982).

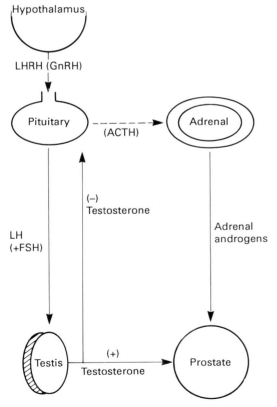

Figure 9.3 Hormonal regulation of androgen secretion (Courtesy of *British Journal of Sexual Medicine*)

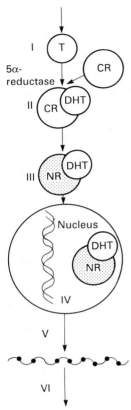

I   Transposition of testosterone (T) into the cell

II Reduction of testos-terone to dihydrotestos-terone (DHT) by the enzyme 5α-reductase. DHT is bound to cyto-plasmic receptors (CR)

III Transformation of the cytosol into the nuclear receptor (NR)

IV Translocation of the androgen receptor complex into the cell nucleus and interaction with the genome (chromatin) or acceptor

V   Activation of RNA poly-merase and synthesis of mRNA (= transcription)

VI Synthesis of specific proteins or enzymes in the ribosomes (= translation)

Figure 9.4 Molecular mechanism of action of androgens – both testosterone and adrenal androgens are converted to active form, DHT, by action of 5α- reductase. (From Neumann and Schenck, 1984, by permission)

LHRH analogues

LHRH is a peptide releasing hormone, which stimulates release of both LH and follicle-stimulating hormone (FSH) from the anterior pituitary (Harris, 1961). While synthetic analogues of the LHRH octopeptide initially stimulate the pituitary, the release of LH then is inhibited so that testosterone, after a transient rise, falls into the castrate range. Hence, these agents can be used to treat prostatic cancer (Waxman *et al.*, 1983).

A number of different LHRH analogues have been developed. At first they could only be given as a daily injection. This severe restriction on their use has been overcome in two ways. Buserilin can be administered as a nasal snuff (Waxman *et al.*, 1983) but a better solution is a depot preparation. Zoladex, the first of these to be granted a product licence, consists of a polyglycolic acid pellet which releases the drug as it is absorbed (Beacock *et al.*, 1987) and is injected monthly.

A potential problem is temporary stimulation of tumour growth during the initial period of increased testosterone secretion. Complications from this tumour 'flare' have been documented (Waxman *et al.*, 1985), and some authorities recommend covering this period with an anti-androgen. This is not universally accepted, and perhaps is only necessary in selected patients, for example those with extensive spinal metastases, stimulation of which could cause cord compression.

Anti-androgens
Peripheral blockage of androgen activity at the target organ is an attractive concept were it not for blockade also occurring at the pituitary, interfering with negative feedback (Neumann, 1983). Thus a drug acting purely as an anti-androgen might, after initial benefit, cause a rise in serum LH and testosterone levels sufficient to overcome the competitive inhibition in the prostate. With the steroidal anti-androgen cyproterone acetate this is not a problem since it is also a progestagen which blocks LH secretion centrally (Neuman and Schenck, 1984). For this reason, cyproterone acetate is an effective single agent therapy.

Flutamide and anandron are non-steroidal drugs which act purely as anti-androgens. As monotherapy, flutamide may be as effective as oestrogen, but without affecting potency (Lund and Rasmussen, 1988). However, in many studies, toxicity has been a problem (Lundgren, 1987), and the number of patients withdrawn makes it difficult to determine whether the relapse to be expected from interference with hormone feedback does indeed occur. A real role for these compounds will depend either on the confirmation that total androgen ablation improves response to hormonal therapy, or a demonstration of useful results in relapsed patients. New non-steroidal anti-androgens which may be less toxic are under development, and may be more useful. Disappointingly, ICI's promised selective drug which does not block pituitary feedback in animals has not behaved in this advantageous way in early human studies. Mention must also be made of a new group of drugs which inhibit 5α-reductase and which may have a very selective effect on the prostate.

Total androgen ablation
Hormonal manipulation by orchiectomy, oestrogens or LHRH analogues although reducing *testosterone* levels into the castrate range has no effect on adrenal androgens, interference with which will produce a more profound reduction of androgenic drive. Adding an anti-androgen to standard therapy will do this and, it is suggested, increase the proportion of tumours responding to therapy with prolongation of survival (Labrie *et al.*, 1983). Labrie's uncontrolled clinical results were impressively better than the accepted figures for standard treatment (Labrie *et al.*, 1984) but judgement on this line of treatment has been suspended pending the results of a number of controlled trials currently being performed. Although only preliminary results are available, it would certainly seem unlikely that any benefit from total androgen ablation will be as great as that suggested by the original reports, and may have to be balanced against the troublesome side-effects of currently available anti-androgens.

Which is the best treatment?
Ignoring the question of total androgen ablation, the practical choices available are oestrogen therapy, orchiectomy, cyproterone acetate or a depot preparation of an LHRH analogue. Clinical trials indicate these treatments, in therapeutic terms, to be equally effective (Smith, 1987), but with regard to tolerance, acceptability, convenience and cost no treatment will score in all categories.

Reluctance to use oestrogens because of cardiovascular toxicity results from experience with doses of DES of 3 mg or more per day. However, even if 1 mg daily is satisfactory, I would be reluctant to use it in a man with a history of cardiovascular disease, excluding a significant proportion of men with prostatic cancer. Excitement over new developments should not be allowed to cloud the benefits of orchiectomy, preferably the subcapsular operation, in the elderly patient. This is a once and for all treatment which places the patient under no obligation to remember to take tablets or attend for regular injections. With proper counselling, in my experience most men accept orchiectomy but there has perhaps been too little research into the psychological effects of the operation *per se*, and some trials have suggested that depot LHRH analogue injections could be more acceptable to some patients (Parmar *et al.*, 1987). Either CPA or an LHRH analogue can be used where the operation is inappropriate for some reason, or as a preliminary 'test' of hormone sensitivity preceding an irreversible orchiectomy. Before the LHRH analogues were available, most patients on CPA had few problems, but a monthly injection might be more convenient than regular tablet taking. Placed in perspective, new developments in hormonal therapy have provided helpful alternatives rather than caused a revolution.

The outcome of hormonal therapy

It is commonly held that hormonal therapy benefits about 75% of men with advanced prostatic cancer. If objective disease remission is sought, the response rate falls well below 50% but only a minority will get no symptomatic relief. Response is inevitably temporary, and those with metastatic disease usually relapse within 2 years. Hormonal therapy can only be considered as a palliation, and this perhaps is reason alone for reserving this, the only realistic hope of modifying the course of the disease, until unquestionable indications arise (Kirk, 1985).

Treatment of the relapsed patient

The rewarding outcome of hormonal therapy in most patients only highlights the problem presented by those who fail to respond or have relapsed. Relapse usually proceeds rapidly towards death (Beynon and Chisholm, 1984), although there is a particularly distressing group of men with unresponsive painful skeletal metastases who seem otherwise to be relatively unaffected by their disease. They contrast with other men who are ill, often anaemic and probably have extensive bone marrow involvement. Recent improvements in imaging of bone marrow may be useful in distinguishing such patients (Haddock *et al.*, 1989).

Secondary hormonal manipulation

Changing to another primary treatment occasionally is beneficial and possibly a successful orchiectomy in these circumstances may imply poor compliance with drug treatment. However, second-line hormonal therapy mainly is directed against residual androgens. These mainly come from the adrenal, and can be reduced at source, as with aminoglutethimide therapy (Harnett *et al.*, 1987), or blocked with the anti-androgens, either using CPA (Wein and Murphy, 1973), or flutamide (Labrie *et al.*, 1988). The drugs used, with the possible exception of CPA, are fairly toxic, and secondary hormonal therapy risks increasing side-effects for decreasing benefit (Harnett *et al.*, 1987; MacFarlane and Tolley, 1985).

High-dose oestrogen therapy

In the VACURG studies the cancer death rate in patients treated with larger doses of oestrogens was reduced, but the complimentary increase in cardiac mortality negated any benefit. It is possible that oestrogens in high dosage have a direct effect on the tumour independent of testosterone suppression and their use in relapsed patients has been suggested (Susan, Roth and Adkins, 1976).

Cytotoxic drugs

Chemotherapy is disappointing in advanced prostatic cancer. Few of the available agents have much effect on this tumour, and elderly unfit patients do not tolerate the side-effects of chemotherapy well. The cause of chemotherapy has not been helped by the NPCP studies in the USA which reported apparently useful response rates which were heavily dependent on disease 'stabilization'. Of currently available drugs, mitomycin-C (Jones *et al.*, 1986) and doxorubicin (Torti *et al.*, 1983) and its derivitive epirubicin, seem most promising. However, the benefits of cytotoxic drugs in prostatic cancer currently seem so small that it is difficult to recommend their use outside the confines of a clinical trial (Gibbons, 1987).

Estramustine phosphate

This drug is a combination of an oestrogen and a nitrogen mustard which is broken down in the prostatic tumour cell, so that it acts both as oestrogen and cytotoxic (Muntzing *et al.*, 1974). Not very popular as primary treatment in the UK, it remains an option in relapsed patients (Walzer, Oswalt and Soloway, 1984), and currently forms a 'control' arm in an EORTC trial against which mitomycin-C is being tested. In the high doses recommended in relapsed patients it might be acting merely as a source of high-dose oestrogen (Daehlin *et al.*, 1986), rather than as a cytotoxic treatment.

Radiotherapy

Although purely a palliative measure, valuable relief of symptoms is achieved by local irradiation of painful metastases, and paraplegia can be prevented or reversed by prompt treatment where spinal compression is threatened. Unfortunately, such metastases rarely are solitary and usually further painful lesions occur. Low dose half/whole body irradiation probably is underused, as it can produce dramatic responses in men able still to have a worthwhile life were it not for the pain (Rowlands *et al.*, 1981). A similar effect may be achievable with radio-isotopes such as phosphorus-32 or strontium-89 (Robinson, 1986). The latter is a very promising development. Initially used as second-line treatment in those relapsing following conventional radiotherapy, strontium-89 now is being investigated as an alternative to external beam treatment.

Palliation

Active therapy for men with relapsed advanced carcinoma of the prostate often has very little to offer and many men will be as well managed by careful regulation of analgesia, blood transfusion for those who are anaemic and other supportive measures. A man in this situation challenges medical practice at its highest level. The urologist who can develop a close liaison with a pain clinic, a sympathetic radiotherapist and a hospice, especially one with home care and day hospital facilities, can find the management of these patients among the most rewarding part of his practice.

How should prostatic cancer be treated?

In 1982, Stamey stated that he did not know how to treat prostatic carcinoma. Those who are familiar with the practice of most British urologists might wonder whether accounts of its management in the American literature (e.g. Catalona and Scott, 1986) were decribing the same disease. The aggressive approach to early prostatic tumours which they described may be correct. Indeed I feel that we in the UK are too conservative, although to change this will require a re-evaluation of how we diagnose the disease and where the patients are treated. We really don't know. The reason for this is the rarity of the well-designed large-scale controlled trial despite the enormous literature on prostatic cancer. We need only consider the certainties about hormonal therapy which were dispelled by the VACURG trials. A major reason why British urologists should start to practise radical prostatectomy is perhaps that it is in the UK that a trial to determine the value of the operation could be performed.

Prostatic cancer – the future

At the outset, this chapter posed a number of questions. The answers are overshadowed by the possibly unique natural history of a tumour which can be shown to have a ubiquitous prevalence in the elderly population and affects largely those who may well succumb to other conditions. Thus only those with a good prognosis are suitable for radical surgery, and judgement on alternative methods of local 'curative' treatment must be suspended. Hormonal therapy now is recognized as able to provide a useful but temporary remission in symptomatic patients, with a question remaining as to its correct timing in others. In either case, its effect on the survival of those who live long enough for their disease to reach its full course is dubious. Unless total androgen ablation should prove the advance its advocates believe, we can expect little more from androgen deprivation. Once the patient has relapsed, although second-line hormonal therapy and chemotherapy can be tried, in the majority of patients little benefit will occur, and such men can expect a short survival, although radiotherapy and other palliative measures will be able to help a substantial number.

Can we cure prostatic cancer? Until there are dramatic improvements in chemotherapy, the answer for patients with advanced disease in 'no'. Indeed in the elderly population afflicted by prostatic cancer, is this a realistic aim? Local tumour control and prevention of symptoms for his remaining life would probably be all the patient would ask. Could screening detect the patient's disease before it reached this stage? Trans-rectal ultrasonography identifies lesions in the prostate which are not clinically detectable. However, even assuming that all those men who now present with advanced disease at some time have had such a localized and thus 'curable' tumour, we also know that the majority of men with such lesions may well not develop clinical prostatic cancer within their lifespan. This paradox might be resolved if McNeal's observations are correct (McNeal et al., 1986). The assurance that a lesion less than 1 ml in volume will not metastasize would allow smaller tumours to be observed, and only those enlarging towards this size need be treated.

Such an approach presents formidable problems: not only would a screening programme, compounded by the need for follow-up, require considerable resources, but how acceptable would most men find trans-rectal ultrasonography as a screening technique, especially if the finding of a tumour was not immediately followed by therapy? Even then, it would be many years before the benefits could be assessed. However, it is in the area of early detection where some improvement seems possible, and its exploitation at least offers hope in a disease where the progression of the last 40 years can be measured more in terms of realism about our limitations than in dramatic therapeutic advance.

Acknowledgements

I should like to thank my colleague Professor James McKillop for providing the bone scan (Figure 9.2), and Mrs J. Breakey for secretarial assistance.

References

Bagshaw, M. A., Ray, G. R. and Cox, R. S. (1985) Radiotherapy of prostatic cancer: long or short term efficacy. *Urology*, **25**, Suppl. 17–23

Barnes R. W. (1969) Prostate cancer. Survival with conservative therapy. *Journal of the American Medical Association*, **210**, 331–332

Beacock, C. J., Buck, A. C., Zwinck, R. *et al.* (1987) The treatment of metastatic prostatic cancer with the slow release LR-RH analogue Zoladex ICI 118630. *British Journal of Urology*, **59**, 436–442

Beynon, L. L. and Chisholm, G. D. (1984) The stable state is not an objective response in hormone-escaped carcinoma of the prostate. *British Journal of Urology*, **56**, 702–705

Beynon, L. L., Busuttil, A., Newsam, J. E. and Chisholm, G. D. (1983) Incidental carcinoma of the prostate: selection for deferred treatment. *British Journal of Urology*, **55**, 733–736

Bishop, M. C., Hardy, J. G., Taylor, M. C. *et al.* (1985) Bone imaging and serum phosphatases in prostatic carcinoma. *British Journal of Urology*, **57**, 317–324

Byar, D. P. (1973) The Veterans Administration Cooperative Urological Research Group's studies of cancer of the prostate. *Cancer*, **32**, 1126–1130

Byar, D. P. and Corle, D. K. (1981) VACURG randomised trial of radical prostatectomy for stages I and II. *Urology*, **17**, Suppl. 2, 7–11

Catalona, W. J. and Scott, W. W. (1986) Carcinoma of the prostate. In *Campbell's Urology* (ed. P. C. Walsh, R. E. Gittes, A. D. Perlmutter and T. A. Stamey), Saunders, Philadelphia, pp. 1463–1534

Daehlin, L., Damber, J.-E., von Schoultz, B. and Bergman, B. (1986) The oestrogenic effects of polyoestradiol phosphate and estramustine phosphate in patients with prostatic carcinoma. *British Journal of Urology*, **58**, 412–416

Ferro, M. A., Barnes, I., Roberts, J. B. M. and Smith, P. J. B. (1987) Tumour markers in prostatic carcinoma. A comparison of prostate-specific antigen with acid phosphatase. *British Journal of Urology*, **60**, 69–73

Ford, T. F., Butcher, D. N., Masters, J. R. W. and Parkinson, M. C. (1985) Immunocytochemical localisation of prostate-specific antigen: specificity and application to clinical practice. *British Journal of Urology*, **57**, 50–55

Ford, T. F., Cameron, K. M., Parkinson, M. C. and O'Donoghue, E. P. N. (1984) Incidental carcinoma of the prostate: treatment selection by second look TURP. *British Journal of Urology*, **56**, 682–686

Forman, J. D., Order, S. E., Zinreich, E. S. *et al.* (1986) The correlation of pretreatment transurethral resection of prostatic cancer with tumour dissemination and disease-free survival. A univariate and multivariate analysis. *Cancer*, **58**, 1770–1778

Franks, L. M. (1954) Latent carcinoma of the prostate. *Journal of Pathology and Bacteriology*, **68**, 603–616

Fraser, K. S. (1985) Prostatic carcinoma. *British Medical Journal*, **290**, 1824

Gaeta, J. F. (1981) Glandular profiles and cellular patterns in prostatic cancer grading. *Urology*, **17**, Suppl. 1, 33–37

Gibbons, R. P. (1987) Prostate cancer chemotherapy. *Cancer*, **60**, 586–588

Gleason, D. F., Mellinger, G. T. and the Veterans Administration Cooperative Urological Research Group. (1974) Prediction of prognosis for prostatic adenocarcinoma by combined histological grading and clinical staging. *Journal of Urology*, **111**, 58–64

Goodman, C. M., Cumming, J. A., Ritchie, A. W. S. and Chisholm, G. D. (1989) Raised acid phosphatase does not imply bony deposits in prostate cancer. Paper read at Annual Meeting of British Association of Urological Surgeons, St. Helier, Jersey, 22nd June

Gothlin, J. H. (1976) Post-lymphographic percutaneous fine-needle biopsy of lymph node guided by fluoroscopy. *Radiology*, **120**, 205–207

Grayhack, J. T. and Bockrath, J. M. (1981) Diagnosis of carcinoma of the prostate. *Urology*, **17**, Suppl. 1, 54–60

Grossman, H. B., Batata, M., Hilaris, B. and Whitmore, W. F. Jr (1982) ^{125}I implantation for carcinoma of prostate. Further follow-up of first 100 cases. *Urology*, **20**, 591–598

Haddock, G., Gray, H. W., McKillop, J. H. *et al.* (1989) ^{99m}Tc-nanocolloid bone marrow scintigraphy in prostatic cancer. *British Journal of Urology*, **63**, 497–502

Hald, T. and Rasmussen, F. (1980) Extraperitoneal pelvioscopy: a new aid in staging of lower urinary tract tumours. A preliminary report. *Journal of Urology*, **124**, 245–248

Handley, R., Carr, T. W., Travis, D. *et al.* (1988) Deferred treatment for prostate cancer. *British Journal of Urology*, **62**, 249–253

Hanks, G. E., Leibel, S. and Kramer, S. (1983) The dissemination of cancer by transurethral resection of localised advanced prostate cancer. *Journal of Urology*, **129**, 309–311

Harnett, P. R., Raghavan, D., Caterson, I. *et al.* (1987) Aminoglutethimide in advanced prostatic cancer. *British Journal of Urology*, **59**, 323–327

Harris, G. W. (1961) The pituitary stalk and ovulation. In *Control of Ovulation* (ed. C. A. Villee), Pergamon Press, New York, pp. 56–74

Hastak, S. M., Gammelsaard, J. and Holm, H. H. (1982) Ultrasonically guided transperineal biopsy in the diagnosis of prostatic carcinoma. *Journal of Urology*, **128**, 69–71

Herr, H. H. (1980) Iodine-125 implantation in the management of localized prostatic carcinoma. *Urologic Clinics of North America*, **7**, 605–613

Hillyard, J. W. (1987) Bacteraemia following perineal prostatic biopsy. *British Journal of Urology*, **60**, 252–254

Holm, H. H., Juul, N., Pedersen, J. F. *et al.* (1983) Transperineal ^{125}iodine seed implantation in prostatic cancer guided by transrectal ultrasonography. *Journal of Urology*, **130**, 283–286

Huggins, C. and Hodges, C. V. (1941) Studies on prostate cancer. 1. The effect of castration of oestrogen and of androgen injection on serum phosphatases in metastatic carcinoma of the prostate. *Cancer Research*, **1**, 293–297

Jewett, H. J. (1970) The case for radical prostatectomy. *Journal of Urology*, **130**, 195–199

Jewett, H. J. (1975) The present status of radical prostatectomy for stages A and B prostatic cancer. *Urological Clinics of North America*, **2**, 105–124

Jobsis, A. C., De Vries, G. P., Anholt, R. R. H. and Sanders, C. T. B. (1978) Demonstration of the prostatic origin of metastases. *Cancer*, **41**, 1788–1793

Jones, W. G., Fossa, S. D., Bono, A. V. *et al.* (1986) Mitomycin-C in the treatment of metastatic prostate cancer: report on an EORTC phase II study. *World Journal of Urology*, **4**, 182–185

Kaufman, J. J., Ljung, B. M., Walther, P. and Waiman, J. (1982) Aspiration biopsy of prostate. *Urology*, **19**, 587–591

Killian, C. S., Yang, N., Emrich, L. J. *et al.* (1985) Prognostic importance of prostate-specific antigen for monitoring patients with stages B_2 to D_1 prostate cancer. *Cancer Research*, **45**, 886–891

Kirk, D. (1985) Prostatic carcinoma. *British Medical Journal*, **290**, 875–876

Kirk, D. (1987a) Trials and tribulations in prostatic cancer. *British Journal of Urology*, **59**, 375–379

Kirk, D. (1987b) Princip. ᶠpatient management: immediate or deferred treatment. *British Journal of Clinical Practice*, **41**, Supp. ᶦ8, 84–87

Labrie, F., Belanger, A., Dupont, A. *et al.*, (1984) Combined treatment with LHRH agonist and pure anti-androgen in advanced carcinoma of prostate. *Lancet*, **ii**, 1090

Labrie, F., Dupont, A., Belanger, A. *et al.* (1983) New approach in the treatment of prostate cancer: complete instead of partial withdrawal of androgens. *The Prostate*, **4**, 579–594

Labrie, F., Dupont, A., Giguere, M. *et al.* (1988) Important benefits of combination therapy with flutamide in patients relapsing after castration. *British Journal of Urology*, **61**, 341–346

Lee, K., Gray, J. M., McLeary, T. R. *et al.* (1985) Transrectal ultrasound in the diagnosis of prostate cancer: location, echogenicity, histopathology, and staging, *The Prostate*, **7**, 117–129

Lindholt, J. and Hansen, P. T. (1986) Prostatic carcinoma: complications of megavoltage radiation therapy. *British Journal of Urology*, **58**, 52–54

Loening, S. A., Beckley, S., Brady, M. F. *et al.* (1983) Comparison of estramustine phosphate, methotrexate and cis-platinum in patients with advanced, hormone refractory prostate cancer. *Journal of Urology*, **129**, 1001–1006

Lund, F. and Rasmussen, F. (1988) Flutamide versus stilboesterol in the management of advanced prostatic cancer. A controlled prospective study. *British Journal of Urology*, **61**, 140–142

Lund, F., Smith, P. H., Suchu, S. *et al.* (1984) Do bone scans predict prognosis in prostatic cancer? A report of the EORTC protocol 30762. *British Journal of Urology*, **56**, 58–63

Lundgren, R. (1987) Flutamide as primary treatment for metastatic prostatic cancer. *British Journal of Urology*, **59**, 156–158

MacFarlane, J. R. and Tolley, D. A. (1985) Flutamide therapy for advanced prostatic cancer: a phase II study. *British Journal of Urology*, **57**, 172–174

McKillop. J. H. (1986) Radionuclide bone imaging for staging and follow-up of secondary malignancy. *Clinics in Oncology*, **5**, 125–139

McNeal, J. E. (1969) Origin and development of carcinoma in the prostate. *Cancer*, **23**, 24–34

McNeal, J. E. (1981) Normal and pathological anatomy of the prostate. *Urology*, **17**, Suppl. 1, 11–16

McNeal, J. E., Bostwick, D. G., Kindrachuck, R. A. *et al.* (1986) Patterns of progression in prostate cancer. *Lancet*, **i**, 60–63

McNicholas, T. A., Carter, S. StC., Wickham, J. E. A. and O'Donoghue, E. P. N. (1988) YAG laser treatment of early carcinoma of the prostate. *British Journal of Urology*, **61**, 239–243

McNicholas, T. A., Charig, C., Dickinson, I. K. *et al.* (1989) Total prostatectomy for localized prostatic carcinoma: early experience. Paper read at Annual Meeting of British Association of Urological Surgeons, St. Helier, Jersey, 22nd June

Meacham, R. R., Scardino, P. T., Hoffman, G. S. *et al.* (1989) The risk of distant metastases after transurethral resection of the prostate versus needle biopsy in patients with localized prostate cancer. *Journal of Urology*, **142**, 320–325

Moon, T. (1985) Prostatic carcinoma. *British Medical Journal*, **290**, 1824

Muntzing, J., Shukla, S. K., Chu, T. M. *et al.* (1974) Pharmacological study of oral estramustine phosphate (Estracyt) in advanced carcinoma of the prostate. *Investigative Urology*, **12**, 65–68

Nesbit, R. M. and Baum, W. C. (1950) Endocrine control of prostatic cancer. Clinical survey of 1818 cases. *Journal of the American Medical Association*, **143**, 1317–1320

Nesbit, R. M. and Plumb, R. T. (1946) Prostatic carcinoma. A follow-up on 795 patients treated prior to the endocrine era and a comparison of survival rates between these and patients treated by endocrine therapy. *Surgery*, **20**, 263–272

Neumann, F. (1983) Different principles of androgen deprivation for palliative treatment of prostatic cancer. In *Androgens and Anti-androgens* (ed. F. Schroeder), Schering, Weesp, pp. 97–114

Neumann, F. and Schenck, B. (1984) Pharmacological principles and rationale of the various methods of endocrine therapy. In *The Therapy of Advanced Carcinoma of the Prostate* (ed. H. Klosterhalfen), Schering AG, West Germany, pp. 15–23

Parker, M. C., Cook, A., Riddle, P. R. *et al.* (1985) Is delayed treatment justified in carcinoma of the prostate? *British Journal of Urology*, **57**, 724–728

Parmar, H., Edwards, L., Phillips, R. H. *et al.* (1987) Orchiectomy versus long-acting D-Trp-6-LHRH in advanced prostatic cancer. *British Journal of Urology*, **59**, 248–254

Paulson, D. F. and Cox, B. E. (1987) Does transurethral resection of the prostate promote metastatic disease? *Journal of Urology*, **138**, 90–91

Paulson, D. F., Lin, G. H., Hinshaw, W. *et al.* (1982) Radical surgery versus radiotherapy for adenocarcinoma of the prostate. *Journal of Urology*, **128**, 502–504

Pollen, J. J. (1981) Bone scanning in prostatic cancer. *Urology*, **17**, Suppl. 1, 31–32

Pontes, J. E., Choe, B. K., Rose, N. R. *et al.* (1981) Clinical evaluation of immunological methods of detection of serum prostatic acid phosphatase. *Journal of Urology*, **126**, 363–365

Prout, G. R., Griffin, P. P., Daly, J. J. and Shipley, W. U. (1981) Nodal involvement as a prognostic indicator in prostatic carcinoma. *Urology*, **17**, Suppl. 1, 72–79

Resnick, M. I. (1985) Ultrasound in evaluating prostatic cancer. *Journal of Urology*, **134**, 314

Ritchie, A. W. S., Smith, G., Preston, C. *et al.* (1985) Prediction of response to radiotherapy for localised prostatic cancer. *British Journal of Urology*, **57**, 729–732

Robinson, R. G. (1986) Radionuclides for the alleviation of bone pain in advanced malignancy. *Clinics in Oncology*, **5**, 39–49

Rowlands, C. G., Bullimore, J. A., Smith, P. J. B. and Roberts, J. B. M. (1981) Half-body irradiation in the treatment of metastatic prostatic carcinoma. *British Journal of Urology*, **53**, 628–629

Schmidt, J. D. (1981) Indications and surgical approaches for prostatic cancer. *Urology*, **17**, Suppl. 2, 4–6

Sheldon, C. A., Williams, R. D. and Fraley, E. E. (1980) Incidental carcinoma of the prostate: a review of the literature and critical appraisal of classification. *Journal of Urology*, **124**, 626–631

Smith, P. H. (1987) Medical management of prostatic cancer: single or combination therapy? *British Journal of Clinical Practice*, **41**, Suppl. 48, 105–111

Stamey, T. A. (1982) Cancer of the prostate: an analysis of some important contributions and dilemmas. *Monographs in Urology*, **3**, 65–96

Stamey, T. A. and Kabalin, J. N. (1989) Prostate specific antigen in the diagnosis and treatment of adenocarcinoma of the prostate. I. Untreated patients. *Journal of Urology*, **141**, 1070–1075

Stamey, T. A., Kabalin, J. N. and Ferrari, M. (1989) Prostate specific antigen in the diagnosis and treatment of adenocarcinoma of the prostate. III. Radiation treated patients. *Journal of Urology*, **141**, 1084–1087

Stamey, T. A., Kabalin, J. N., Ferrari, M. and Yang, N. (1989a) Prostate specific antigen in the diagnosis and treatment of adenocarcinoma of the prostate. IV. Anti-androgen treated patients. *Journal of Urology*, **141**, 1088–1090

Stamey, T. A., Kabalin, J. N., McNeal, J. E. *et al.* (1989b) Prostate specific antigen in the diagnosis and treatment of adenocarcinoma of the prostate. II. Radical prostatectomy treated patients. *Journal of Urology*, **141**, 1076–1083

Susan, L.P., Roth, R. B. and Adkins, W. C. (1976) Regression of prostatic cancer metastases by high doses of diethyl stilboestrol diphosphate. *Urology*, **7**, 598–601

Tolley, D. A. and Robinson, S. M. (1984) Attitudes towards the management of prostatic cancer – results of a postal survey. Paper read at Annual Meeting of British Association of Urological Surgeons: Dublin

Torti, F. M., Aston, D., Lum, B. L. *et al.* (1983) Weekly doxorubicin in endocrine refractory carcinoma of the prostate. *Journal of Clinical Oncology*, **1**, 477–482

Tunn, U. W., Graff, J. and Senge, T. H. (1983) Treatment of inoperable prostatic cancer with cyproterone acetate. In *Androgens and Anti-androgens* (ed. F. Schroeder), Schering, Weesp, pp. 149–159

Wajsman, Z. (1981) Lymph node evaluation in prostatic cancer: is pelvic lymph node dissection necessary? *Urology*, **17**, 1, 80–82

Wallace, D. M., Chisholm, G. D. and Hendry, W. F. (1975) TNM classification for urological tumours (UICC) – 1974. *British Journal of Urology*, **47**, 1–12

Walsh, P. C. (1986) Radical retropubic prostatectomy. In *Campbell's Urology* (ed. P. C. Walsh, R. E. Gittes, A. D. Perlmutter, and T. A. Stamey), Saunders, Philadelphia, pp. 2754–2775

Walsh, P. C. and Lepor, H. L. (1987) The role of radical prostatectomy in the management of prostatic cancer. *Cancer*, **60**, 526–537

Walsh, P. C., Lepor, H. and Eggleston, J. C. (1983) Radical prostatectomy with preservation of sexual function: anatomical and pathological considerations. *The Prostate*, **4**, 473–485

Walzer, Y., Oswalt, J. and Soloway, M. S. (1984) Estramustine phosphate – hormone, chemotherapeutic agent, or both? *Urology*, **24**, 53–58

Waxman, J. H., Man, A., Hendry, W. F. *et al.* (1985) Importance of early tumour exacerbation in patients treated with long-acting analogues of gonadotrophin releasing hormone for advanced prostatic cancer. *British Medical Journal*, **291**, 1387–1388

Waxman, J. H., Wass, J. A. H., Hendry, W. F. *et al.* (1983) Treatment of advaced prostatic cancer with buserelin, an analogue of gonadotrophin releasing hormone. *British Journal of Urology*, **55**, 737–742

Wein, A. J. and Murphy, J. J. (1973) Experience in the treatment of prostatic carcinoma with cyproterone acetate. *Journal of Urology*, **109**, 68–70

Whitmore, W. F. Jr (1956) Hormone therapy in prostatic cancer. *American Journal of Medicine*, **21**, 697–713

Young, H. H. (1905) The early diagnosis and radical cure of carcinoma of the prostate. *Bulletin of the Johns Hopkins Hospital*, **16**, 315–321

Zincke, H., Utz, D. C., Benson, R. C. and Patterson, D. E. (1984) Bilateral lymphadenectomy and radical retropubic prostatectomy for stage C carcinoma of prostate. *Urology*, **24**, 532–539

Chapter 10

Testis cancer

S. B. Kaye

Introduction

Although testicular cancer is uncommon it is of major interest to clinicians and scientists involved in cancer. The reason is that even at an advanced stage the disease is curable with chemotherapy, and this phenomenon is rare for any disseminated solid tumour. Moreover, the tumour usually produces biochemical tumour markers which allow more accurate assessments of response to treatment than are generally possible. The reason for this exquisite sensitivity is not known, but presumably it is related to the biological nature of the cancer which generally arises in pluripotential germ cells.

Incidence and aetiology

Testicular cancer is an uncommon disease, although it does represent the most common form of cancer in young men because of its age-specific incidence (Figure 10.1). The incidence is increasing in many countries; in Scotland, for example, the frequency has risen from 2.5 per 100 000 males to 5.0 per 100 000 males in the past 20 years. This rise is accompanied by a change in histological distribution, whereby teratoma is increasing in incidence relative to seminoma (Figure 10.1). This is

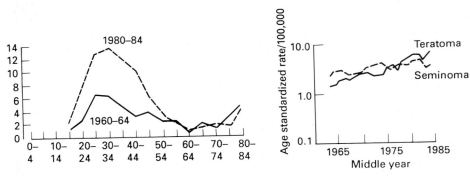

Figure 10.1 Left, Age-specific incidence rates per 100 000 of testicular cancer in Scotland in 1960–1964 and 1980–1984. Right, Testicular cancer incidence rate per 100 000 in Scotland for males age 15–44, by histological type (Courtesy of Pergamon Press)

accompanied by a downward shift in the peak age incidence, but there is still a distinct difference between the peak age incidence for teratoma (20–30 years) and that for seminoma (30–50 years) (Boyle, Kaye and Robertson, 1987).

The reasons for the increased incidence are unknown, although it is of interest that testicular cancer remains more common in men in social classes I and II than in classes IV and V. Epidemiological studies are proceeding, but at present the only established predisposing factor for testicular cancer is the presence of an undescended testis. Men with a history of cryptorchidism have a 14-fold increase in incidence of testicular tumours compared with normals; early prophylactic surgery (orchidopexy) may reduce this risk to some degree.

This association with cryptorchidism, as well as with congenital inguinal hernia, suggests that prenatal factors may be important as regards aetiology. Recently, exogenous hormone (oestrogen) use by the mother during pregnancy has been implicated, as has excessive nausea during pregnancy, since elevated levels of free endogenous oestrogen have been detected in women with hyperemesis. The hypothesis is that these hormonal abnormalities *in utero* cause maturation arrest of fetal germ cells in males. Then at puberty these arrested primitive cells are stimulated to become active (by FSH) and malignant instead of normal germ cells develop.

Experimental data in mice support this hypothesis, and do confirm that high levels of maternal oestrogen prevent testicular descent in male fetuses. They also show that testosterone protects against this effect, and it is of great interest that pregnant black women have recently been shown to have higher serum testosterone levels than white women, since testicular cancer continues to be much less common in young black males compared to white males. These recent findings may lead to an explanation for the increasing incidence of the disease and may even give rise to some rational ideas for prevention (Henderson, Ross and Bernstein, 1988).

Pathology

Testicular tumours can be divided into germ-cell tumours, which comprise the great majority, and non-germ-cell tumours, which are rare. Non-germ-cell tumours include lymphoma (usually large-cell lymphoma and seen mainly in older age groups), gonadal stromal tumours (including Leydig and Sertoli cell tumours), adenocarcinoma of the rete testis, and mesenchymal tumours (including paratesticular rhabdomyosarcoma).

Germ-cell tumours comprise one or more of five major cell types. Frequently several cell types coexist within one tumour, but the histological label given to an individual tumour refers to the predominant cell type. The five cell types are listed in Table 10.1. Although they have been given different titles by pathologists in

Table 10.1 Histological classification of testicular germ-cell tumours

British testicular tumour panel	*USA classification*
Malignant teratoma undifferentiated (MTU)	Embryonal carcinoma
Malignant teratoma intermediate (MTI)	Teratocarcinoma
Malignant teratoma trophoblastic (MTT)	Choriocarcinoma
Teratoma	Teratoma
Seminoma	Seminoma

Great Britain and North America, there is general agreement about the nature of each cell type.

The relative incidence of teratoma in comparison to seminoma appears to have increased in recent years, and overall they each now constitute approximately almost half of the total number of germ-cell tumours. For the purposes of therapy tumours which contain both teratoma and seminoma (10–15% of total) are treated along the lines of teratoma (see below).

With respect to teratoma, and before the introduction of effective chemotherapy for advanced disease, the histological subtype of primary tumour carried significant prognostic implications. Recent experience in the treatment of metastatic disease has resulted, however, in the identification of other prognostic factors, such as tumour bulk and levels of tumour markers (MRC Working Party in Testicular Tumours, 1985); thus, in advanced disease the specific histological subtype of teratoma is unlikely to be an independent prognostic variable. It is in fact possible for patients to harbour one predominant cell type in the primary site, and other cell types in metastatic sites, as judged by tumour markers.

The major prognostic implications of the histological subtype relate to patients with Stage I disease, in whom the risk of relapse can be directly related to histological features in the primary tumour (see below).

Since the majority of germ-cell tumours produce either human chorionic gonadotrophin (HCG) or alphafetoprotein (AFP) or both, and since these proteins are expressed on the cell surface, immunohistochemistry using antibodies directed against these antigens may be a useful additional technique in diagnosis of difficult cases. These may include patients with extragonadal germ-cell tumours which can arise in the retroperitoneum, mediastinum, or pineal gland, and which require an approach to treatment similar to that used for testicular tumours.

The major characteristics of the five subtypes of germ-cell tumours are as follows, although it should be emphasized that elements of the different subtypes often coexist in a single tumour.

Malignant teratoma undifferentiated (MTU)

Macroscopically these often contain areas of necrosis and haemorrhage, with a firm nodular texture. Histologically, large anaplastic cells are generally seen, with eosinophilic cytoplasm and nuclei of widely differing shapes. A degree of differentiation may be seen, and a glandular pattern may be visible, although less so than in MTI.

Malignant teratoma intermediate (MTI)

Macroscopically, MTI has a characteristic nodular appearance, with a gritty texture in sectioning because of the presence of bone or cartilage. A wide variety of germ-cell types are seen, including bone, cartilage, smooth muscle and gastrointestinal or respiratory-type epithelial cells. The presence of yolk sac elements in the tumour is recognized by the appearance of characteristic Schiller–Duval bodies.

Malignant teratoma trophoblastic (MTT)

Tumours which comprise predominant elements of MTT are uncommon, although teratomas may often contain a minor trophoblastic element. The histological appearances of cytotrophoblasts and/or syncytiotrophoblasts are distinctive, and the tumours are often markedly haemorrhagic.

Teratoma differentiated (TD)

Minor elements of TD are often seen among other components in malignant teratoma, but tumours comprising entirely this type of tumour are unusual. The pattern is of fully mature or differentiated elements, including bone, cartilage, bone marrow and other elements. Although such primary tumours may be considered to have limited malignant potential, it should be noted that they may coexist with metastatic disease containing frankly malignant teratoma, e.g. MTU. Mature teratoma may also be seen in specimens resected following chemotherapy, and this is considered more fully later in the chapter.

Seminoma

Macroscopically, seminoma may differ from teratoma in possessing a pale cut surface with little haemorrhage or necrosis. Microscopically, large round cells with clear cytoplasm, and large nuclei with conspicuous nuclei, are seen, together with a variable lymphocytic infiltrate.

Disease spread

Metastases from the testis are detected in the majority of patients with testicular germ-cell tumours, lymphatic spread being the major means by which this occurs. This generally occurs via the spermatic cord to para-aortic, retroperitoneal and retrocrural lymph nodes, then through the thoracic duct to the posterior mediastinum and supraclavicular lymph nodes (usually left-sided). In addition, vascular spread may occur, usually to involve the lungs as well as lymph nodes.

Malignant teratoma and seminoma differ in their biological behaviour with respect to patterns of spread, in that vascular spread in addition to lymphatic metastases occurs earlier and more frequently in teratoma than in seminoma. This difference has important therapeutic implications, as discussed later in this chapter.

Vascular spread to the liver and brain occurs infrequently, generally in patients with advanced disease elsewhere and more often in cases of malignant teratoma trophoblastic. Metastases to bone are unusual, occurring more regularly in advanced seminoma than teratoma.

Clinical features

Testicular cancer presents generally with a mass in the testis, which is painless in 75% of patients. It is distinguished by its characteristic hard texture, and the suspicion of malignancy is raised by the difficulty in palpating the mass separately from the testis. The differential diagnosis includes infection involving the testis, torsion of the appendix of the testis (which is characteristically painful and tender), and epididymitis (which should respond to antibiotics). The failure of antibiotics to resolve the swelling completely is an important indication for surgical referral.

A coexistent (secondary) hydrocele may occur in 10–15% of patients and a further difficulty occasionally encountered is the presence of an anteverted testis when the epididymis lies in front of the testis rather than its usual posterior position.

Patients usually detect the mass by self-examination, and programmes of education to improve awareness of the importance of this may be of benefit in reducing the length of history to diagnosis, thereby improving the results of treatment, at least in theory.

Symptoms of metastases are uncommon and patients will usually have no other symptoms of ill health. However, specific questions should be asked at presentation. These include an enquiry regarding low back pain which is the most common early symptom of retroperitoneal lymph node spread. Symptoms such as anorexia, weight loss and dyspnoea indicate more advanced disease, while gynaecomastia is an indication that metastatic disease is present and is likely to be predominantly trophoblastic in nature.

Clinical examination should include a careful search for any evidence of lymph node spread, to sites such as supraclavicular fossae. A palpable abdominal mass indicates significant spread to retroperitoneal lymph nodes. Metastases to inguinal nodes are rare, although the primary tumour occasionally presents in the inguinal canal if the affected testis has remained undescended.

Diagnosis and investigation

The finding of a suspicious mass should result in prompt referral to a surgeon. In doubtful cases a testicular ultrasound may be useful, but this generally adds little information to clinical findings, and if clinical suspicion of malignancy remains, the patient should be prepared for orchiectomy. Preoperative investigations should include serum estimation of alphafetoprotein (AFP) and human chorionic gonadotrophin (HCG), as well as chest X-ray. In about 70% of cases of teratoma AFP will be detectable in the serum, and in 60% HCG will be detected. Either marker will be present in about 85% of patients at diagnosis.

Orchiectomy should always be performed by the inguinal approach, with the internal spermatic ring exposed and retractors placed therein to visualize the cord. Scrotal orchiectomy should be avoided because of the potential for trans-scrotal spread of tumours and subsequent inguinal node involvement. Although biopsies with frozen sections are sometimes performed these are only helpful in exceptional circumstances, and radical orchiectomy is generally preferable.

Once the diagnosis of a testicular malignancy has been made histologically, whether this proves to be malignant teratoma or seminoma, subsequent management depends on the result of staging investigations which comprise chest X-ray, serial measurements of tumour markers, and a CT scan of the chest and abdomen. The CT scan has become mandatory since it provides information which cannot be obtained by other imaging techniques. This includes the detection of small peripheral pulmonary deposits, and the visualization of retroperitoneal tumour, sometimes adjacent to the kidneys, which would not be detected by lymphangiography.

In studies which have included surgical data, a false-negative rate of 25% for CT scans of the abdomen has been reported (Lien et al., 1986). This raises the question of the role of lymphangiography: however, data suggest that this investigation adds very little information in the presence of a normal CT, and its use in this context has largely been discontinued. If the CT scan of the chest and abdomen are normal, the determination of the initial stage of the disease rests with the measurement of serum tumour markers, i.e. AFP and HCG, since the trend in levels measured at weekly intervals following orchiectomy accurately reflects disease stage. Rising tumour markers postorchiectomy are a reliable indication of metastatic spread, indicating the need for further therapy irrespective of results of radiological investigations. In the absence of disease spread outside the testis tumour markers will fall to normal level in the weeks following orchiectomy; the rate of fall approximates to the half-life of the marker, i.e. 30 hours of HCG and 5 days of AFP. Failure of marker levels to fall to normal following orchiectomy indicates that disease spread has indeed occurred (Figure 10.2).

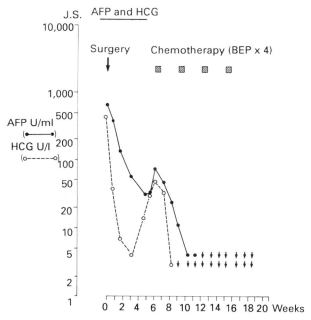

Figure 10.2 Serial tumour markers (AFP and HCG) following orchiectomy for testicular teratoma. The rising levels after 4 weeks define the need for chemotherapy which returns markers to undetectable levels

The value of serial estimations of tumour markers in testicular seminoma is less well established. If detectable levels of AFP are seen in a patient whose primary tumour contains only seminoma it is assumed that any metastatic disease contains teratoma, and the patient is managed accordingly. If detectable HCG is noted in serum from patients with a primary seminoma its significance depends on the level. An HCG level of up to 200 i.u./L in such a patient is compatible with a diagnosis of metastatic seminoma, since this tumour is known occasionally to be associated with low level HCG secretion. Higher levels of HCG, however, are taken to indicate that metastases in such a patient are likely to contain metastatic trophoblastic teratoma rather than seminoma, and again management is along the lines recommended for teratoma.

Recent data reported for a new tumour marker, placental alkaline phosphatase (PLAP) are promising in that up to 70% of patients with seminoma have detectable levels present in the serum, and correlation with disease state has been confirmed (Tucker *et al.*, 1985). However, at present PLAP estimation is not yet established as routine in seminoma to the extent of HCG and AFP monitoring in teratoma.

As a result of the investigations outlined above, patients with testicular malignancies, either teratoma or seminoma, may be assigned a clinical stage of disease, and various classifications have been proposed. In Great Britain the most widely used of these is the one evolved at the Royal Marsden Hospital, and it is outlined in Table 10.2. It is emphasized that this represents clinical staging, in

Table 10.2 Staging of testicular tumours (teratoma and seminoma)

Stage	I	Tumour confined to testis (CT scan, lymphography, tumour markers – all normal)
Stage	IM	No radiological evidence of metastases, but persistently elevated tumour markers (AFP and/or HCG) post-orchidectomy
Stage	II	Tumour in retroperitoneal lymph nodes, visualized at CT scan and/or lymphography
	IIa	Maximum (transverse) diameter of largest node mass less then 2 cm
	IIb	Maximum diameter of 2–5 cm
	IIc	Maximum diameter of 5–10 cm
	IId	Maximum diameter of greater than 10 cm
Stage	III	Mediastinal and/or supraclavicular lymph node spread
	IIIa–d	According to maximum diameter as in Stage II
Stage	IV	Extralymphatic spread
	IV L1	Lung metastases, less than 4 in number, all less than 2 cm in diameter
	IV L2	Lung metastases, 4 or more in number all less than 2 cm in diameter
	IV L3	Lung metastases, 4 or more in number, one or more being 2 cm or larger in diameter
	IV H	Hepatic metastases

contrast to pathological staging which is commonly performed in the United States and elsewhere, where retroperitoneal lymph node dissection is routinely carried out in patients who have clinical Stage I disease. When such patients are found to have microscopic evidence of retroperitoneal lymph node spread (observed in about 20% of cases) they are classified as pathological Stage II disease. Patients with clinical Stage I disease in Great Britain do not routinely undergo surgical evaluation in this way, and their management is discussed below.

Management

Malignant teratoma

Following the introduction of cisplatin into the chemotherapeutic management of metastatic teratoma in the mid-1970s it became apparent that the disease was curable in the majority of patients (Einhorn, 1981). Thus chemotherapy has become the major modality used in the treatment of patients with metastatic disease. The use of chemotherapy for patients without overt metastatic disease is currently being evaluated (see below).

Stage 1

A total of 20–30% of patients fall into this category, and the management of Stage I teratoma has been a controversial issue. Until recently many patients in Great Britain were treated with prophylactic radiotherapy to para-aortic lymph nodes; however, data on relapses in patients treated this way (10–20% of total) indicated that a significant proportion relapsed outside the treated field, particularly in the lungs; moreover, chemotherapy in such patients was made more difficult because of prior radiotherapy. Accordingly the value of radiotherapy in Stage I teratoma has been questioned. A recent retrospective study conducted by the Medical Research Council in Great Britain examined those factors which might predict relapse in a total of 259 patients managed by a policy of surveillance only in several referral centres. The overall 2-year relapse rate for all patients was 26% and all but 3 of the relapse patients were successfully treated with chemotherapy. Within this group it was possible to identify a subgroup of patients with a much higher rate of relapse (58% at 2 years). These patients had characteristic histological features in the primary tumour, including the pattern of undifferentiated malignant teratoma, vascular or lymphatic invasion, and the absence of yolk sac elements in the tumour (Freedman *et al.*, 1987).

These data may make it possible to select patients with Stage I disease who are at high risk of relapse, and who might therefore best be treated with immediate chemotherapy. Such a study is currently being formed by the Medical Research Council. The remaining, larger group of patients with Stage I disease may then be managed by surveillance only, although it is still the policy of some clinicians to treat such patients with abdominal radiotherapy.

As noted previously the management of clinical Stage I disease differs further in centres outside Great Britain. Retroperitoneal lymph node dissection is routinely performed by many urologists, and if microscopic disease spread is detected most patients will then receive a course of chemotherapy. It has been established that in this situation, two courses of platinum-combination chemotherapy is sufficient to ensure that the likelihood of disease relapse is minimal (Williams *et al.*, 1987b). The disadvantage of this approach is that patients are subjected to the morbidity of surgery which is not necessarily required in offering them the best prospect of cure. A bilateral retroperitoneal lymph node dissection will inevitably cause retrograde ejaculation which would be a significant problem for young men wishing to father children. The recent modification of the operation in a nerve-sparing approach has considerably reduced the incidence of this complication (Donohue, 1988), but the value of this approach remains uncertain, and most British urologists agree that it is probably unwarranted, because of the very high probability of cure of patients in this disease category with chemotherapy alone in selected cases according to the guidelines described above.

Stages II–IV

A total of 70–80% of patients fall into this category, and their management involves combination chemotherapy for all stages. The use of radiotherapy for Stage II disease is no longer appropriate, for the reasons outlined above, and because chemotherapy can be expected to be curative in the majority of patients (Figure 10.3).

The initial observations by Li and Samuels that metastatic teratoma could respond, albeit temporarily to chemotherapy, were made in 1968 and 1971, but it was in 1977 that Einhorn published data on the incorporation of cisplatin into

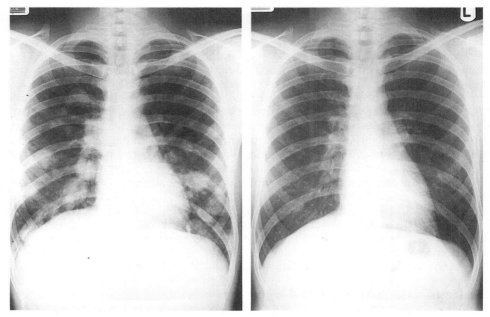

Figure 10.3 Chest X-ray showing multiple metastases from testicular cancer (Stage IV L3) before, and after completing 3 months of combination chemotherapy

combination chemotherapy, and for the first time durable complete remission of metastatic disease was observed in more than half of the treated patients (Einhorn and Donohue, 1977). The Einhorn schedule, comprising platinum, vinblastine and bleomycin (PVB) has been superseded by the introduction of another new drug etoposide (VP16), which has replaced vinblastine in a 3-drug combination, with the eponym BEP (bleomycin, etoposide, platinum) which is used in several centres (Williams *et al.*, 1987a). This combination can be expected to yield overall complete response rates of about 80% in patients with metastatic teratoma, and since only a small minority will subsequently relapse, this figure approximates to a cure rate. The use of this 3-drug schedule is associated with a degree of toxicity, although most patients tolerate treatment reasonably well once the curative aim of therapy is appreciated. The major acute side-effects are nausea and vomiting, attributable to the cisplatin, and hair-loss due to etoposide. Myelosuppression is also attributed mainly to etoposide, and the schedule often used involves a 3-week cycle, with chemotherapy given over 5 days. Although generally given for 4 cycles, a recent study has shown that in certain patients, 3 cycles of treatment are just as effective (Einhorn *et al.*, 1989).

Bleomycin can give rise to allergic reactions, and skin and pulmonary toxicity is sometimes a problem. Current European studies are addressing the issue of whether bleomycin is an essential component of therapy, at least in those patients with the lower metastatic load.

Major long-term side-effects are unlikely to occur. Although initial azoospermia is universal, recovery of sperm production and fertility is observed after 3–5 years in more than half of the patients receiving the drugs mentioned above, and there is no evidence of an increased frequency of abnormalities in the children fathered by treated patients. Recovery of fertility cannot be guaranteed, however, and pretreatment sperm storage is therefore sometimes appropriate.

Cisplatin is a nephrotoxic drug, and careful hydration at the time of administration is required to avoid acute renal toxicity. Current investigations are examining the possibility that subclinical long-term renal damage might occur, and might predispose to subsequent cardiovascular disease (Bosl *et al.*, 1988). However, present experience suggests that this is unlikely to be a major problem.

A variety of treatment schedules have been adopted in different centres, but they are based on the use of the same group of drugs. The major principles of treatment include careful monitoring of tumour marker levels, since complete remission of disease can only be considered possible once levels have become undetectable (Figure 10.2). At that stage, generally after about three months of chemotherapy, repeat radiological assessment may reveal persistent mass lesions, either in the retroperitoneum or in the lungs. These masses may comprise necrotic or scar tissue, or mature differentiated teratoma, or persistent malignant teratoma with features similar to the primary tumour. More recently, a further unusual variation in the histological appearance of resected masses has been described, as 'immature' teratoma, in which non-germ-cell elements with malignant characteristics are seen (Davey *et al.*, 1987).

Surgical evaluation of residual masses following chemotherapy for malignant teratoma forms an essential part of the management of these patients. The reason is that current non-invasive investigations do not distinguish between the possible components of these masses as outlined above, and the management of patients is significantly different according to the findings. Patients whose masses contain persistent frankly malignant teratoma do require further chemotherapy using alternative drugs, and their outlook is rather uncertain, although long-term survival is still possible. Fortunately the proportion of cases found to be in this category is falling (probably now less than 20%), and this reflects the increased effectiveness of initial chemotherapy. On the other hand, an increasing proportion of patients are found to harbour mature (differentiated) teratoma in residual masses following chemotherapy (about 40% in several series), and their outlook is excellent.

A correlation has been found between the presence of elements of mature teratoma in the primary tumour and in resected lesions following chemotherapy, and it is probable that the lesion arises because other histological elements of metastatic lesions have been eradicated by chemotherapy. The other possible mechanism by which teratoma might arise is through differentiation induced by cytotoxic drugs, although there are few data available in support of this hypothesis (Oosterhuis *et al.*, 1983). Whichever mechanism applies, it is clear that mature (and immature) teratoma represents a form of disease which cannot be eradicated by further chemotherapy or radiotherapy.

The major reason for recommending surgery for residual masses is the uncertainty about the long-term biological behaviour of these lesions. Mature teratoma does have the capacity to grow over a period of years, sometimes locally when it adopts a cystic appearance, but occasionally more widely when a relapse of frankly malignant teratoma occurs. It is conceivable that this is more likely to occur with immature teratoma, although longer follow-up of patients with this histological variant is required (Loehrer, Hin and Clark, 1988). For these reasons complete surgical excision of lesions which might contain mature teratoma is recommended. Such lesions may lie in the retroperitoneum, mediastinum or lungs, and removal may even involve a combined thoraco-abdominal approach and a prolonged surgical procedure, but present information indicates that this is justified. The aim of future studies will be to identify those patients whose post-chemotherapy masses are extremely unlikely to contain mature teratoma, and who might therefore be spared surgical excision (Donohue et al., 1987).

The results of chemotherapy for Stages II to IV testicular teratoma, followed when necessary by surgery, indicate that the majority of patients, about 80%, experience long-term survival and probably cure (although a small fraction may relapse over a period of years following treatment) (Roth et al., 1988). It is now possible to predict more accurately the outcome of treatment, by analysis of the pre-treatment characteristics of patients with metastatic disease, and as a result two broad groups of patients have been identified, based on the size of metastatic lesions and the levels of tumour markers.

1. 'Low volume' patients, with the minimal or moderate tumour bulk (i.e. less than 20 lung metastases, or abdominal masses less than 10 cm in diameter, with lower levels of HCG and AFP), have an expected cure rate of over 90%. This includes 65–75% of the total number of patients.
2. 'High volume' patients, with larger tumour masses (or more lung metastases) or higher levels of HCG and AFP, with an expected cure rate of 40–70%. This group comprises 25–35% of the total number of patients.

These data have encouraged some centres to begin treating these two categories of patients with metastatic disease with schedules of combination chemotherapy of differing intensity. In each case, bleomycin, cisplatin and etoposide are generally used, but it is possible that the intensity with which treatment is given can be adjusted according to the prognostic category. In particular, 'high volume' patients are receiving more intensive chemotherapy, using higher drug doses, shorter treatment intervals, or additional new drugs such as the cyclophosphamide analogue, ifosfamide, in an attempt to improve their outlook, even though greater toxicity from treatment would be anticipated. On the other hand, treatment for 'low volume' patients who have an excellent prognosis, may comprise 3 rather than 4 cycles of chemotherapy or may involve the deletion of drugs such as bleomycin, or the substitution of less toxic analogues of cisplatin, such as carboplatin. The aim in this case is to maintain efficacy but reduce toxicity if possible. These adjustments to the patterns of treatment require carefully controlled clinical studies to ensure that the present overall excellent results are maintained, and for this reason referral of patients with metastatic testicular cancer to specialist centres is mandatory (Graham et al., 1988).

Seminoma

The principles of management of seminoma differ from those which apply to malignant teratoma because of its different pattern of spread and predictable biological behaviour as discussed previously. As a result of the exquisite radiosensitivity of seminoma, radiotherapy to the retroperitoneal area is accepted as a standard form of therapy for many patients with this disease, whereas it is much less commonly used in patients with malignant teratoma.

Stages I and IIA
Over 80% of patients with seminoma fall into these disease categories, their long-term prognosis is excellent and the recommended therapy for them is

radiotherapy. For patients with Stage I disease the treatment can be regarded as prophylactic and some centres have demonstrated that surveillance only (as in Stage I teratoma) is a valid option, since those patients who relapse (10–20%) can generally be treated successfully with radiotherapy. However, this policy has not been widely accepted in the UK, for the reasons outlined above, which emphasize the differences in behaviour between teratoma and seminoma. A typical treatment programme would involve a total dose of 30 Gy delivered by anterior and posterior fields over a 3-week period, usually using daily fractions, to para-aortic and ipsilateral pelvic lymph nodes. Ipsilateral inguinal nodes and the scrotal sac are also included if a scrotal operation has been done. 'Prophylactic' radiotherapy to the mediastinum and supraclavicular nodes was part of standard therapy, but is now included less frequently because of the advent of very effective chemotherapy for patients with bulky lesions. Radiotherapy given in this context is generally carried out on an out-patient basis and the toxicity is mild. Some patients develop nausea and diarrhoea is also sometimes seen. There are no significant long-term sequelae, although irradiation of bone marrow within the radiotherapy field leads to enhanced myelosuppression in the small proportion of patients who are treated with chemotherapy as a result of subsequent disease relapse. Lead shielding of the contralateral testis is routinely done, so that there is minimal risk of impaired fertility from scatter of radiation. With this form of treatment the relapse rate of Stages I and IIA disease does not exceed 10% (Thomas, Rider and Dembo, 1982). If relapse does occur, generally within two years, chemotherapy is usually given and often results in eradication of disease.

Stage IIB

Only a small percentage of patients fall into this category, in which retroperitoneal lymph node metastases, greater than 2 cm, but smaller than 5 cm in diameter are found. Standard therapy comprises radiotherapy to involved nodes, and this eradicates the disease in about 70% of cases. Relapsing patients may be successfully treated with chemotherapy, although this may prove difficult because of compromised bone marrow function. For this reason initial chemotherapy may be a valid alternative for this subgroup (as in the more advanced subgroups discussed below). The disadvantage of increased toxicity compared with radiotherapy is balanced by a greater likelihood of eradication of disease, occurring in about 90% of cases.

Stages IIC, III and IV

Only a minority of patients with metastatic seminoma fall into these categories (probably less than 20%). The results of treatment with radiotherapy are less satisfactory. Prior to the introduction of chemotherapy less than 50% of patients treated with radiotherapy alone experienced long-term survival. However, it has now become clear that seminoma is at least as sensitive to the same group of cytotoxic drugs as teratoma, cisplatin forming the basis of all schedules used in this context. Thus the use of combinations of drugs used in teratoma will result in disease eradication in the majority of patients with advanced seminoma with cure rates in the range of 80–90%. Following chemotherapy, residual lesions may remain in sites such as the retroperitoneum and they may regress over a period of many months after treatment is completed. The most appropriate management of such patients is controversial. The use of surgical excision, as in patients with residual lesions following treatment for teratoma, has been questioned because these lesions have proved much more difficult to resect, and surgical morbidity is higher. Alternative approaches include a period of observation only, perhaps followed by radiotherapy to a lesion which is not continuing to regress (Peckham, Horwich and Hendry, 1985).

References

Bosl, G., Geller, N. L., Bajorin, D. *et al.* (1988) A randomised trial of etoposide and cisplatin versus vinblastine + bleomycin + cisplatin + cyclophosphamide + dactinomycin in patients with good prognosis germ cell tumours. *Journal of Clinical Oncology*, **6**, 1231–1238

Boyle, P., Kaye, S. B. and Robertson, A. G. (1987) Changes in testicular cancer in Scotland. *European Journal of Cancer and Clinical Oncology*, **23(6)**, 827–830

Davey, A. D., Ulbright, T. M., Loehrer, P. J. *et al.* (1987) The significance of atypia within teratomatous metastases after chemotherapy for malignant germ cell tumour. *Cancer*, **9**, 533

Donohue, J. P. (1988) Preservation of ejaculation following nerve-sparing retroperitoneal lymphadectomy. *Journal of Urology*, **139**, 206a

Donohue, J. P., Rowland, R. G., Kopecky, K. *et al.* (1987) Correlation of CT-changes and histological findings in 80 patients having radical retroperitoneal lymph node dissection after chemotherapy for testis cancer. *Journal of Urology*, **137**, 1176–1179

Einhorn, L. H. (1981) Testicular cancer as a model for curable neoplasm. *Cancer Research*, **41**, 3275–3280

Einhorn, L. H. and Donohue, J. (1977) Cisplatin, vinblastine and bleomycin combination chemotherapy in disseminated testicular cancer. *Annals of Internal Medicine*, **87**, 293–298

Einhorn, L. H., Williams, S. D., Loehrer, P. J. *et al.* (1989) Evaluation of optimal duration of chemotherapy in favourable-prognosis disseminated germ cell tumours: A South Eastern Cancer Study Group Protocol. *Journal of Clinical Oncology*, **7**, 387–391

Freedman, L. S., Parkinson, M. C., Jones, W. G. *et al.* (1987) Histopathology in the prediction of relapse of patients with stage I testicular teratoma treated by orchidectomy alone. *Lancet*, **ii**, 294–298

Graham, J., Harding, M., Mill, L. *et al.* (1988) Results of treatment of non-seminomatous germ cell tumours: 122 consecutive cases in the West of Scotland, 1981–5. *British Journal of Cancer*, **57**, 182–185

Henderson, B. E., Ross, R. and Bernstein, L. (1988) Oestrogen as a cause of human cancer. *Cancer Research*, **48**, 246–253

Lien, H. H., Stening, A. E., Ous, S. and Fossa, S. D. (1986) Influence of different criteria for abnormal lymph node size on reliability of computed tomography in patients with non-seminomatous testicular tumour. *Acta Radiologica Diagnosis (Stockholm)*, **27**, 199–203

Loehrer, P. J., Hin, S. and Clark, S. (1988) Teratoma following cisplatin-based combination chemotherapy for non-seminomatous germ cell tumours: a clinicopathological correlation. *Journal of Urology*, **135**, 1183–1189

MRC Working Party in Testicular Tumours (1985) Prognostic factors in advanced non-seminomatous germ-cell tumours: results of a multi-centre study. *Lancet*, **i**, 8–12

Oosterhuis, J. W., Suurmeyer, A. J. H., Sleyfer, D. T. *et al.* (1983) Effects of multiple-drug chemotherapy (cis-diamine-dichloroplatinum, bleomycin and vinblastine) on the maturation of retroperitoneal lymph node metastases of nonseminomatous germ cell tumours of the testis. *Cancer*, **51**, 408–416

Peckham, M. J., Horwich, A. and Hendry, W. F. (1985) Advanced seminoma; treatment with cisplatin-based combination chemotherapy or carboplatin. *British Journal of Cancer*, **52**, 7–12

Roth, B. J., Greist, A., Kubilis, P. S. *et al.* (1988) Cisplatin-based combination chemotherapy for disseminated germ cell tumours: long term follow-up. *Journal of Clinical Oncology*, **6**, 1239–1247

Thomas, G. M., Rider, W. D. and Dembo, A. J. (1982) Seminoma of the testis, results of treatment and patterns of failure. *International Journal of Radiation Oncology, Biological Physiology*, **8**, 165–174

Tucker, D. F., Oliver, R. T., Travers, P. and Bodner, W. F. (1985) Serum marker potential of placental alkaline phosphatase-like activity in testicular germ cell tumours. *British Journal of Cancer*, **51**, 631–639

Williams, S. D., Birch, R., Einhorn, L. H. *et al.* (1987a) Treatment of disseminated germ cell tumours with cisplatin, bleomycin and either vinblastine or etoposide. *New England Journal of Medicine*, **316**, 1435–1440

Williams, S. D., Stablein, D. M., Einhorn, L. H. *et al.* (1987b) Immediate adjuvant chemotherapy versus observation with treatment at relapse in pathological stage II testicular cancer. *New England Journal of Medicine*, **317**, 1433–1438

Chapter 11

Tumours of the head and neck

Ian A. McGregor

Skin tumours

The malignant skin tumours regularly seen in the facial skin are basal-cell carcinoma, squamous carcinoma and malignant melanoma.

Both basal-cell carcinoma and squamous carcinoma arise in two clinical forms — as a *single lesion* in apparently normal skin, and as *multiple lesions* arising on a background of abnormal skin. The single tumour arising in a background of normal skin has the appearance and behavioural characteristics of the lesion as it is classically described in surgical textbooks, in terms of its clinical appearance, pattern of local infiltration and metastatic potential. The multifocal lesion seldom has a completely typical appearance and the more abnormal the surrounding skin the less typical is the tumour both in appearance and in behaviour. Various aetiological factors are regularly cited in textbooks of pathology and surgery, particularly in relation to squamous carcinoma, but today much the most frequent causal factor with both in creating the background skin abnormality is solar radiation, the fraction of the spectrum close to the ultraviolet band being responsible.

The type of skin most susceptible to such damage is the fair, freckled skin, often referred to as 'Celtic skin'. The skin of such individuals tans with difficulty or not at all. The comparative absence of melanin in their skin, normally concentrated in the supranuclear cap of the basal layer of the epidermis, leaves the cell open to damage to its DNA. The end result of such damage over a lifetime of exposure, even in a temperate climate, is widespread dysplastic changes in the exposed skin, with the frequent development of focal areas of frank neoplasia. Both the epithelial cells and the population of melanocytes are affected by these changes, the epithelial neoplasms which develop being squamous carcinoma and basal-cell carcinoma, the melanocytic neoplasm being lentigo maligna melanoma. Fortunately the evolution of the sequence to fully developed invasive tumour is extremely slow both in the epithelial and melanocytic cell lines and the neoplasms which develop are themselves usually equally slow in their growth, infiltration and metastasis.

Basal-cell carcinoma

This is the most common neoplasm to arise in facial skin. It predominantly affects the older age group and when it arises in the patient under 25 years of age it is almost invariably found to have arisen in an organoid naevus (sebaceous naevus of

Jadassohn). Occurring as multiple lesions it is also the most conspicuous element of the much more rare Gorlin–Goltz syndrome. As a tumour it is slow growing, spreads locally but virtually never metastasizes. Whether it is capable of metastasis at all is doubtful. Reports of metastasizing 'basal-cell carcinoma' are regularly found in the literature but it is increasingly recognized that the reported instances are either tumours of the adnexal structures of the skin or are a variant of basal-cell carcinoma, the metatypical basal-cell carcinoma, a tumour type recognized to be capable of metastasis.

Most basal-cell carcinomas are localized and have well-defined margins both clinically and histologically but a proportion have a much more infiltrative pattern of spread. These are referred to as *morpheic* and their excision provides more problems for the surgeon than the usual localized lesion. The problems arise predominantly in three anatomical areas — the inner canthal area, the alar base, and around the pinna and external acoustic meatus. Although many basal-cell carcinomas of the face are treated successfully by radiotherapy, it is increasingly recognized that this method of treatment is better avoided in these three sites because of the recognized difficulty of achieving cure by surgical means if tumour recurs after radiotherapy has been used. Even in the absence of previous radiotherapy, basal-cell carcinomas in these sites, particularly if they exhibit a morpheic pattern, require to be treated more radically than in most other areas and followed-up more carefully.

Squamous carcinoma

Arising as a single tumour this tumour is very rare on the face. In the form of multiple actinically-induced lesions it is extremely common. The precursor premalignant lesion, actinic keratosis, generally shows as a focal area with a covering scale whose removal leaves a temporarily weeping surface. Progress of such a lesion to invasive squamous carcinoma is slow and not inevitable. Such areas often respond well to fluorouracil, and particularly if they are multiple, the method may be preferable to surgery. It can be most effective where there is a mixture of areas of actinic damage, actinic keratosis, and squamous carcinoma and it is difficult to distinguish between them. With the fluorouracil the first two resolve, allowing the areas of carcinoma to be recognized and treated surgically. With the background of skin damage from actinic radiation, such lesions are not suitable for radiotherapy. The presence of a nodule, or a warty patch is usually indicative of infiltrating squamous carcinoma and the development of a plaque of keratin in the form of a horn is also a form which the tumour can take. Such tumours are generally low-grade, remaining localized and metastasizing only very rarely. Treated surgically it is usually possible to carry out excision and suture. Wide clearance is not often required.

Specific sites often involved are the pinna and the vermilion of the lower lip. *In the pinna* the condition is virtually confined to the male, the longer hair of the female protecting the ear from the sun. *In the lower lip* the vermilion which is exposed is frequently the site of actinic damage over its entire length, angle to angle, showing as persistent scaling. Actinic damage in this form can be present on its own or as the premalignant background to an obviously invasive squamous carcinoma. In such circumstances the carcinoma tends to be slow growing, though not as slow as in the face and scalp in general. Metastasis is rare but when it occurs the submandibular group of nodes is the one involved. The submental nodes are described in anatomical texts as draining lymph from the lower lip but in clinical practice they are virtually never the site of metastasis.

Diffuse premalignancy of the lower lip, even in the absence of an overt malignant focus, is best treated by prophylactic stripping of the exposed vermilion, the so-called 'lip-shave'. The defect is most often closed by advancing the mucosa lining the lip. Squamous carcinoma of the lip is regularly associated with premalignancy of the adjoining vermilion and in such circumstances it is often necessary to resect the carcinoma in continuity with a 'lip-shave' as a combined excision.

Malignant melanoma

Although nodular and superficial spreading melanomas regularly arise in the skin of the face the tumour type which is virtually confined to that site is lentigo maligna melanoma. This variant is much slower in its evolution than the other forms. It typically arises in the cheek or temple of an elderly patient whose skin is already actinically damaged. Its precursor state is lentigo maligna — a pigmented macule which exhibits radial growth, slowly increasing in area and often becoming darker in colour. Histologically, the melanocytes are increased in number, extending down the hair follicles but remaining confined to the epidermis. The individual melanocytes show dysplastic changes of considerable severity, but confined to the epidermis. In the macular background of such a lentigo maligna the appearance of a nodule indicates the development of a vertical growth phase and the change to invasive malignancy — lentigo maligna melanoma. The sequence from initial appearance of the pigmented macule to the development of invasive tumour is extremely slow, taking up to 20 years and more often than not is never completed. It has generally been considered to be a relatively benign form of malignant melanoma, rarely metastasizing and responding well to local excision but some doubt has recently been cast on this. In the other forms of melanoma Breslow thickness is accepted as the best prognostic indicator, and evidence has been presented which suggests that it is also relevant in lentigo maligna melanoma.

Oral premalignancy and malignancy

Leukoplakia is a condition on which the surgical literature is extremely vague, particularly in relation to the malignant potential of its various clinical forms. The term literally means a white plaque. Keratin becomes white when it is wet, and in the moist environment of the mouth patches of oral epithelium which have a sufficient increase in keratinization to show clinically as white areas against the surrounding mucosa have the name leukoplakia applied to them. The great majority of such patches which are seen in clinical practice have no malignant potential but a small proportion, in the region of 5%, are premalignant and left untreated for sufficiently long become malignant.

Both of these forms have a roughly similar clinical appearance and both have the term leukoplakia applied to them despite the fact that their pathology, proper therapy and prognosis are quite different. The term should be regarded as a clinically descriptive one with implications which require to be investigated to ascertain their significance in pathological terms. The word has no place in the vocabulary of the pathologist. He is concerned, not with the presence of keratinized surface epithelium, but with the cells which underlie the keratinized layer, the normality or otherwise of their maturation, and the severity of any dysplasia which may be present.

Leukoplakia can take several clinical forms and these forms vary in their neoplastic potential. It may present as an area of soft, white, velvety mucosa, as a patch or fleck of white 'paint' on the mucosa, often with a slightly wrinkled surface which does not amount to wartiness, or as a diffuse area where the pink sheen of the normal mucosa is replaced by a slight but distinct pallor and changes in surface characteristics, for example the way in which light is reflected. There is an absence of inflammatory reaction in and around the affected area and an absence of induration so that the area cannot be detected by touch alone. This type of leukoplakia has been referred to as *leukoplakia simplex*. An area of leukoplakia with these clinical findings is seldom associated with significant dysplasia. It represents a lesion which is unlikely to become malignant unless some change in its clinical character takes place to bring it into one of the categories described below. The forms of leukoplakia which are much more likely to be in the category of premalignant are *verrucous leukoplakia* and *leukoerythroplakia*.

Verrucous leukoplakia occurs in two different forms depending on whether or not the chewing of tobacco is a factor in its aetiology. When the patient chews tobacco the verrucous leukoplakia which develops at the site where the quid is held in the mouth is the starting point on the road to its ultimate neoplastic end-point – verrucous carcinoma. Tobacco chewing is uncommon in the UK and this form of verrucous leukoplakia is correspondingly rare.

When there is no history of tobacco chewing, verrucous leukoplakia has a different pattern of behaviour. In its mildest form the patch of mucosa has a diffusely fine warty surface and is slightly indurated. Its epithelium is likely to show some signs of dysplasia, though hyperkeratosis is the most striking feature histologically. All gradations can occur from such a minor wartiness of the surface up to the markedly indurated plaque with a coarse warty surface. The clinical picture of gradation is paralleled microscopically with mild dysplasia at one extreme and carcinoma-in-situ at the other. The development of ulceration in such an area is strong presumptive evidence of invasive tumour.

Although a proportion of such patches do progress towards frank neoplastic change and some develop invasive carcinoma, this is not inevitable. More often than not the condition remains static, particularly when the patch is at the minor end of the spectrum of activity.

Leuko-erythroplakia occurs as an irregular mixture of white areas associated with areas of inflamed reddened mucosa, often with a velvety appearance. The proportion of the two surfaces, white and red, can vary considerably. The red areas are usually level with the surrounding mucosa and may even show a slight depression, indicative of the mucosal atrophy so often associated with severe dysplasia. As a rule induration is absent.

The presence of such areas of reddened mucosa is referred to as eythroplakia, but it is uncommon for it to occur on its own — the mixture of leukoplakia and erythroplakia being much the commoner, meriting the term leuko-erythroplakia. This mixture is to be regarded as having considerable malignant potential. In considering leukoplakia and its neoplastic potential, the area which needs to concern the clinician in the great majority of instances because it represents the site of the most severe dysplasia is the area of erythroplakia rather than the area of leukoplakia. It has been shown in studying early asymptomatic oral squamous carcinoma that an erythroplakic component can be found in over 90% of instances. With growth of the tumour this evidence of a precursor state is lost.

Aetiological factors

Premalignant change in the oral mucosa in the form of leukoplakia or erythroplakia has a basic incidence in the general population, for the most part with an unknown aetiology. To this basic incidence must be added a further incidence confined to particular populations in different parts of the world. In these, aetiological factors are clear and relate particularly to tobacco. In India the chewing of tobacco with lime, together with betel nut, as a quid wrapped in betel leaf is responsible for leukoplakia in the vicinity of the lower buccal sulcus, in the cheek or behind the lip, depending on where the quid is held. A similar clinical pattern is found in those parts of the United States where tobacco chewing is also common.

The clinical problem

Confronted with an area inside the mouth suspected of being premalignant, the degree of neoplastic activity should be established by carrying out a biopsy. Where the clinical appearance of the entire area is uniform a representative sample is adequate. If the area shows variation, as it usually does when an accurate pathological appraisal matters most, it is essential to sample the most active part. In the absence of erythroplakia the site of greatest induration should be sampled. If erythroplakia is present the sample should include it, for it will be the area of most severe dysplasia — the area on which the treatment required depends. It is also desirable to include in any biopsy a sample of the adjoining normal mucosa for comparison.

Patient management

The patient with a patch of leukoplakia which shows little or no evidence clinically of activity and on biopsy a virtual absence of dysplasia, can safely be reassured and no treatment is required. He might reasonably be warned to have the state of his mucosa reviewed afresh if there is any change in the appearance of the lesion. At the same time he can be reassured that such change is unlikely.

The patient with verrucous leukoplakia should have a biopsy carried out, sampling the most verrucous element, to establish the severity of any dysplastic changes. In the presence of a clear background of local trauma, it may be sufficient to eliminate the cause and follow-up the patient to see whether the condition regresses, remains static or progresses. Progress is likely to take the form of an increase in induration and wartiness, with a coarsening of its pattern. Such change would call for a further biopsy. Verrucous leukoplakia related to tobacco chewing requires immediate and permanent elimination of the causative factor. Management thereafter will depend on the extent of the area involved and how far the condition is judged to have progressed towards carcinoma.

The patient with leuko-erythroplakia requires an urgent biopsy and a diagnosis of carcinoma-in-situ if not early invasive cancer is probable. With either of these diagnoses excision of the entire area is called for. Radiotherapy has to be considered in treatment but it has little to offer such patients, particularly when, as is often the case, several sites are involved in different areas of the mouth.

Squamous carcinoma

Of the various tumour types which arise in the mouth squamous carcinoma is much the most common, accounting for approximately 90% of all intraoral malignancies. It typically occurs as a single tumour. Any mucosal surface within the mouth can be involved but it does have a predilection for the areas in which the saliva tends to pool, the floor of mouth and neighbouring sites such as the side of tongue and retromolar trigone. Many of the patients in whom squamous carcinoma of the oral cavity arises are elderly and they tend to have certain characteristics in common — a fondness for tobacco, smoked or chewed, for alcohol, usually but not invariably in the form of spirits, and poor oral hygiene. Carcinoma does, of course, also arise in non-smoking, teetotallers with excellent oral hygiene, but the occurrence is rare.

A further form which squamous carcinoma takes is as a multifocal tumour with pre-existing multiple areas of leuko-erythoplakia in which the malignancy develops. Fortunately this form is very rare since it is extremely difficult to treat.

In the average patient the clinical picture is dominated throughout by local disease with neighbouring structures being infiltrated by tumour. Metastasis to neck nodes also occurs and much less often systemic metastases. The different sites in the mouth vary greatly in the incidence of these three types of spread, but the majority of patients who die of intraoral cancer die with their disease still confined above the clavicle.

Longer survival of patients with oral cancer, the result of more effective treatment, is bringing to light the fact that such patients have an increased likelihood of developing a second, quite independent, primary squamous carcinoma. Such second tumours may arise in the symmetrical area of the mucosa on the opposite side of the mouth as well as in other areas inside the mouth. A higher-than-expected incidence of subsequent tumours arising in the oesophagus and bronchi is also recognized.

A factor in the incidence of such second tumours has been considered to be the continuation of smoking. More recent studies have not confirmed this and it is now considered that the entire mucosa is probably primed for neoplasia before the first clinical cancer appears.

The surgical approach to the mouth

The majority of intraoral cancers arise from sites within the concavity of the body of the mandible and it acts as a barrier to access for surgical resection. In the past hemi-resection of the mandible was part of the standard resection for tumours of the tongue and floor of mouth even though in many instances the bone was free of tumour. With removal of the hemimandible in this way access presented no difficulty. Today mandibular resection cannot be justified unless involvement by tumour is suspected and access has become a problem. The open mouth provides the basis of the various surgical approaches to tumours in the anterior part of the oral cavity, and if the access which this provides is inadequate it is generally added to by splitting the lower lip in the mid-line.

In its classic form the lip-splitting incision divides the entire thickness of the lip in the mid-line, continuing down over the symphysis of the mandible. If the intraoral resection is being combined with a neck dissection the incision becomes continuous with the submandibular component of a neck dissection incision. While this is an

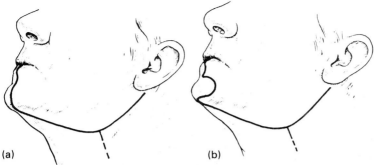

Figure 11.1 The classical lip-splitting incision (a), in which lip and chin are divided by a mid-line vertical incision, and the modified incision (b), in which the lower part encircles the chin prominence. Both incisions can be continued into the submandibular component of a neck dissection incision. (From McGregor and McGregor, *Cancer of the Face and Mouth,* Churchill Livingstone, by permission)

adequate incision the cosmetic result achieved by lip splitting can be considerably improved if the incision is modified (Figure 11.1).

In the modified version the upper part of the lip is split vertically in the mid-line, but the incision halts at the deepest part of the hollow between the lip and the chin prominence. Thereafter its line follows a circular curve at the base of the chin prominence, beginning in the mid-line and encircling the prominence to reach the mid-line below it. From that point, it can also be continued to meet the submandibular component of the neck dissection incision. By following the contour of the chin in this way the incision leaves a scar which is less obtrusive, becoming largely invisible in many instances.

Once the lip has been divided, the steps taken to provide further exposure depend on whether or not the mandible is being retained or resected. *When the mandible is being resected* an incision is made backwards along the lower buccal sulcus as far as the line of the bony resection. Extension of exposure backwards intraorally in this way is almost always accompanied by a submandibular incision even if a neck dissection is not being performed, and the elevation of a submandibular flap as far as the lower border of the mandible. *When the mandible is not being resected* an osteotomy of the bone is carried out and the hemimandible on the side of the resection is swung laterally to allow access to the floor of mouth and tongue, the 'mandibular swing' approach. The bone can be sectioned either at the symphysis or in the body between the mental foramen and the insertion of the anterior belly of the digastric. The symphyseal site is probably the one most widely used, but it has the disadvantage that the tongue muscle, genioglossus, has to be divided in addition to geniohyoid, mylohyoid and the anterior belly of digastric in order to allow the swing to take place. If the site immediately anterior to the mental foramen is used (Figure 11.2), the only muscle which requires to be divided in order to allow the mandibular body to swing laterally is mylohyoid because the osteotomy site is lateral to the origin of the tongue musculature.

The exposure which is provided by the mandibular swing approach is excellent and it allows a much greater precision in intraoral resection.

With resection of the tumour and reconstruction of the defect completed it becomes necessary to reduce and fix the osteotomy, and several techniques have been developed to achieve this — direct wiring, a combination of direct wiring and

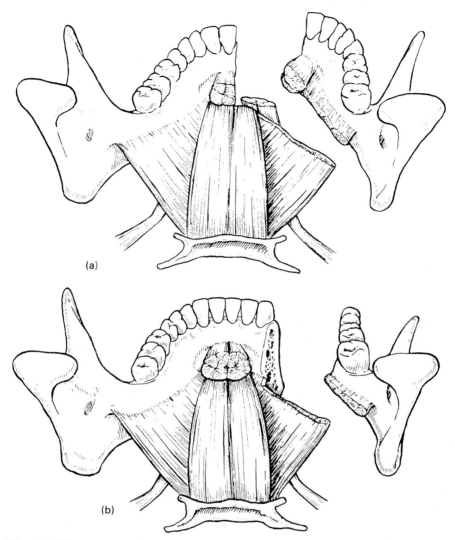

Figure 11.2 The structures divided in carrying out an osteotomy to allow the body of the mandible to 'swing' laterally. In (a), the symphyseal site, the main attachment of the tongue to the mandible, genioglossus, is divided together with geniohyoid, the anterior belly of digastric, mylohyoid and the mucous membrane of the floor of the mouth. In (b), the site between the mental foramen and the insertion of the anterior belly of digastric, the only structures divided are mylohyoid and the floor of mouth mucosa. (From McGregor and McGregor, *Cancer of the Face and Mouth,* Churchill Livingstone, by permission)

K-wire transfixion, and compression plating. Direct wiring does not provide good stability unless it is combined with stepping of the osteotomy cut and such a cut is not readily applicable to the dentate mandible. The stability which a K-wire transfixing the osteotomy adds to the direct wire (Figure 11.3) makes it possible to

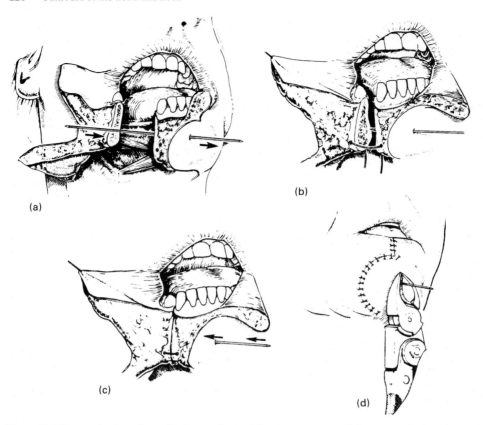

Figure 11.3 Reconstitution of mandibular continuity following osteotomy. Prior to carrying out the osteotomy, drill holes are bored on each side of the site selected, in preparation for interosseous wiring. The short K-wire, sharp at both ends, is driven into the symphyseal side of the osteotomy and emerges through the skin (a). It is then pulled through until its tip is just visible at the cut end of the bone (b). The bone ends are then wired together (c), held steady in correct alignment and the K-wire is driven across the osteotomy site, engaging the bone opposite and stabilising it. The K-wire is cut short (d), leaving the end palpable under the skin for easy subsequent removal. (From McGregor and McGregor, *Cancer of the Face and Mouth,* Churchill Livingstone, by permission)

use the technically easier and generally applicable straight bone cut. For those familiar with the technique of compression plating in other surgical contexts the method provides very positive stabilization of the osteotomy.

Management of the postexcisional defect

Over the past 25 years management of the defect after an intraoral resection has changed radically. From a situation where the defect was closed directly, largely ignoring the functional and cosmetic defects which almost invariably resulted, it is now routine for the defect to be reconstructed so that the intraoral structures left are restored as far as possible to their original site. The structure which has benefited most from this has been the tongue, in terms both of its contribution to speech and the part it plays in disposing of saliva and the manipulation of food.

The techniques used have evolved also and today the methods used to reconstruct major defects make use either of *myocutaneous flaps* or of *free flaps*.

Myocutaneous flaps exploit the fact that the skin in certain body sites is effectively perfused via the muscle immediately underlying it to the extent that it will survive even if isolated from all other vascular sources. Also in those muscles whose entry point of blood supply is concentrated in a neurovascular hilum it is possible to elevate the muscle, centred on the hilum as a pivot point, and transfer it to a new position, as a muscle flap, or, incorporating an island of the skin overlying it, as a myocutaneous flap. Pectoralis major has such a neurovascular hilum, sited 2 cm medial to the coracoid process, and with an island of the skin overlying the muscle medial and just below the nipple the composite of skin and muscle has been elevated and transferred using the hilum as its pivot point into the mouth in order to reconstruct a postexcisional defect, passing under the skin flaps of a neck dissection — the pectoralis major myocutaneous flap. Other myocutaneous flaps have been described for this purpose but at present the pectoralis major flap is the one most frequently used.

Free flaps make use of the fact that an island of skin, in this clinical context on the forearm, can be raised along with its underlying superficial and investing layer of fascia, together with its perfusion source, the radial artery and its venae comitantes. The vessels can then be divided leaving the hand to be perfused by the ulnar arteriovenous system and the flap moved *en masse* to the intraoral site and sutured to the defect, the radial vessels being anastomosed to suitable vessels in the neck, for example, the superior thyroid artery and the external jugular vein — the radial forearm flap.

In the absence of the microsurgical expertise necessary for successful use of a free flap, the myocutaneous flap is the method routinely used. Where the choice exists the comparative indications are clear-cut and relate to the matching of the characteristics of the defect in relation to those of the flap. When the defect is large in volume in relation to its mucosal area, as when a segment of mandible has been resected, the myocutaneous flap is more likely to match the defect in volume in relation to the area of its skin surface. When the mandible has not required resection, the myocutaneous flap is liable to be too large in volume to be ideal. The free flap with its comparatively small volume in relation to its skin surface will give a better result.

In its transfer to the mouth the muscle of the pectoralis major myocutaneous flap comes to overlie the major vessels of the neck and in this respect is capable of providing a protective cover for them when the neck has been previously been irradiated and they are judged to be at risk of rupture should the neck wound break down. In the post-radiotherapy situation this virtue might be seen as an indication for using it in preference to a free flap.

Neck dissection

The principle of resecting the lymph nodes of the neck as an important element in the surgical management of head and neck cancer was consolidated in a definitive manner by Hayes Martin as a *radical neck dissection*. The margins of such a dissection are: inferiorly, the clavicle, superiorly, the lower border of the mandible, anteriorly, the midline and posteriorly, the anterior border of trapezius. Within these boundaries the posterior triangle is cleared of its contents, sternocleidomastoid and the internal jugular vein with its associated chain of nodes are resected, and above the hyoid bone the submandibular salivary gland with associated nodes are removed.

Neck dissection is sometimes extended and this can take various forms and be required for various reasons:

1. Intermediate node groups, such as the occipital, post- and preauricular, not normally resected in the standard neck dissection, may be involved by tumour. It is then usual to resect the involved group of nodes in continuity with the deep jugular group as an extended dissection. The parotid group is the one most frequently involved in this situation.
2. The primary tumour may be so close to the jugular or submandibular nodes that it is not practical to resect both it and the nodes other than in continuity. An example of such a situation would be the extensive squamous carcinoma of the pinna with positive neck nodes, calling for amputation of the ear as an extension of the standard neck dissection.
3. Part of the exposure required for the neck dissection and for excision of the primary tumour may be common to both procedures. This situation arises when the primary tumour is in the vicinity of the floor of the mouth, in the floor itself, in the tongue, lower alveolus or faucial area. Exposure of such a tumour, if it is extensive, involves opening the submandibular triangle. In these circumstances, dissection of the neck nodes is frequently extended to be made continuous with the resection of the tumour at the primary site. The submandibular triangle having once been opened, the best chance the surgeon has of achieving a technically and pathologically clean resection in mouth and neck lies in doing both together. This may mean carrying out the neck dissection prophylactically, that is, in the absence of palpable nodes in the neck. This is one of the few situations where a prophylactic neck dissection is standard clinical practice.

Radical neck dissection has proved an extremely effective therapeutic measure and at present it is probably the surgical procedure most frequently used in managing metastatic tumour in neck nodes. In recent years, however, experienced head and neck surgeons have increasingly recognized that in certain circumstances radical neck dissection sacrifices structures unnecessarily and in an unselective manner. The structures concerned are the accessory nerve, sternocleidomastoid and the internal jugular vein. Of these, the accessory nerve is the most important functionally, its resection resulting in drooping of the shoulder from loss of upper trapezius function as a consequence of which many patients, particularly in the older age group, complain of shoulder stiffness and aching. The modified versions of radical neck dissection devised as part of the reappraisal are collectively referred to as 'functional' neck dissections.

Functional neck dissection

The accepted form of this modification of radical neck dissection has not been clearly defined. Common to all versions is removal of the deep jugular chain of nodes together with the submandibular salivary gland and its associated nodes, while preserving the accessory nerve and in most instances sternocleidomastoid, and sometimes also the internal jugular vein. The variations concern the possible extensions beyond this common denominator, extensions whose justification depends on the known geographical distribution of nodal metastases in the neck from different primary tumour sites, in particular the contrasting patterns from sites within the oral cavity and the laryngopharyngeal sites. The versions which have been described are:

1. The procedure corresponding to a radical neck dissection, except that the accessory nerve is dissected free throughout its course in the neck and preserved.
2. The procedure corresponding to a radical neck dissection except that the accessory nerve, sternocleidomastoid and internal jugular vein are retained.
3. The procedure corresponding to a radical neck dissection except that the accessory nerve, sternocleidomastoid and internal jugular vein are retained, and the nodes of the posterior triangle are not resected.
4. Resections corresponding to (2) or (3), but in addition the internal jugular vein is removed.

The rationale of functional neck dissection

Probably the most controversial factor separating the different versions of functional dissection concern the circumstances in which it is safe to leave the posterior triangle with its content of nodes undisturbed without compromising the pathological basis of the procedure. If its role in cancer of the oral cavity is being considered it is essential to establish the frequency with which tumour spreads from the oral cavity to the nodes of the posterior triangle, and if such metastasis does occur, in which circumstances it does so. The incidence of metastatic involvement of the nodes in the posterior triangle, both in the irradiated and in the non-irradiated neck, has been investigated in several studies, and the universal finding has been that there is an absence of involvement of these nodes in patients whose tumour was viewed as operable. If these findings are to be used as a guide to clinical practice, it is reasonable to assume that if the neck dissection is viewed by the surgeon as prophylactic, the submandibular triangle having been opened for the reason described above, the likelihood of the posterior triangle nodes being involved by tumour is remote. The probability of posterior triangle node involvement by tumour one would expect to increase with an increasing number of clinically positive nodes elsewhere in the neck.

The influence of preserving the accessory nerve on the outcome of a functional neck dissection involves considering its anatomical pathway through the neck (Figure 11.4) and the probability of its being involved by tumour in the different parts of its course. As already demonstrated the probability of tumour being present in the nodes in the posterior triangle is extremely small and the segment of the accessory nerve in that triangle is equally unlikely to be involved. Sternocleidomastoid is only involved by tumour infiltrating locally and the presence of such infiltration implies grossly advanced disease. In the absence of such infiltration preservation of the muscle could be justified on pathological grounds and if this is so, preservation of the segment of the nerve within muscle can equally well be justified. It is the length of the nerve between its emergence from the jugular foramen and its disappearance into sternocleidomastoid which is most likely to be involved by tumour because of its close proximity to the deep jugular nodes high in the neck. The crucial question is in what clinical circumstances the nerve in this area can be dissected free and still allow an effective node clearance.

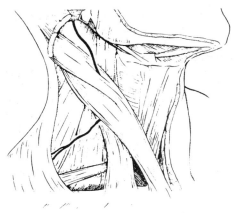

Figure 11.4 The accessory nerve, showing the three parts of its course: from skull base to sternocleidomastoid, within sternocleidomastoid, and in the posterior triangle. (From McGregor and McGregor, *Cancer of the Face and Mouth,* Churchill Livingstone, by permission)

In the case of a prophylactic neck dissection there would seem to be little objection on pathological grounds to functional neck dissection replacing radical neck dissection, since the likelihood of extracapsular or obviously permeative spread of tumour is remote. The combination of palpable submandibular nodes with clinically negative deep jugular nodes provides a clinical situation where the decision is more difficult to reach. The deep jugular nodes may contain tumour in such circumstances though they are clinically negative. Equally they may not and there is no foolproof way of making the distinction before or during the neck dissection. In either event, any metastasis is likely to be early, with little likelihood of significant extracapsular spread. The question is one to which, in our present state of knowledge, an absolute answer cannot be provided with certainty, though many surgeons would consider functional dissection acceptable in such a clinical situation. A much more acute dilemma arises where deep jugular nodes are palpable, particularly in the upper neck, for the established effectiveness of radical neck dissection is then being exchanged for the dubious therapeutic status of functional neck dissection. There are no studies which can provide figures to justify the use of functional neck dissection in such a clinical situation and in view of the fact that even with radical neck dissection the dissection towards the skull base, if it is to be suitably radical, can be extremely difficult technically it would be difficult to justify the use of functional neck dissection in such circumstances.

The form which the functional neck dissection should take in managing an intraoral primary is not established in a manner comparable to radical neck dissection but, having regard to the arguments advanced above, a rational approach could be the removal of the deep jugular group of nodes from an arbitrary line 2 cm behind the internal jugular vein. Anterior to that line the dissection would proceed exactly as for the radical neck dissection, but preserving sternocleidomastoid and the accessory nerve.

Salivary tumours

The majority of salivary tumours arise in the parotid gland and in that site usually present either as a localized painless mobile nodule or as a harder, more diffuse and less mobile swelling. The tumour with the first type of clinical presentation was called, until comparatively recently, a mixed parotid tumour and was regarded as basically benign. The second was malignant. This simple concept is unfortunately no longer adequate.

In the parotid, hardness, diffuseness, lack of mobility, and involvement of facial nerve are still recognized as indicative of malignancy. The change in attitude has been with respect to the localized mobile nodule. It is now recognized that such a nodule does not represent a single tumour type but represents a group of tumours which, although they share their initial mode of presentation, have a distinctive histology, behaviour pattern and prognosis. As a result of correlating histological pattern and clinical behaviour, categories of salivary tumours have been introduced by the World Health Organisation and these are generally accepted today.

The epithelial tumours of salivary origin which occur with any frequency are grouped thus:

1. Adenoma (a) Monomorphic (b) Pleomorphic
2. Mucoepidermoid tumour
3. Carcinoma (a) Adenoid cystic carcinoma (b) Adenocarcinoma (c) Squamous carcinoma (d) Anaplastic carcinoma (e) Carcinoma in pleomorphic adenoma

Monomorphic adenoma

The only monomorphic adenoma which occurs with any frequency is adenolymphoma. This benign tumour is virtually confined to the parotid gland and its immediate environs. It is unusual in having two tissue elements which coexist within it — glandular tissue and lymphoid tissue with germinal centres. This association of tissue has been explained on the basis of the common finding of islets of salivary tissue within the lymph nodes in and around the parotid salivary gland, and adenolymphoma has actually been seen developing in a lymph node containing a salivary tissue inclusion. The glandular element alone is considered to be neoplastic. Although it is well encapsulated it can arise multifocally and this probably explains its unexpectedly high 'recurrence' rate.

Pleomorphic adenoma

This tumour is still called a mixed parotid tumour by many surgeons. At one time the term 'mixed' implied a dual origin, with epithelial and mesodermal elements, but the tumour is now recognized to be epithelial and the term is now used in the sense of indicating its morphological complexity. The tumour is characterized by the presence of epithelial tissue surrounded by a mixture of chondroid or mucoid stroma, and the proportions of the two vary very considerably in different examples.

It is when the tumour arises in the parotid gland that problems of recurrence arise. The reason for this lies in the fact that the branches of the facial nerve run through the substance of the gland and these restrict the surgeon's freedom of action since it is regarded as essential to maintain the structural integrity of the nerve, despite the fact that its branches are often found to be stretched over the capsule of the tumour with virtually no tissue between. To remove the tumour complete and intact without damage to the nerve can be extremely difficult technically. The tumour can also vary in its site within the parotid, superficial to the nerve, deep to the nerve though within the main part of the gland, or in the plane of the nerve, separating its branches widely (Figure 11.5). Very rarely, growth of the tumour in the deep lobe medially through the gap between the mandible and the styloid process, the stylomandibular tunnel (Figure 11.6), into the parapharyngeal space (Figure 11.7), gives rise to the classic picture of a deep lobe tumour. Such a tumour is often noticed by the patient only when it presents as a swelling intraorally, most often in the tonsillar region. In that site its slow increase in size allows the patient to accommodate to the swelling and most are large before their presence is recognized.

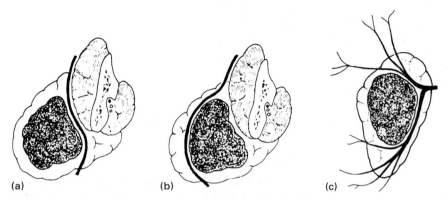

(a)   (b)   (c)

Figure 11.5 Variations in the site of a tumour within the parotid gland in relation to the facial nerve: (a) superficial to the nerve; (b) deep to the nerve; (c) in the plane of the nerve, separating its branches widely (From McGregor and McGregor, *Cancer of the Face and Mouth,* Churchill Livingstone, by permission)

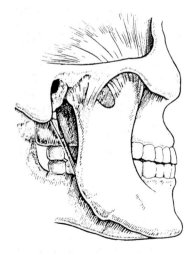

Figure 11.6 The stylomandibular tunnel, its margins formed by the ascending ramus of the mandible, the styloid process, and the stylomandibular ligament joining them. (From McGregor and McGregor, *Cancer of the Face and Mouth,* Churchill Livingstone, by permission)

The established pleomorphic adenoma has a nodular surface with a fibrous covering capsule — thinnest over the convexities and thickest in the hollows between the nodules, bridging them with a screening cover which makes the tumour appear smoother than it is in reality. Although the nodules in most instances are sessile the occasional nodule is pedunculated, to the extent that it

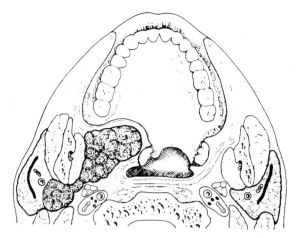

Figure 11.7 Deep lobe tumour, showing extension medially through the stylomandibular tunnel into the parapharyngeal space. (From McGregor and McGregor, *Cancer of the Face and Mouth,* Churchill Livingstone, by permission)

almost appears to be an independent tumour. Serial sections of such examples almost invariably show continuity between the nodule and the main tumour at some point.

Recurrence of pleomorphic adenoma is the result of incomplete removal and it can occur in one of two ways. 'Seeding' of tumour fragments can take place when rupture of the capsule with spillage occurs during removal; alternatively, a lobule of tumour may inadvertently be left behind. When the tumour has ruptured with spillage, recurrence takes the form of multiple tumour nodules within the operative field, pleomorphic adenoma seeming to have a peculiar capacity for successfully implanting in those circumstances.

Although it is a simple tumour, pleomorphic adenoma carries potential for malignancy. In such instances the tumour has usually been present over a very long period and it would appear that the longer a pleomorphic adenoma is left untreated, the greater is the likelihood of malignancy occurring. The onset of malignancy is usually heralded by a sudden increase in size and speed of growth and in the characteristics of the nodule, which becomes harder and more diffuse and which may begin to involve the facial nerve. Such a tumour tends to behave like anaplastic carcinoma with rapid growth and a poor prognosis.

Mucoepidermoid tumour

Despite the recognition of this tumour type as an entity with a distinctive behaviour pattern and prognosis, the slight vagueness of the title and the failure to indicate its degree of malignancy would suggest that views still differ concerning it. Within the tumour type there appears to be a spectrum from low grade to high grade so far as malignancy is concerned, but there is also a large intermediate group between the two extremes. The problem of assessment exists at a histological level as well as clinically and attempts to relate histological appearance to clinical behaviour are not convincing. The tumour considered to have low-grade malignancy is likely to have been diagnosed clinically as a pleomorphic adenoma and, properly treated as one, should carry an equally good prognosis. High-grade mucoepidermoid tumours are more likely to be diagnosed as carcinoma, the points of distinction between the two forms, low- and high-grade, concerning such matters as speed of growth of the swelling, the degree of induration and lack of mobility, both factors which result from the absence of a capsule and the presence of local infiltration. The majority of mucoepidermoid tumours in the major glands behave in a manner similar to pleomorphic adenomas. In the minor glands they are more apt to behave like high grade tumours.

Adenoid cystic carcinoma

This tumour has a distinctive histological appearance and an equally distinctive clinical pattern of behaviour. Its histological characteristic is of clumps of small tumour cells with numerous spaces, the resulting appearance being referred to as the 'Swiss cheese' pattern. The margins of the tumour are ill-defined with narrow columns of cells streaming off from the main mass along tissue planes, between muscle fasciculi, and, most markedly, along perineural spaces. The characteristics unique to adenoid cystic carcinoma are an extremely slow rate of growth for a carcinoma, an absence of tissue response to the tumour, a striking tendency of the tumour to infiltrate locally in tissue planes and between muscle fasciculi well beyond the naked eye tumour, in bone as well as soft tissue, and a marked proneness to infiltrate and spread along perineural spaces. Although the 'Swiss cheese' pattern with its spaces is considered typical, some tumours contain areas where spaces are not present. This pattern resembles that of basal-cell carcinoma and is referred to as 'basaloid'. It is considered to represent areas of less well differentiated tumour. There is evidence that the presence of basaloid areas is associated with a poorer than average prognosis in terms of speed of growth. Whether the 'Swiss cheese' form with its slower growth pattern is any less lethal in the long run is extremely doubtful.

The striking clinical feature of the tumour throughout is of infiltration and extension locally, though pulmonary metastases are recognized to occur. Even when tumour is widespread in the lungs it is remarkable how fit the patient may remain, despite the presence of little apparently normal lung tissue. The initial presentation of adenoid cystic carcinoma, particularly when it arises in one of the major glands, is not unlike that of pleomorphic adenoma. When first seen the tumour is nearly always uninodular; recurrences are almost invariably multinodular. The slow but inexorable course of the disease can be judged from the fact that in one series the survival rate which at 5 years was 71%, fell to 13% by 20 years.

The treatment of adenoid cystic carcinoma is essentially surgical and the excision has to be extremely radical if it is to be effective. In practice the prognosis is very bad even from the outset, and recurrent tumour is very rarely operable. There is some evidence that radiotherapy delays the appearance of recurrent tumour but it does not prevent it.

Adenocarcinoma, squamous carcinoma and anaplastic carcinoma

These tumours, though each has a distinctive histological picture, behave in a similar manner clinically. When they arise in the parotid the initial swelling has clinical characteristics not unlike those of a pleomorphic adenoma, though growth is likely to have been faster and the swelling itself tends to be harder in consistency. At the early stage of development it is rarely possible to make an absolute clinical distinction between the carcinoma and the adenoma but the differences become increasingly obvious as the tumour enlarges and local infiltration leads to tumour fixation and involvement of the facial nerve.

Management of parotid tumours

In managing a tumour of the parotid gland the diagnosis is frequently only a clinical one, and a biopsy is not possible because it would breach the capsule of the gland with all that this would mean in terms of cell spillage. The tumour which is clearly malignant clinically does not pose the real problem. The difficulty in practice arises from the need to separate from one another pleomorphic adenoma, mucoepidermoid tumour, adenoid cystic carcinoma and the other rarer tumours, all of which present in the first instance as an asymptomatic mobile swelling in an otherwise normal gland but whose management and prognosis are so very different.

The use of aspiration needle biopsy which has proved extremely effective in other surgical contexts has been criticized on the grounds of possible cell implantation along the needle track. Implantation is an undoubted danger when a wide-bore needle is used but with a finer needle, e.g. a 22 gauge, the likelihood is exceedingly small. A more valid criticism is the inadequacy of the sample obtained and it is this which markedly reduces its value in practice.

In the parotid approximately 80% of tumours are either a pleomorphic adenoma or an adenolymphoma and in practice most tumours presenting as an asymptomatic mobile swelling in the gland are managed on the assumption that they are one or other of these. Enucleation, at one time the treatment method used, has been replaced by excision of the 'lobe' containing the tumour. When the superficial lobe is the site of the tumour, a superficial lobectomy, leaving the facial nerve intact, is appropriate; the deep lobe tumour is managed by total parotidectomy preserving the facial nerve. With such uncertainty of diagnosis, the surgeon, in carrying out his resection, should be constantly on the look-out for any suggestion of infiltration so that he can take steps to widen his margin of clearance. In such circumstances it is usually possible to preserve the facial nerve though local infiltration may occasionally make resection of one or more branches necessary.

The clinically malignant tumour is treated by radical parotidectomy *en bloc* with no attempt to preserve the facial nerve. If at the time of initial treament neck nodes are palpable a dissection of the nodes in continuity with the parotidectomy is appropriate treatment. Such an occurrence is not common, however, and the status of prophylactic node dissection is not clear-cut. The main advantage of the neck dissection in such a clinical situation may well be that it allows ready access to the lower pole of the parotid and to its deep lobe, in this way making a radical resection easier. The striking characteristic of most salivary tumours is of local recurrence rather than of metastasis to lymph nodes and failure to cure the patient is usually due to inadequate local excision. This fact should make node dissection take second place in the surgeon's mind to radical local excision.

When a tumour which was considered clinically to be a pleomorphic adenoma and at operation showed no signs of infiltration is found by the pathologist to be a mucoepidermoid tumour a careful follow-up is probably adequate, but when the tumour is reported as an adenoid cystic carcinoma management becomes totally different. Immediate further surgery of the most radical kind is called for. Its extent will be determined by the clinical situation, taking account of the tumour's characteristic of local spread along tissue planes, perineural spaces, between muscle fasciculi and through bone. As a minimum, a radical parotidectomy is essential, removing the facial nerve from the stylomastoid foramen to the anterior margin of the gland. Such an approach may appear to be unduly aggressive but in the light of the recognized fact that a recurrent adenoid cystic carcinoma is seldom cured it is clear that only the most radical local primary surgery holds out any hope of success.

The place of radiotherapy

Salivary tumours are in general among the less radiosensitive and the surgeon who designs his surgery on the assumption that radiotherapy is not available as a back-up is the one most likely to be most effective. In general, radiotherapy should be considered only after the surgery which is appropriate to the clinical and pathological problem has been properly carried out. The problem is likely to arise in its most acute form in managing adenoid cystic carcinoma where the surgeon, inexperienced in managing this tumour and seeing the innocuous manner of its initial clinical presentation, is unwilling to contemplate the radical surgery necessary to meet the situation and takes refuge in radiotherapy, thereby postponing but not preventing the inevitable, and generally ultimately fatal, recurrence.

Facial nerve grafting

A consequence of a percentage of properly carried out lobectomies or parotidectomies will be a facial palsy, partial or total. This is an extremely disabling sequel but it is one which can be mitigated in a considerable proportion of patients by the use of facial nerve grafting. The technique, if it is to be effective, is a demanding one, making use of the operating microscope. During the resection, the ends of the divided nerves are tagged with black silk for ready identification. The local nerve source which has been most often used as the graft is the great auricular; the usual distant source is the sural nerve. An important point of technique concerns the orientation of the graft. Once cut the graft has no directional orientation and its distal end should be sutured to the proximal stump of the facial nerve to ensure that any regenerating axons are not side-tracked into a branch of the graft instead of reaching the distal stump of the facial nerve. Surgical effort is usually concentrated on restoring continuity of the branches to the eyelids and mouth. Even with good restoration of facial movement the pattern rarely takes on the involuntary quality of facial expresson in concert with the innervated side which constitutes complete normality. Despite this the result is a considerable improvement on the otherwise inevitable palsy, and with greater experience in more accurately linking proximal to distal axons in terms of the intraneural topography of the nerve a more normal play of emotional expression is increasingly being achieved.

Salivary tumours are comparatively rare and the surgery involved in their management is among the more demanding in the field of head and neck surgery. If improvement is to be achieved in terms of lower recurrence rates and better functional and cosmetic results there is much to be said for concentrating the management of such patients in the hands of a few surgeons in a particular area, so that the necessary experience and expertise can be built up.

Chapter 12

Management of cutaneous malignant melanoma

Rona M. MacKie

Introduction

Twenty to thirty years ago cutaneous malignant melanoma was a malignancy which was rare and usually fatal. In the past two decades, however, the incidence of melanoma has risen rapidly in all parts of the world in which figures are available, including Scotland (MacKie *et al.*, 1985) Scandinavia (Magnus, 1981) and Australia (Green and Siskind, 1983). In all these three areas the incidence has doubled in the past 10 years and for example, melanoma is now much commoner than Hodgkin's disease in Scotland. A high proportion of patients who develop malignant melanoma are otherwise healthy and are relatively young, under the age of 50 years at presentation.

Clinical features

It is common current practice to divide malignant melanoma into four main subsets on clinicopathological grounds. These are superficial spreading melanoma which accounts for approximately 50% of UK cases, lentigo maligna melanoma, nodular melanoma and acral lentiginous melanoma.

Superficial spreading melanoma is seen most commonly on the calf in women and the trunk in men. Clinically it presents as a new or growing pigmented lesion with an irregular outline and variegate central pigmentation. Mild itch and crusting or oozing may be present.

The nodular melanoma is usually a dark red or black, sharply demarcated, elevated lesion, and the lentigo maligna melanoma is commonly seen on the cheek of elderly individuals as a slowly expanding irregular lesion which may remain as a melanoma *in situ* confined to the epidermis for many years. At this stage the term lentigo maligna or Hutchison's melanotic freckle is appropriate. In time, however, a central nodule may develop in this area which indicates that dermal invasion has begun. The acral lentiginous melanoma is seen clinically as an irregularly shaped pigmented lesion on the palm or sole. Personal experience is that these lesions are 8 times as common on the soles as on the palms.

Pathology

The essential and diagnostic pathological feature of malignant melanoma is the presence of malignant melanocytes invading the papillary dermis and deeper tissues. Malignant melanocytes may also be seen moving upwards through the epidermis from their normal position adjacent to the dermoepidermal junction.

In the case of the superficial spreading melanoma, the characteristic feature is the presence of malignant melanocytes both singly and in clusters above the invasive component. The nodular melanoma has a very abrupt transition between normal skin and invasive melanoma, and the lentigo maligna melanoma is associated with striking actinic damage in the surrounding dermal collagen.

Clinical and pathological prognostic features

The most important prognostic feature for patients with malignant melanoma is the thickness of their primary tumour measured in millimetres from the granular layer in the epidermis to the deepest underlying tumour cell in the dermis. The importance of measurement was established by the late Alexander Breslow and it is therefore often referred to as the Breslow or tumour thickness (Figure 12.1) (Breslow, 1970). Five-year survival figures for patients with malignant melanoma

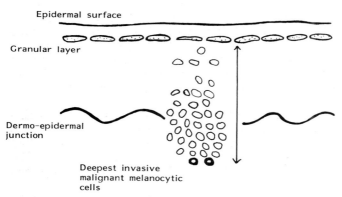

Figure 12.1 Malignant melanoma thickness measurement (Breslow)

are directly and inversely proportional to this measurement. It is common practice, to divide patients with malignant melanoma into three categories: those with thin good prognosis tumours 0–1.49 mm thick, those with medium thickness intermediate prognosis tumours 1.5–3.5 mm thick, and those with poor prognosis tumours thicker than 3.5 mm. Five-year survival in the UK (MacKie *et al.*, 1985) for patients in these three categories are 95%, 67% and 38% respectively. The very great difference in survival prospects for patients with thin and thick tumours illustrates the importance of having the Breslow thickness figure available when discussing the outlook with a patient or relative. Early papers on the importance of Breslow thickness and prognosis stated that tumours less than 0.76 mm never metastasized. This statement appears in most series to have been confirmed.

Assessment of Clark levels of invasion is a similar approach to tumour thickness in assessing the depth to which the malignant cells have penetrated into the skin. These are: level 1 *in situ* melanoma only, level 2 invasion into the papillary dermis by small numbers of cells, level 3 melanoma cells filling and expanding the papillary dermis, level 4 invasion into the reticular dermis, and level 5 invasion into subcutaneous fat.

The presence of malignant melanoma cells in vascular channels is an indication that metastatic spread is relatively likely (Clark *et al.*, 1969).

Balch *et al.* (1980) has also suggested that ulceration is a poor prognosis feature independent of Breslow thickness, but not all subsequent studies have confirmed this.

Clinical features shown to be of prognostic significance include the sex of the patient (females tend to do better than males), and the site of the lesion (lesions on the lower leg tend to have a better prognosis than lesions on the trunk).

In any new publication of prognostic features in malignant melanoma it is, however, essential to check that the author has carried out the appropriate statistical tests to control for Breslow thickness, as in the past a number of prognostic variables have been suggested to be of significance, but have subsequently been shown merely to be indirect measures of tumour thickness.

Establishing the diagnosis

If malignant melanoma is suspected on clinical grounds, histological confirmation of the diagnosis is essential. There have in the past been many arguments about the advisability of an incisional biopsy because of the possible risk of dissemination of tumour cells into vascular channels near the site of the incisional biopsy. Opinions are still divided as to whether or not this is a real rather than a theoretical risk, and for this reason an excisional rather than an incisional biopsy is recommended for diagnostic purposes whenever possible.

A further possible hazard in obtaining a biopsy is encountered when considering anaesthesia. There are theoretical grounds for believing that infiltration with local anaesthetic adjacent to the tumour could cause an increase in fluid pressure and thus dislodge friable tumour cells into lymphatic channels. For this reason the infiltration of the local anaesthetic at a relatively distant site from the suspected melanoma, or a ring block is recommended.

It is strongly recommended that the surgeon who will be responsible for the definitive surgical therapy carries out the biopsy or at least sees the patient prior to biopsy so that he can site the incision appropriately. All biopsies of pigmented lesions suspected of being melanoma should be by scalpel excision. Punch biopsies, and shave or curette biopsies are contraindicated. This is because there are usually two points to be established from such biopsies. The first is whether or not the lesion is melanoma, and the second is the tumour thickness. Shaves and curettings will make determination of the latter impossible, and punch or curette procedures could actually push tumour cells deeper into the dermis.

While pathological confirmation that a pigmented lesion is malignant melanoma may be required rapidly, a frozen section of the lesion is not usually recommended in the UK although large centres in Australia which see many melanomas report satisfactory results. This is because a number of benign melanocytic lesions may histologically be very similar to malignant melanoma, and the subtle features which allow the experienced pathologist to make a differential diagnosis between melanoma and lesions such as a benign Spitz naevus (benign so-called juvenile melanoma) or a dysplastic naevus may be lost on frozen sections. Because of this the tissue is usually fixed in formalin and processed in the usual way. Modern laboratory techniques are such that a report can be obtained on a sepcimen processed in this manner in less than 24 hours. If it is decided that a frozen section should be requested, it should be remembered that there will be a lack of the shrinkage of tissue associated with formalin fixation, and that the tumour thickness measurement will be greater than if the specimen had been processed in the standard manner.

It is important that the tissue is examined by a pathologist with experience in malignant melanoma. Melanoma is still a relatively rare tumour, and many district general hospitals see less than six primary melanomas annually. If there is any pathological doubt the specimen should be referred to a pathologist with experience in the recognition of these lesions.

Staging of melanoma

A number of staging systems are in current use and care should therefore be taken to check which is in use when reading a paper on this. A common system in the UK at present is Stage I primary tumour only, Stage IIa tumour recurrence between the primary site and the draining lymph nodes, Stage IIb tumour in the lymph nodes, and Stage III tumour detected beyond the draining lymph nodes.

First-line treatment

Once primary malignant melanoma is histologically confirmed the definitive treament is surgical and should be carried out within a week of a diagnostic biopsy. In the past the standard surgical approach has been wide excision with 3–5 cm of normal skin in all directions around the tumour and the closure of the resulting deficit with a skin graft. Full-thickness grafts are usually required for the face, using tissue from behind the ear or the axilla, and split-skin grafts used in all other sites. With the work of Alexander Breslow and the recognition that the outlook for melanomas of different thicknesses was very different a more logical approach to the extent of surgery required for primary malignant melanoma has developed. A common current approach is to consider that 1 cm clearance of normal skin around the primary tumour is required for each millimetre of depth of the primary tumour (Taylor and Hughes, 1985). Thus a primary melanoma which is only 1 mm in thickness requires only a margin of 1 cm of normal skin around the lesion. Experts on the management of melanoma in both the UK and Australia currently manage patients in this way, but do not believe that tumours thicker than 3 mm require a margin of greater than 3 cm in all directions. This is because these patients tend to have a poor prognosis irrespective of the margin of excision as indicated above, and problems arise not with local recurrence but with distant dissemination.

A World Health Organisation trial is currently in progress comparing both survival and disease-free interval in patients with primary malignant melanomas less than 2 mm in thickness treated with surgical excision with a margin of either 1 cm or 3 cm of normal skin. Three hundred patients have been entered into each arm of this study and at 3-years follow-up the disease-free intervals and survival in the two groups are identical with 94% survival disease free in each case (WHO Melanoma Programme Trial 10). Thus for the patients with a thin melanoma less than 1 mm in thickness, local excision and direct closure of the wound is adequate treatment (Veronesi et al., 1988).

If an excision biopsy confirms that the lesion is a melanoma less than 1 mm in thickness, and if 1 cm of normal skin has been included in the excision biopsy sample, no further surgical treatment may be required, but if the melanoma is thicker than 1 mm, wider excision and possibly skin grafting may be indicated. Provided that this is carried out within one week of the first surgery, there is no evidence that this two-stage procedure in any way alters the patient's prognosis.

Clearly this approach may involve an increase in theatre time required for some patients because of the two-stage procedure required in thicker tumours. This is, however, balanced by the minor out-patient surgery and lack of requirement for in-patient treatment for those with thinner tumours.

Until recently it has been common practice to take the skin for a split-skin graft required for a leg lesion from the opposite limb, but Flook *et al.* (1986) have challenged this habit and produced logical reasons for using skin from the ipsilateral limb.

A further area of surgical controversy has been the decision as to whether or not to excise the deep fascia (Olsen, 1964). The current view is that this is only necessary when the depth of excision required by the Breslow thickness is such that it would form a natural part of the excision specimen (Kenady, Brown and McBride, 1982). Clearly this will vary with different body sites, and deep fascia proper is only found on the limbs and neck. In situations where the deep fascia forms part of a muscle insertion, it should not be excised as to do so would increase morbidity. Patients should be warned before surgery that some depth of tissue will require to be removed. Personal experience has been confirmed by psychological studies that patients readily accept a long linear scar, or graft area of moderate proportions, but are distressed by the depression under the graft (Cassileth, Luck and Tenaglia, 1983).

For subungual lesions, it is usual to carry out a partial amputation of the affected digit. In the case of the thumb or first finger as much functional digit should be preserved as is practical.

Despite the recent development of the use of free flaps and tissue transfer to create a cosmetically more acceptable result, these are used rarely in the initial management of primary melanoma. This is because of fear of recurrent disease being hidden under the flap, but those who do use flaps for primary closure state that this worry has been found to be without foundation. A common current practice is to close the primary defect with a skin graft, and offer the patient wound revision with a flap if indicated after 2–3 years follow-up. In the event, many patients who were initially distressed by their graft site adjust well and decline the offer of such revisions.

Once a thin primary melanoma has been excised and pathological examination shows that excision in depth and at the margins is complete, the patient should be followed-up at appropriate intervals for at least 5 years. In many centres this will involve return visits at 3-monthly intervals for the first 2 years and at 6-monthly intervals thereafter. Approximately 5% of all patients with primary malignant melanoma develop a second primary tumour, and therefore patients should be taught to recognize the features of early melanoma in order that they may recognize a secondary primary tumour at a very early growth stage. There is currently discussion over the value of longer-term follow-up on the grounds that the intervals between visits are so lengthy that patients will self-diagnose any recurrence between visits, and that very prolonged follow-up creates large and unwieldy review clinics. Against this argument it should be considered that if recurrence does develop in patients who have had thin primary tumours, it is not uncommonly seen between 5 and 10 years after surgery to the primary lesion. It should also be noted that the policy of well-established services such as the Sydney Melanoma Clinic is to follow up all patients indefinitely.

Prophylactic node dissection or not?

For patients with thicker primary tumours arising on the limbs there is controversy about the advantage to the patient of prophylactic lymph node dissection of the draining groin or axillary region. The logic of this approach is based on the fact that a number of patients will have subclinical involvement of their draining nodes, and that removal of these nodes before they are palpable will reduce mortality more effectively than by waiting until lymph nodes are clinically involved by which time micrometastases may have spread beyond the nodes.

There are striking differences in the frequency with which prophylactic lymph node dissection is carried out in Europe and North America. In Europe the general approach is not to carry out prophylactic lymph node dissection but to follow-up the patient as detailed above and remove lymph nodes only when they are clinically enlarged. In the USA the trend is to carry out prophylactic node dissections much more readily. The more conservative European approach has been supported by the results of a World Health Organisation trial in which therapeutic versus prophylactic dissection was compared (Veronesi et al., 1977). This study has been criticized on the grounds that the majority of patients are females with relatively good prognosis lesions on the lower limbs.

Results of other published series do not offer definitive evidence that one approach is statistically significantly better than the other, although there are a number of publications, including a large series from Sydney, Australia, which suggest that for patients with tumours in the intermediate thickness category 1.5–3.5 mm thick the prophylactic lymph node approach does offer an advantage (Milton et al., 1982).

In contrast those with thicker tumours do not benefit and this may be because at the time of the prophylactic node dissection the disease is already disseminated. Thus, the prophylactic lymph node approach may offer a survival advantage to a small proportion, approximately 15% of patients with tumours in this thickness category, but lymph node dissection does carry some morbidity and a proportion of patients subjected to this extensive surgical procedure will not in fact benefit.

Adjuvant limb perfusion

A further surgical approach to the management of poor prognosis primary melanoma of the limbs is the technique of adjuvant arterial perfusion of the affected limb with a cytotoxic drug, usually melphalan. Adjuvant limb perfusion has been practised in a small number of centres for over 20 years, notably in New Orleans and Groningen (Krementz, 1983). Until recently, however, no randomized controlled trial of lymph node perfusion following surgical excision of the primary tumour versus surgical excision alone had been reported. At present one such study is in progress, conducted jointly by the World Health Organisation and European

Organisation for the Research and Treatment of Cancer. This study should prove whether or not this approach is of survival advantage to the affected patient.

Treatment of recurrent malignant melanoma

Management of recurrent disease between the primary site and the local draining lymph node basin — Stage IIa disease

This problem can be divided into three situations: local recurrence, satellitosis, and in-transit metastases. Local recurrence is commonly defined as disease recurring within 5 cm of the excision margins of the primary lesion. This is best treated by wide local excision and grafting. The area excised should allow for the fact that there may well be additional subclinical metastatic deposits in the area. Some surgeons would consider that local recurrence would justify a prophylactic node dissection, but there are no published studies to support this approach. Similarly, centres in which arterial limb perfusion with cytotoxic agents is available may include this situation in their indications for perfusion.

The terms 'satellitosis' and 'in-transit metastases' cover overlapping clinical situations. Satellitosis is usually used to describe the situation of large numbers of subcutaneous or intradermal secondary tumour deposits on the affected limb, and in-transit metastases used to describe a situation in which subcutaneous metastases develop in a more linear fashion, presumably originating from tumour cells in the draining lymphatics. The leg is most commonly affected, and may present a considerable management problem because of oedema, and sometimes breakdown of the skin overlying the deposits with resulting ulceration and secondary infection. This type of tumour spread is much more distressing for the patient than non-visible tumour spread.

There is no universally agreed best method of managing this situation. It is important to stage the patient in whom this development has occurred and investigate for any evidence of lung, liver or cerebral spread. If any of these are found, clearly a more palliative approach is indicated, but if the only evidence of recurrent disease is in the originally affected limb, a more radical surgical approach including possibly amputation may be considered. Unfortunately, personal experience of observing a small number of patients suggests that these patients do have occult metastases elsewhere in the body, and that amputation is not a curative procedure. Arterial limb perfusion can bring about dramatic but temporary shrinkage of this type of tumour recurrence. Although melanoma is not generally considered radiosensitive, high dose fractions of radiation may also give worthwhile palliation. If the lesions are not too numerous, local excision of individual lesions, or even cryotherapy may improve the appearance of the limb and be of help to the patient, although clearly neither method will be curative.

Management of clinically involved draining regional lymph nodes — Stage IIb

When the draining lymph nodes become palpable in a patient with previous primary melanoma, it is highly likely that this is due to metastatic disease, and many surgeons would proceed directly to node dissection. If the quality of the enlargement suggests that it could be due to infection, a needle aspiration node biopsy and cytology should be arranged.

If positive, this is a situation in which a CT scan is justified to establish whether or not there are extensive metastases in other organs such as liver and lung. Clearly, if this is the case a more palliative approach to management of the nodes may be justified. If, however, the only evidence of metastatic spread is to the lymph nodes, it is considered that every effort should be made to carry out a full anatomical node dissection with the aim of removing all tumour cells. Five-year survivals after positive lymph node dissection from the major centres are in the 20–25% range.

An ilio-inguinal node dissection should include the femoral triangle, femoral nodes, the iliac nodes, the obturator nodes and the node of Cloquet. Detailed operative procedure is beyond the scope of this chapter but every effort should be made to avoid any potential seeding of tumour cells from the lymph nodes draining the previously affected limb into the operative cavity. Many surgeons at the end of deep ilio-inguinal lymphadenectomy will incise the peritoneum and check the abdomen and periaortic nodes for involvement. Patients are usually mobilized 24–48 hours after ilio-inguinal node dissection and drains are removed at 6–8 days. Postoperative limb oedema can be a problem and a surgical stocking can be ordered and used immediately after surgery. Bilateral ilio-inguinal node dissections should be avoided if at all possible as this can give rise to extremely distressing genital oedema.

An axillary node dissection should be complete and include nodes deep to the pectoralis muscle. Cervical node dissection can be radical or modified, sparing the spinal accessory nerve and sternomastoid muscle. In situations where a cervical node dissection is needed, the parotid nodes may also require to be removed.

If only one node contains tumour on pathological examination, the prognosis for the patient is little different from the prognosis related to the Breslow thickness of his primary tumour. Four or more nodes histologically involved with tumour is, however, a poor prognostic sign, as is the presence of tumour cells outwith the capsule of the lymph node (Balch et al., 1981). It is therefore important to ask the reporting pathologist for these details. As at present there is no established chemotherapy for advanced malignant melanoma, there is no regime which is of proven value in an adjuvant setting after full anatomical dissection.

Stage III disease

Malignant melanoma is a relatively insensitive tumour to chemotherapy and for this reason there is at present no regime which confers a proven survival advantage for treating patients with advanced disease. Single agents which have been used with a 20–25% response rate include DTIC (Carter et al., 1976) and vindesine (Retsas et al., 1980) and quadruple chemotherapy regimes include bleomycin, vindesine or vinblastine, lomustine and DTIC. This combination regime gives a slightly higher response rate of 30–40% partial and complete responses (Young et al., 1985) but responses are relatively short lived, and very few patients are alive 1 year after commencing chemotherapy.

Radiotherapy is of limited value in malignant melanoma but can be of value in palliating advanced disease. Two situations in which it is of particular value are in relieving symptoms from cerebral metastases, and the relief of pain from bony metastases.

It will be apparent that once malignant melanoma has spread from the primary site the prospects of a cure are almost nil. For this reason it is essential that all medically qualified individuals are aware of the features of malignant melanoma at its earliest recognizable growth phase on the skin. It is also important that members of the public, particularly those in high-risk groups are aware of these features to allow for rapid excision of melanoma at a curable stage.

References

Balch, C. M., Soong, S. J., Murad, T. M. *et al.* (1981) A multifactorial analysis of melanoma 3. Prognostic factors in patients with lymph node metastases (Stage II). *Annals of Surgery*, **183**, 377–382

Balch, C. M., Wilkerson, J. A., Murad, T. M. *et al.* (1980) The prognostic significance of ulceration of cutaneous melanoma. *Cancer*, **43**, 3012–3017

Breslow, A. (1970) Thickness, cross-sectional area, and depth of invasion in the prognosis of cutaneous melanoma. *Annals of Surgery*, **172**, 902–906

Carter, R. D., Krementz, E. T., Hill, G. J. and Metter, G. E. (1976) D T I C and combination therapy for melanoma. *Cancer Treatment Reports*, **60**, 601–605

Cassileth, B. R., Lusk, E. J. and Tenaglia, A. N. (1983) Patients' perceptions of the cosmetic impact of melanoma resection. *Plastic and Reconstructive Surgery*, **71**, 73–75

Clark, W. H. Jr, From, L., Bernardino, E. A. and Mihm, M. C. (1969) The histogenesis and behaviour of primary human malignant melanoma of the skin. *Cancer Research*, **29**, 705–712

Flook, D., Horgan, K. Taylor, B. A. and Hughes, L. E. (1986) Surgery for malignant melanoma: from which limb should the graft be taken? *British Journal of Surgery*, **73**, 793–795

Green, A. and Siskind, V. (1983) Geographic distribution of cutaneous melanoma in Queensland. *Medical Journal of Australia*, **1**, 407–410

Kenady, D. E., Brown, B. W. and McBride, C. M. (1982) Excision of underlying fascia with primary malignant melanoma. Effects on survival and recurrence rates. *Surgery*, **92**, 615–618

Krementz, E. T. (1983) Chemotherapy by isolated regional perfusion for malignant melanoma of the limbs. Recent results. *Cancer Research*, **86**, 193–201

MacKie, R. M., Smyth, J. F., Soutar, D. S. *et al.* (1985) Malignant melanoma in Scotland 1979–1983. *Lancet*, **ii**, 858–861

Magnus, K. (1981) Habits of sun exposure and risks of melanoma. *Cancer*, **48**, 2329–2335

Milton, G. W., Shaw, H. M., McCarthy, W. H. *et al.* (1982) Prophylactic lymph node dissection in clinical stage I cutaneous malignant melanoma. Results of surgical treatment in 1319 patients. *British Journal of Surgery*, **69**, 108–114

Olsen, G. (1964) Removal of fascia. Cause of more frequent metastases of malignant melanoma of the skin to regional lymph nodes? *Cancer*, **17**, 1159–1163

Retsas, S., Peat, I., Ashford, R. *et al.* (1980) Updated results of vindesine as a single agent in the therapy of advanced malignant melanoma. *Cancer Treatment Reviews* (Suppl.) **7**, 87–90

Taylor, B. A. and Hughes, L. E. (1985) A policy of selective excision for primary cutaneous melanoma. *European Journal of Surgical Oncology*, **11**, 7–13

Veronesi, U., Adamus, J., Bandiera, D. C. *et al.* (1977) Inefficiacy of immediate node dissection in Stage I melanoma of the limbs. *New England Journal of Medicine*, **297**, 627–630

Veronesi, U., Hunter, J. A. A., Mackie, R. M. *et al.* (1988) Thin Stage I primary cutaneous malignant melanoma. Comparison of excision with margins of 1 or 3 cm. *New England Journal of Medicine*, **318**, 1159–1162

Young, D. W., Lever, R. S., English, J. S. C. *et al.* (1985) The use of BELD combination chemotherapy in advanced malignant melanoma. *Cancer*, **55**, 1879–1881

Chapter 13

Bone and soft tissue

J. Pooley

In a book on surgical oncology a section entitled 'Bone and Soft Tissue' deals, of course, with tumours of the musculoskeletal system. In such a book written more than ten years ago these tumours were placed firmly within the province of the orthopaedic surgeon who may then have enlisted the help of a radiotherapist. The topic inevitably made depressing reading with the term 'poor prognosis' used frequently and was perhaps summarized by Illingworth and Dick (1968) who observed, 'some sarcomata, notably those arising in bone are almost always uniformly fatal'. The main decision a surgeon was required to make concerned the level of an amputation and it was generally concluded that the only good thing to be said about these tumours was that they are relatively uncommon.

The incidence of tumours of the musculoskeletal system remains unchanged but their importance has increased during the last decade in proportion with the significant advances in their management made during this time. The evolution of effective chemotherapy regimens for some tumours has led to the increased probability of a patient's long-term survival. This in turn has led to the development of techniques and equipment which now allow a surgeon to consider treating certain malignant tumours within a limb by resection and reconstruction rather than to proceed automatically to primary amputation.

Even today, however, some orthopaedic surgeons are perhaps not fully aware of the procedures now available for the management of a patient with a tumour of the musculoskeletal system while others remain unconvinced that any surgical procedure other than the amputation of a limb can be safely recommended. The aim of this chapter is to describe a plan of management into which any patient who presents with a musculoskeletal tumour can be included and to present the treatment options currently available which will enable a surgeon, in consultation with his patient, to make the most appropriate choice.

It will become evident that some of the surgical treatments require the use of techniques more familiar to the vascular surgeon or plastic surgeon than the orthopaedic surgeon. Furthermore, firm diagnosis and surgical planning depend upon the skills of the pathologist and diagnostic radiologist and improvement in long-term survival is due almost entirely to treatment supervised by the oncologist. The importance of a 'team' approach to the treatment of a patient with a malignant musculoskeletal tumour has been stressed (Sim, 1983) and cannot be over-emphasized. It is therefore stated categorically here that the definitive surgical operation represents only an incident in the overall management of these patients and that the timing of surgery and even the choice of the procedure must be a team decision. The effective treatment of patients with musculoskeletal tumours has now transgressed the boundaries of general orthopaedic practice and increasingly therefore a case is being made for the management of these patients to be undertaken in centres which are staffed and equipped to offer the comprehensive service necessary to ensure that the improvement in results continues.

Before proceeding to discuss the management of a patient who presents with a tumour of the musculoskeletal system it is necessary to define the groups of tumours to be included and to consider their behaviour.

Tumour types

The tissues comprising the musculoskeletal system develop from primitive mesenchyme and can be divided into two broad groups: (a) connective tissues, and (b) haematopoietic and reticuloendothelial tissues. Tumours originating from connective tissues vary in their degree of malignancy from the undoubtedly benign to the highly malignant. Tumours derived from haematopoietic and reticuloendothelial tissues tend to exhibit varying degrees of malignancy. Any malignant tumour of mesenchymal origin is of course designated a 'sarcoma'.

It is the patients who present with tumours of connective-tissue origin, which include the relatively well-known osteosarcoma and chondrosarcoma who in general are regarded as 'bone tumour patients' and for whom surgery plays a major role in treatment. Most of the forthcoming discussion will relate to patients who present with this type of tumour.

Tumours derived from haematopoietic and reticuloendothelial tissues which include the leukaemias, lymphomas and plasmacytoma differ substantially in their natural history and response to treatment from tumours of connective-tissue origin. As the management of patients suffering from tumours of the haematopoietic and reticuloendothelial system is primarily medical, discussion will in the main be confined to the place of surgery in diagnosis and the treatment of complications. Nevertheless, it should be recognized that within the context of musculoskeletal tumours these neoplasms are relatively common, in fact plasmacytoma has the distinction of being the commonest malignant primary bone tumour of all.

Certain carcinomas characteristically, and all too frequently, metastasize to the skeleton. As sarcomas in general are rare in comparison with carcinomas, this accounts for the fact that in the adult a destructive lesion within a bone is much more likely to be a secondary deposit from a carcinoma than a primary bone tumour. Although surgery for the treatment of secondary deposits within bone is palliative it has much to offer patients who frequently are suffering considerable pain, and this justifies its inclusion here.

Tumours of connective-tissue origin

Incidence

It is not possible to give an accurate figure for the incidence of all tumours which occur within the musculoskeletal system as many benign tumours, such as lipomas, remain unbiopsied. Although sarcomas usually come to medical attention, difficulties in reaching a specific diagnosis complicates the interpretation of figures, and data collected from the major tertiary referral centres are subject to inevitable bias. However, it is well recognized in surgical practice that tumours of the musculoskeletal system are comparatively rare. According to the National Cancer Institute's Third National Survey performed in the USA in 1976, 4500 new cases of soft-tissue sarcoma and 1900 new cases of malignant bone tumours occurred, which can be compared with 93 000 cases of lung cancer and 88 700 cases of breast cancer. Furthermore, it has been calculated that primary bone tumours account for only 1% of deaths from malignant disease. In the UK approximately 150 new cases of osteosarcoma, the commonest primary bone tumour of connective-tissue origin, present each year.

The significance of those figures can perhaps be better appreciated when one considers that it has been estimated that the number of patients presenting with a primary bone tumour of an extremity, and therefore more amenable to surgical treatment, provides approximately 1 case/year/two-man orthopaedic group in the USA. This therefore, strengthens the case mentioned above for central referral of these patients for treatment.

Classification

Despite their comparative rarity, a comprehensive list of all the types of primary tumours which have been found within the musculoskeletal system would be long.

Table 13.1 A classification of musculoskeletal tumours by tissue of origin

Tissue of origin	Benign	Malignant
Haematopoietic and reticuloendothelial		Plasmacytoma (myeloma) Lymphosarcoma Leukaemias Reticulum-cell sarcoma
Cartilage	Osteochondroma Chondroma Chondroblastoma Chondromyxoid fibroma	Chondrosarcoma and its variants
Bone	Osteoid osteoma Osteoblastoma	Osteosarcoma and its variants
Synovium	Giant-cell tumour of tendon sheath	Synovial sarcoma
Uncertain origin	Giant-cell tumour Fibrous histiocytoma	Malignant giant-cell tumour Malignant fibrous histiocytoma Ewing's sarcoma Adamantinoma
Fibrous tissue	Non-ossifying fibroma Desmoplastic fibroma	Fibrosarcoma
Muscle	Leiomyoma Rhabdomyoma	Leiomyosarcoma Rhabdomyosarcoma
Fat	Lipoma	Liposarcoma
Nerve	Neurilemmoma Neurofibroma	Neurosarcoma
Notochordal		Chordoma
Vascular	Haemangioma	Haemangioendothelioma Haemangiopericytoma

Indeed Enzinger and Weiss (1983) classified more than 150 types and variants of soft-tissue tumours alone. A comprehensive list would, however, be of little relevance to surgical practice. Classification of these tumours is, nevertheless, important as this facilitates selection of the appropriate treatment for a given patient and allows comparisons to be made between groups of patients receiving different treatments. The system originally proposed by Lichtenstein (1951) in which tumours are listed by tissue of origin, and classified into benign or malignant on histological grounds, has provided a practical framework for the classification of bone tumours and is widely used. Table 13.1 has been constructed by using this method of classification expanded to include the more common soft-tissue tumours.

Natural history

The natural history of tumours derived from the connective tissues is now recognized to be the same whether they arise within bone or the surrounding soft tissues. Enneking (1986) succinctly stated that 'a fibrosarcoma behaves as a fibrosarcoma whether it arises in bone and invades the soft tissues or vice versa'. It follows that the investigation and management of these tumours should follow the same principles. This fact is not yet widely appreciated and there is still a tendency for malignant soft-tissue tumours to be treated by a less than adequate surgical procedure.

The principles of surgical treatment may be more readily appreciated by considering the types of lesion which can arise and their subsequent behaviour. Although, for clarity, the widely used classifications of musculoskeletal tumours divide these into benign or malignant, depending upon whether or not a given tumour will give rise to metastases, in fact a spectrum of behaviour is observed ranging from the undoubtedly benign to the highly malignant. This has led to the identification of a number of groups into which an individual tumour may be placed. For practical purposes, however, three main patterns of behaviour are observed. This enables a given tumour to be placed in one of the following groups.

1. Benign tumours: Examples of these are the osteoid osteoma involving bone, or lipoma, more usually found in the soft tissues. These tumours are normally amenable to local surgical excision which is curative.
2. Locally aggressive or low-grade malignant tumours: These tumours either rarely metastasize or do so after an interval of some years. An example is the giant-cell tumour which characteristically recurs locally if a complete surgical excision is not achieved and microscopic remnants of tumour are left behind. It is in this group of tumours that inadequate excision of the original lesion and subsequent local recurrences carries the risk of changing the nature of the tumour into one of higher grade malignancy with a risk of metastasis.
3. High-grade malignant tumours: The classical 'central' osteosarcoma is the commonest tumour in this group. These tumours are characterized by rapid growth, destruction rather than displacement of local tissues and a tendency to metastasize early. Blood-borne spread is the usual method of metastasis, with the lungs being the commonest site of secondary tumours. Less commonly, metastases may appear in other bones and occasionally in the regional lymph nodes.

The patients with a tumour in the last group therefore have the poorest prognosis. They require a more extensive surgical procedure and this may be combined with chemotherapy or radiotherapy. Although the results of combined treatment appear to be improving, this is the area which has aroused most controversy and in which the most careful judgement is required to ensure the safe treatment of a tumour and yet retain the optimum function of a limb.

Irrespective of the type of tumour, successful treatment depends upon a surgeon performing an adequate surgical procedure. The question in any individual case is, what constitutes an adequate surgical procedure? Is it safe to remove the tumour piecemeal, shell it out or should it be excised *en bloc* with a margin of normal tissue? If the latter is selected, how wide should the margin be?

If we consider the behaviour of each of the above three groups of tumours, then the problems facing a surgeon will become apparent. The reader is referred to the text book entitled *Musculoskeletal Tumour Surgery* by W. F. Enneking (1983) for an illustrated detailed account of the behaviour of musculoskeletal tumours within the tissues.

As the tumour grows within the compartment in which it originates, for example marrow cavity, muscle group or subcutaneous tissue, the normal connective tissue within that compartment is compressed to form a distinct capsule of mature fibrous connective tissue around the tumour. The presence of the tumour also incites a reaction in the zone of adjacent normal tissue enveloping it. This 'reactive zone' which forms between the compressed fibrous capsule and the surrounding normal tissue has three components:

1. A proliferation of mesenchymal cells which form fibrous tissue, cartilage or bone depending upon their environment.
2. A proliferation of new blood vessels.
3. An infiltration of inflammatory cells.

The relationship of the tumour to its capsule and reactive zone reflects the degree of malignancy of the lesion. This is illustrated in Figure 13.1.

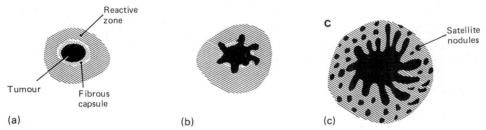

Figure 13.1 Diagram to illustrate the interface between benign, locally aggressive and malignant tumours with the host tissues: (a) benign, (b) aggressive, (c) high-grade malignant

Figure 13.1a is a diagram illustrating the characteristics of a benign tumour. It is well encapsulated by a thin mature fibrous border. There is a relatively narrow reactive zone in which there would be little or no evidence of blood vessel proliferation and few inflammatory cells. Such tumours, of which the simple lipoma is a good example, being well encapsulated can be excised intact locally. A plane of cleavage is found between the reactive zone and the surrounding normal tissue.

Locally aggressive tumours are by implication more invasive and this behaviour is reflected at their interface with the surrounding normal tissues. The features of a locally aggressive tumour are illustrated in Figure 13.1b. Characteristically the edge of the tumour is more irregular than that of a benign lesion and its compressed fibrous capsule thinner. Of more significance is the tendency for finger-like processes to protrude from the main body of the tumour through the capsule and into the reactive zone. The reactive zone is thicker than that surrounding benign tumours and histological examination reveals a proliferation of new blood vessels in this region. Within the reactive zone an inflammatory response is more in evidence.

The presence of finger-like processes of tumour extending into the reactive zone which surrounds a locally aggressive lesion must be considered when planning a surgical excision. If the plane of dissection is carried through the reactive zone there is a risk of leaving microscopic extensions of tumour behind which would then give rise to local recurrence of the lesion. An adequate surgical procedure therefore requires an excision to be performed by dissection through normal tissue beyond the extensions of tumour into the reactive zone.

There is a difference between the behaviour of locally aggressive tumours which do not metastasize, and those of low-grade malignancy which do. In the reactive zone of lesions of low-grade malignancy, nodules of tumour are found which appear to have separated off from the protruding processes of the main body of the tumour. These nodules are called 'satellites'.

In the high-grade malignant tumour illustrated in Figure 13.1c numerous satellite nodules are seen to extend deep into the reactive zone. These tumours characteristically destroy the host tissues and undermine attempts at encapsulation. Little or no fibrous tissue can therefore be found to represent a capsule around the tumour. The reactive zone is much wider than that of locally aggressive and low-grade malignant sarcomas and a proliferation of new blood vessels is a prominent feature of this region. In particular the presence of large thin-walled vascular channels into which buds of tumour can be seen to be growing are a disturbing feature of the reactive zone surrounding sarcomas of high-grade malignancy. An inflammatory response is usually seen in the reactive zone but is variable in its intensity. Another disturbing finding in high-grade sarcomas is the presence of satellite nodules *beyond* the reactive zone in apparently normal tissue. An adequate surgical procedure, therefore, would require excision of the tumour by dissection through normal tissue well away from the edge of the reactive zone. The presence of distant satellites, however, makes the outcome of such surgery less certain in tumours of high-grade malignancy.

Staging

It is evident from the above discussion that it is only after considering the behaviour of a tumour within the tissues that an operative procedure can be chosen which would ensure the complete removal of a primary lesion whilst avoiding unnecessarily extensive surgery. Before deciding the surgical procedure appropriate to an individual case it is therefore necessary first to determine the degree of malignancy of the primary tumour.

A fundamental concept was expressed by Enneking (1986) who pointed out that the significant changes observed in the biological behaviour of the various musculoskeletal tumours progressed through a series of stages from benign, through locally aggressive, low-grade malignancy, and high-grade malignancy, to the presence of metastatic disease. Furthermore, each of these progressions has distinctive clinical, radiological and histological features which Enneking and his colleagues have used as the basis of a staging system.

This staging system, which can be used for any musculoskeletal tumour of connective-tissue origin, whether the tumour arises within bone or the surrounding soft tissues, takes into account the surgical grade (G), the site and local extent of the tumour (T), and the presence or absence of metastasis (M).

The surgical grade (G) is a measure of the overall biological aggressiveness of a lesion. It is arrived at by not only considering the histological features of the tumour, such as the degree of cellular differentiation or amount of mitotic activity, but also by taking into account its clinical and radiological features. The rapidity of the clinical course and the degree of bone destruction demonstrated on an X-ray may be of more importance than the histological appearances in grading some bone tumours. Conversely, the grading of a soft-tissue fibrosarcoma is more dependent upon its histological appearance.

Tumours are placed into one of three grades: G_0 = benign, G_1 = low-grade malignant and G_2 = high-grade malignant. A simple lipoma would be classified G_0, whereas giant-cell tumours of bone, juxtacortical osteosarcomas and some chondrosarcomas are designated G_1, while the classical (central) osteosarcomas, other chondrosarcomas, fibrosarcomas and rhabdomyosarcomas are G_2 tumours.

The surgical grade (G) is an indication of the biological aggressiveness of a lesion and indicates the magnitude of the surgical margin required for its effective removal. The site and local extent of a tumour (T) indicates the type of procedure required, local excision, wide excision, or radical excision, in order to achieve the necessary surgical margin. The principal determinant of the type of surgical procedure required is whether the tumour is contained within the compartment in which it originated, or whether it has already extended out into neighbouring compartments by the time the patient presents for treatment. Tumours are therefore classified as either intracompartmental (T1) or extracompartmental (T2). The medullary cavity of a bone, a joint cavity, or a muscle group bounded by its fascia are examples of single compartments.

The presence or absence of metastasis (M) is of major prognostic importance and must be taken into account when considering the surgical treatment of a primary lesion.

By combining the surgical grade of a tumour (G), its site and extent (T), and the presence or absence of metastasis (M), Enneking and his colleagues devised the staging system which was later refined (Enneking, 1986) and is summarized in Table 13.2. In this system, lesions are classified as benign or malignant, and the malignant tumours divided into three groups, I = low-grade, II = high-grade, III = low or high grade associated with metastasis. Each of these groups is further divided into subgroups. In subgroup A the tumour is considered to be intracompartmental, in subgroup B extracompartmental extension has occurred.

Table 13.2 Enneking's system for staging malignant musculoskeletal tumours

Stage	Grade	Site
IA	Low (G_1)	Intracompartmental (T_1)
IB	Low (G_1)	Extracompartmental (T_2)
IIA	High (G_2)	Intracompartmental (T_1)
IIB	High (G_2)	Extracompartmental (T_2)
III	Any (G) regional or distant metastasis	Any (T)

This system precisely places tumours in a progressively descending order of prognosis from good to poor and correlates with the appropriate surgical procedures ranging from local excision to radical amputation. It can be appreciated that Stage I lesions have a better prognosis than either Stage II or Stage III lesions, and that the type of surgical procedure required to achieve an adequate surgical margin for a IA lesion (low-grade malignant, intracompartmental) would be much less extensive than for a IIB lesion (high-grade malignant, extracompartmental).

This staging system has now gained wide acceptance and is the basis for the investigation and treatment of musculoskeletal tumours in many major centres. By adhering to this system logical decisions can be made about surgical procedures and adjuvant therapy for any given tumour, and the methods employed and the results obtained in different centres can be compared.

Clinical presentation

In most patients presenting with a musculoskeletal tumour the local symptoms and physical signs are non-specific. Because of this and the relative rarity of these tumours, clinical suspicion is perhaps more important than either a detailed history or physical examination in ensuring their early diagnosis. It is not uncommon for a patient with mild initial symptoms to seek medical advice several months before finally being referred to a surgeon who then confirms the presence of a malignant tumour. An increased awareness of the mode of presentation of the more common musculoskeletal tumours is therefore important as this would shorten referral intervals and consequently improve the results of subsequent treatment.

Soft-tissue tumours

The presence of a soft-tissue tumour is usually heralded by the appearance of a lump or localized swelling which then increases in size. The most common soft-tissue tumour by far is the solitary benign lipoma situated in the subcutaneous tissues. They are often 'confidently' diagnosed on clinical grounds and then effectively treated by local excision. However, it is important to realize that superficially situated sarcomas may present the physical characteristics of a benign lipoma and that the absence of pain or apparent smoothness of the surface of a lesion perceived by palpation does not exclude malignancy. Nevertheless, there are some features of soft-tissue lesions which enable these to be diagnosed as probably benign, or malignant, on clinical grounds.

Rydholm (1983) studied soft-tissue tumours and concluded that, by applying certain clinical criteria, patients who were at risk of having a sarcoma could be selected and referred for further evaluation prior to surgery. He compared simple benign lipomas with sarcomas and found that these lesions differed in the following respects:

Age of patient

Lipomas occurred much more commonly in patients under 60 years of age. Sarcomas were more common in the older age groups.

Duration

Perhaps predictably, the length of time the tumour had been present was found to be greater in the benign lesions. More than two-thirds of the lipomas had been present for one year or longer before the patients presented for treatment. This compares with the sarcomas in which three-quarters had been present for less than one year, and most for less than three months.

Size
Sarcomas were generally larger than lipomas. Ninety-five per cent of lipomas were found to be smaller than 5 cm in diameter, whereas two-thirds of the sarcomas were found to be larger than 5 cm in diameter.

Site
The anatomical locations of the two types of lesion were significantly different. Solitary lipomas were found mainly on the trunk and upper limb. This contrasts with the sarcomas which demonstrated a marked predilection for the lower limb (59%), particularly the thigh in which 36% of the lesions were found.

Relationship to deep fascia
Lipomas were almost always (99%) superficial to the deep fascia, whereas more than half of the sarcomas were located more deeply.

Symptoms
Although lipomas are characteristically painless, the absence of pain did not necessarily indicate the presence of a benign lesion. In a series of 278 patients with a soft-tissue sarcoma, Rydholm (1983) observed that the lesions had been recorded as presenting a painful mass in only 20% and that the finding of a painless mass was recorded positively in 50% of cases.

It would appear therefore that any soft-tissue tumour 5 cm or greater in diameter which has been present for less than one year should be viewed with suspicion, irrespective of its physical characteristics or the absence of symptoms. The occurrence of the lesion in the buttock or lower limb, especially if it is deeply placed and the patient is in the older age groups, should increase the suspicion that it may be a sarcoma.

Bone tumours

Pain associated with a swelling or the occurrence of a pathological fracture is a mode of presentation which is common to both benign and malignant tumours of bone. In these cases a plain X-ray of the involved part will usually reveal the presence and location of the lesion. However, initial symptoms are characteristically mild or even absent. In many instances the more benign lesions are discovered by chance as a result of an X-ray examination performed during an investigation for other unrelated conditions. It is not uncommon in a patient seeking advice about persisting discomfort attributed to the effects of an injury for the presence of an unsuspected bone tumour to be revealed by X-ray examination.

Occasionally, referred pain may delay diagnosis. This is particularly true of lesions around the hip joint which may present solely as pain in the knee and lead to inadequate X-ray examination. An awareness of the site of predilection of the more common tumours together with a knowledge of the age groups involved, for example the occurrence of osteosarcoma in the distal femur during the second decade, should increase clinical suspicion. This would then lead to the prompt referral of patients for further investigation in spite of a paucity of signs and symptoms.

Investigations

Most patients who present with a lesion which appears to be a musculoskeletal tumour require to undergo a series of investigations. The aims of these are to confirm the diagnosis and to stage the lesion. When this has been accomplished the appropriate treatment may then be planned.

Definite confirmation of the diagnosis in the case of most benign and *all* aggressive or malignant tumours requires the microscopic examination of material obtained by biopsy. The other investigations necessary to stage a tumour involve the various imaging techniques used to determine the precise location and extent of the disease. Interpretation of the results of these investigations is complicated by distortion of both the lesion and the adjacent tissues which results from biopsy, irrespective of the technique used. It is therefore better to wait until all other staging investigations have been completed before proceeding to biopsy a lesion.

The assistance of radiological colleagues is helpful in both choosing the most appropriate imaging procedures and interpreting the results. In a team approach to management the radiologists involved are consulted prior to embarking on a programme of investigations.

The plain X-ray

A plain X-ray is usually the first diagnostic imaging procedure to be performed. It is of limited value in the assessment of soft-tissue tumours, although an impression of their extent may be gained from the size of the soft-tissue shadow visible on the radiograph. A benign lipoma appears as a clearly outlined area of radiolucency which is practically diagnostic. A soft-tissue shadow adjacent to an irregular area of bone cortex would suggest that the tumour is probably malignant and destroying adjacent bone.

Calcified phleboliths within a cavernous haemangioma give rise to a unique radiographic appearance which is almost pathognomonic. The calcification which occurs within necrotic areas of some soft-tissue sarcomas may also be visible on the plain X-ray film.

Although the radiological appearances of many bone tumours are non-specific, plain X-ray examination remains the single most informative diagnostic imaging technique. Benign tumours of bone are characteristically clearly delineated with a well-formed margin and tend to produce expansion of the intact bone cortex. These appearances contrast with those of malignant bone tumours which usually appear to be poorly marginated and permeate or destroy the cortical bone. Periosteal new bone formation is often seen at the edges of the bone lesion and radiological evidence of tumour bone formation may also be visible. An associated soft-tissue shadow adjacent to the bone is evidence of extraosseous and therefore extracompartmental extension.

Both the type of bone involved and the site of the radiographic abnormality within a long bone are of considerable value in diagnosis.

In vertebrae, lesions with a benign appearance are likely to be due to osteoid osteoma, osteoblastoma or haemangioma. Malignant lesions of vertebrae are commonly due to myeloma or secondary carcinoma.

In the flat bones, chondrosarcoma, myeloma and metastatic carcinoma predominate.

It is the long bones in which the location of a lesion is of diagnostic significance.

In the epiphysis, a giant-cell tumour and chondroblastoma are found. The metaphyseal region is the usual site of origin of osteosarcoma. Diaphyseal lesions are more commonly due to chondrosarcoma and fibrosarcoma. Ewing's sarcoma also tends to involve the diaphyseal region in common with tumours of reticuloendothelial origin and metatastatic carcinoma.

It must be stressed that although plain X-ray films illustrate the type of bone destruction occurring and demonstrate well the nature of the margin between a bone lesion and normal bone, they are not by themselves diagnostic of either the nature or even the presence of a bone tumour. There are a number of conditions involving bone which are capable of producing lesions whose radiological appearances are indistinguishable from those of primary bone tumours. The principal conditions are listed in Table 13.3. Further staging studies including

Table 13.3 Conditions simulating primary bone tumours

Osteomyelitis
Exuberant callus
Simple (unicameral bone cyst)
Aneurysmal bone cyst
Fibrous dysplasia
Hyperparathyroidism
Bone infarcts
Synovial chondromatosis

Metastatic carcinoma

biopsy should distinguish between these lesions and primary bone tumours. However, relatively common conditions such as osteomyelitis and stress fractures have led to diagnostic difficulties. The radiological appearance of osteomyelitis may closely resemble that of an infiltrating malignant bone tumour and this impression may be reinforced by the histological findings of numerous inflammatory cells associated with areas of bone necrosis and new bone formation. Similarly, the appearance of abundant new bone formation around the shaft of a long bone in the absence of a history of injury may lead to a stress fracture being diagnosed as an osteosarcoma. Furthermore, the histological appearances of fracture callus and those of a well-differentiated (low-grade malignant) osteosarcoma are similar. The inclusion of an experienced osteoarticular pathologist in any team involved in the management of patients with musculoskeletal tumours is therefore self-evident.

Tomography

Tomograms, in general, add little to the information obtained from examining plain X-ray films, although they do occasionally demonstrate the presence of a pathological fracture through a lesion not detectable on the plain radiograph. Tomography is also useful in making a diagnosis of osteoid osteoma by demonstrating the typical small radiolucent nidus within the area of dense reactive bone which surrounds this.

Computed tomography

The images obtained by computed tomography (CT) are inferior to plain radiographs for identifying the precise site and nature of a tumour involving a long bone. However, in other areas of the skeleton, for example the spine and pelvis in which superimposition of the bones are seen on plain radiographs, CT may demonstrate a lesion which is not visible on these. A more important feature of CT in the staging of bone tumours is its ability to demonstrate the extent of the local disease both within the medullary cavity of a bone and out into the soft tissues. In particular, the relationship of extraosseous tumour to major neurovascular structures can be determined, enabling the feasibility of a limb-preserving procedure to be assessed.

The ability of CT to detect metastatic deposits of tumour within the lung fields, too small to be seen on plain radiographs, is now well established. A CT examination of the lungs is now therefore an essential investigation both in the initial staging of a bone tumour and the further follow-up of a patient during and after a course of treatment.

Radio-isotope bone scans

These are obtained after intravenous injection of a bone-seeking radio-isotope. The radio-isotope used most commonly is technetium-99 combined with a polyphosphate compound. Local accumulations of radio-isotope occur in regions of increased vascularity or new bone formation and give rise to areas referred to as 'hot spots' visible on the scan.

Although tumours characteristically destroy normal bone tissue, this always induces a local repair process at the periphery of the lesion and it is the new bone produced in this region which gives rise to a 'hot spot'. Some soft-tissue tumours, notably the liposarcoma, also give rise to areas of increased isotope uptake which is visible on a bone scan. This, however, is a reflection of the vascularity of these lesions as there is no significant mineralization within them.

The major limitation of the radio-isotope bone scan is that it is non-specific. 'Hot' areas may be produced by trauma or other conditions, such as inflammatory joint disease and infection. Nevertheless, when interpreted in conjunction with the other imaging studies, radio-isotope scans may give additional information about the extent of bone involvement by a tumour. Their principal use, however, is in the detection or exclusion of the presence of multiple bone lesions.

Angiography

Opinions differ amongst the major centres about the usefulness of angiography in staging connective-tissue tumours. For example, in the Mayo clinic angiography is usually not employed as it is considered that injection of contrast medium in combination with a CT scan allows the relationship of the tumour to the adjacent major vessels to be adequately assessed. In other institutions, however, angiography is used routinely.

Hudson et al. (1975) reviewed 200 angiograms performed to evaluate both bone and soft-tissue lesions and concluded that the investigation had been useful in planning the appropriate resection or amputation. The angiograms were found to be of particular value in delineating the extent of most malignant soft-tissue tumours. Enneking (1983) has found angiography to be as accurate as lymphangiography in detecting local regional node involvement in malignant fibrous histocytomas.

In the orthopaedic clinic of the University of Vienna angiography is used routinely to assess the response of a tumour to adjuvant therapy prior to surgery (Kotz, personal communication).

Resolution of the neovasculature within the reactive zone of malignant tumours, indicating a favourable response to treatment, may influence the choice of surgical procedure to be used.

Magnetic resonance imaging

The use of magnetic resonance imaging (MRI) for staging musculoskeletal tumours is currently being evaluated. Baker *et al.* (1985) reported their experience in evaluating 44 tumours of varying grades of malignancy. They found that in all cases MRI depicted the extent of the lesion and its distinction from adjacent normal tissue more clearly than the CT scan. In particular they noted that in the presence of a metal prosthesis the CT image was often completely obscured by artefact whereas MRI was only minimally affected.

Experience with MRI is growing and, in a series of more than 400 patients with musculoskeletal tumours investigated at the University of Leiden, MRI has been found to be superior to CT in delineating the extent of the primary lesion (Taminiau, personal communication). It appears probable therefore that MRI will eventually supersede CT in evaluating the local extent of musculoskeletal tumours.

However, at present CT remains superior to MRI in detecting pulmonary metastasis as these lesions are obscured by normal lung movements during the relatively prolonged period of time required to collect the data necessary to form the magnetic resonance image.

Biopsy

The firm diagnosis of a musculoskeletal tumour depends upon its recognition by microscopic examination of material obtained by biopsy. Definitive treatment of a presumed malignant tumour should *never* be carried out until the diagnosis has been confirmed by a pathologist experienced in the recognition of these tumours. Amputations have been inappropriately performed in the past for benign tumour-like lesions because of their alarming X-ray appearances, and it is only if this principle is observed that this tragedy will be avoided.

In addition to confirming the diagnosis, microscopic examination of the biopsy material completes the staging studies as it enables the histological grade (G) of the tumour to be determined. The techniques and problems associated with the biopsy of musculoskeletal tumours were comprehensively reviewed by Simon (1982) who began by stating that biopsy is a crucial, if not the most crucial, procedure in the diagnosis of many musculoskeletal lesions. This is not an overstatement, as unrepresentative material obtained at biopsy may lead to error in diagnosis, and a poorly placed biopsy incision may prevent a subsequent limb-preserving procedure or even a complete radical amputation from being performed successfully.

The team approach to the treatment of musculoskeletal tumours applies equally to the planning of the surgical biopsy. Prior consultation is recommended with the radiologist, oncologist or radiotherapist if appropriate, and certainly the pathologist involved. Furthermore, because the placing of the biopsy incision must integrate with the planned definitive surgical procedure, it is better if the surgeon who intends to perform the definitive procedure also performs the biopsy.

When planning to biopsy a musculoskeletal tumour, the timing of the biopsy as well as the placement of the incision and the technique to be used must be carefully considered.

Timing of biopsy

The accuracy of the various imaging techniques in demonstrating the local extent of a tumour is impaired by distortion of the tissues as a result of surgical biopsy. For this reason it is better to perform the biopsy after the other staging studies have been completed. Furthermore if a firm diagnosis can be made by examination of frozen sections of the biopsy material, then if staging has been completed, the definitive surgical procedure can be carried out under the same anaesthetic. However, most pathologists prefer to examine permanent sections before confirming the diagnosis of a malignant tumour, and many surgeons consider that a definite diagnosis is necessary before they discuss the surgical options with a patient. Nevertheless, because of the risk of disseminating malignant cells by performing a biopsy, the interval between this and the definitive procedure should be kept as short as possible.

Placing the incision

The placement of the biopsy is crucial. As a general rule, the most direct route to the tumour is taken. It is, however, important to consider the surgical alternatives for the definitive treatment prior to making the incision for the biopsy. It is again emphasized that a misplaced biopsy incision which cannot be excised *en bloc* with the tumour may necessitate an amputation when perhaps a limb-saving procedure could have been performed. Even if amputation is considered to be the most appropriate surgical option the placing of the biopsy incision must allow the raising of the required skin flaps at the time of the definitive operation.

When considering the siting of a biopsy incision the following guide lines should be borne in mind:

1. Always use a longitudinally placed biopsy incision in a limb as transverse incisions cannot be excised *en bloc* together with the longitudinally disposed segments of bone and muscle.
2. Avoid approaching the major neurovascular structures in a limb. If these are involved in the biopsy track then they will have to be excised at the time of the definitive surgical procedure.
3. The biopsy track should run through a muscle belly rather than in the plane between muscles as this reduces the chances of tumour spreading along fascial planes.

Biopsy technique

Material may be obtained by either open biopsy or closed (needle) biopsy. Although opinions differ as to which is the better method most surgeons agree that closed biopsy should be reserved for lesions in surgically inaccessible sites such as the spine and pelvis, or for lesions which are thought to be metastasis from a known primary tumour. The small amounts of tissue obtained by this technique may lead to errors in the diagnosis or staging of those tumours which are not homogeneous.

It should be noted that osteosarcoma is a tumour with a variegated histological pattern and if a closed biopsy sampled only a chondroid area this could then lead to a misdiagnosis of chondrosarcoma (Malcolm, 1987).

In general, therefore, open biopsy which allows an amount of tissue to be obtained sufficient to minimize sampling error is considered to be better than closed biopsy for primary tumours involving the limbs. When performing an open biopsy the smallest incision consistent with obtaining adequate amounts of tissue should be used. It should be remembered that the central regions of a tumour are often necrotic and so examination of material from this site may not provide the diagnosis. It is better therefore to biopsy the periphery of a tumour and to include tissue taken from the interface of the lesion and its capsule or pseudocapsule. If a bone tumour extends into the soft tissues, a specimen of the soft-tissue extension rather than of the bone itself should be taken as this would both provide suitable tissue for diagnosis and reduce the risk of pathological fracture should subsequent adjuvant treatment be required.

In order to prevent the local spread of malignant cells within a postoperative haematoma haemostasis must be meticulous following biopsy. It is better to avoid the use of a wound drain as the drain site would then have to be included *en bloc* in any subsequent resection.

Some surgeons routinely perform open biopsy of a tumour within a limb after placing a tourniquet proximally, in order to reduce the risk of disseminating its cells into the blood stream. However, there is no evidence to indicate that this practice improves the survival of patients with malignant tumours. Furthermore, the implication of fibrin clots in the implantation of malignant tumour cells has led some to believe that the congestion produced distal to a tourniquet may have an adverse effect on survival.

There are occasions when even an experienced pathologist may be unable to make a firm diagnosis despite receiving comparatively large amounts of material obtained by open biopsy. Difficulties arise because of the variegated histological patterns demonstrated by many tumours and the wide variations in malignancy between both the tumours of different histological origins and even within the same tumour. For this reason there is now in Great Britain a 'Bone Tumour Panel' of oesteoarticular pathologists who are able to express a collective opinion in difficult cases. Their task is made easier if fresh material obtained by open biopsy is sent immediately to an osteoarticular pathologist who then has an option of using special staining techniques and electron microscopy which would be lost had the biopsy material been immediately fixed in formaldehyde. Diagnosis is therefore more certain in a centre with an osteoarticular pathologist included as part of the musculoskeletal tumour management team.

Treatment

Surgical principles

The principal aim of surgery in the treatment of musculoskeletal tumours is to completely remove the primary lesion. It is important to understand that despite the advances in adjuvant therapy in the treatment of high-grade sarcomas, if complete surgical excision of the primary lesion is not achieved, then long-term survival of the patient is unlikely. A secondary surgical goal is to preserve, as far as possible, the function of an extremity by the use of reconstructive procedures if necessary.

The type of surgical procedure required to achieve the complete removal of the primary lesion depends upon the stage of the lesion determined by the preoperative investigations. Enneking (1986) has graded the types of surgical procedures available on a scale of 1 to 4 in correlation with his staging system for musculoskeletal tumours (Figure 13.2). For most benign and locally aggressive lesions the lower-grade surgical procedures (1 or 2) are usually appropriate, whereas for malignant tumours only the higher grades of surgical procedure (3 or 4) are adequate.

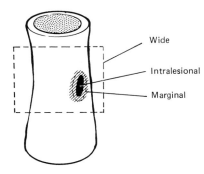

Wide

Intralesional

Marginal

Figure 13.2 Grading of the surgical procedure used to excise a tumour: Intralesional excision = Grade 1; Marginal excision = Grade 2; Wide excision = Grade 3; Radical excision (not shown) = Grade 4

A Grade 1 surgical procedure includes any procedure in which the tumour mass is entered at the time of operation. This would therefore include incisional biopsy.

In the soft tissues, other than for benign latent lesions, a Grade 1 procedure is *never* adequate as microscopic remnants of tumour are always left behind and recurrence is therefore inevitable.

Curettage of a bone lesion is also a Grade 1 procedure. However, by combining curettage and lavage with physical agents toxic to tumour cells, its use is justified in benign and locally aggressive bone lesions. Curettage is particularly indicated in the treatment of tumours situated close to a joint as it allows removal of these whilst preserving the function of the joint. Because of the risk of local recurrence following treatment of a bone lesion by curettage, a careful follow-up of the patient is required. A more radical procedure should be considered if a recurrence does occur, as locally aggressive tumours treated by repeated curettage have been known to become more aggressive and finally frankly malignant.

The risk of recurrence of a benign or locally aggressive bone tumour following curettage is reduced if the operation is performed correctly. There is still, however, a tendency for inadequate curettage to be performed by the introduction of instruments through a small window made in the cortical bone overlying a tumour (Figure 13.3a). Probably the most important factor in performing a successful curettage is the adequate exposure of the tumour. This is achieved by removing a large window of cortical bone in order to exteriorize the tumour cavity which can then be inspected in its entirety (Figure 13.3b). Thorough excision of the tumour tissue should then be possible by using a sharp curette, and the margins of this excision further extended with a dental burr. 'Chemical cautery' of the defect is often employed as phenol has the potential to permeate into the surrounding cortical bone and destroy the microscopic extensions of tumour present in this region. Following this, the cavity in the bone may then be filled with suitable bone graft. The use of methylmethacrylate cement instead of bone graft has been

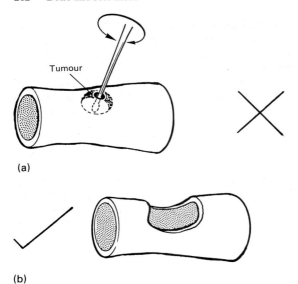

Tumour

(a)

(b)

Figure 13.3 Curettage: (a) attempted curettage through a small window in bone cortex always leaves residual tumour in areas which are inaccessible to the curette; (b) in order for the complete removal of all macroscopic tumour to be achieved by curettage a window in cortical bone must be made which is large enough to allow direct access to the whole cavity occupied by the tumour

advocated by some who consider that the local heat generated whilst the methylmethacrylate cures may help to kill any microscopic remnants of tumour present within the surrounding bone.

A Grade 2 surgical procedure describes an operation in which a tumour is removed intact by dissection through the reactive zone, therefore achieving a 'marginal' excision. For benign lesions which can be readily enucleated through the periphery of their narrow reactive zone, such as a simple lipoma, marginal excision is curative and therefore entirely appropriate.

For aggressive and malignant lesions, in which satellite nodules of tumour are found in the reactive zone, dissection through this region is to be avoided. The marginal excision of malignant tumours, even though the tumour itself may be contained entirely within its pseudocapsule, is inadequate as this procedure leaves microscopic deposits of tumour behind within the tissues and therefore local recurrence is inevitable.

A Grade 3 surgical procedure implies the removal of a tumour and its reactive zone together with a surrounding envelope of normal tissue. The surgical margins obtained by this type of procedure are described as 'wide' and may be achieved by performing either a wide local (*en bloc*) excision or by amputating a limb through the bone proximal to the level of the tumour.

A Grade 4 surgical procedure describes a 'radical resection' or amputation. For a resection to be regarded as radical the excised tissue must include the whole of the bone or muscle compartment in which the tumour originated, together with the whole of the tissues of any other compartment into which the tumour has extended locally. Involved muscle groups must therefore be excised from their origins to insertions together with any neurovascular structures contained within these compartments in order to achieve a 'radical' margin. A radical amputation must also fulfil these criteria. In the case of a lesion involving the bone and soft tissues of the distal thigh this would therefore require amputation by hip disarticulation. For a sarcoma involving the proximal femur a hindquarter amputation is usually required in order to achieve a radical margin.

It should be noted that the term 'radical' surgery used in the context of musculoskeletal tumours is not synonymous with amputation. If a limb is amputated at the level of a tumour then this would correspond to a Grade 1 surgical procedure, and similarly, if the level of amputation transgressed the reactive zone then only a Grade 2 surgical procedure would have been performed. The outcome of these amputations would, of course, be the same as if the surgical margins had been achieved by local excision.

A through-bone amputation performed at a level proximal to a tumour and its reactive zone, for example an amputation through the proximal femur for the treatment of a tumour involving the distal femur, is a Grade 3 surgical procedure and equivalent to a wide local (*en bloc*) excision both in terms of the surgical margins obtained and therefore the ultimate prognosis.

Surgical procedures
Benign and locally aggressive tumours
For the treatment of benign and locally aggressive lesions a Grade 1 or Grade 2 surgical procedure is usually appropriate. More extensive surgery is reserved for treatment of the local recurrences of these lesions should they occur. Occasionally, for those locally aggressive lesions which present with a significant extra-compartmental extension initially, wide local excision, a Grade 3 surgical procedure, is more appropriate primary treatment.

Malignant soft-tissue tumours
In a review of the results of surgery for the treatment of soft-tissue sarcomas of the extremities Simon and Enneking (1976) found that an 'adequate' surgical procedure resulted in a local recurrence rate of 2%, whereas 'inadequate' primary surgery resulted in a local recurrence rate of 100%. These authors pointed out that the behaviour of soft-tissue sarcomas is similar irrespective of their tissue of origin and considered therefore that the treatment of these tumours should follow the same principles. They felt that because some tumours, for example low-grade fibrosarcoma and Grade 1 liposarcoma, were known to metastasize rarely, there was a tendency for their surgical treatment to be less than adequate with resulting high rates of local recurrence.

Although pseudo-encapsulation by surrounding connective tissue is a constant characteristic of soft-tissue sarcomas, the temptation to remove these surgically by 'shelling them out' (a Grade 2 procedure) must be resisted as this of course leaves satellite nodules within the remains of the reactive zone. Local recurrence following such a procedure would be inevitable. Furthermore the local spread of soft-tissue sarcomas is relatively rapid by longitudinal extension both proximally and distally within their compartment of origin. However, these tumours rarely transgress intermuscular septa or spread from one type of tissue to another to extend transversely across a limb. This local behaviour, which is common to all soft-tissue sarcomas, explains the observations of Simon and Enneking (1976) who found that the rate of local recurrence was very low following radical resection of these tumours, but inevitable after more conservative procedures.

It is therefore recommended that any surgical procedure employed for the treatment of a soft-tissue sarcoma in a limb should include excision of all involved muscles from their origin to insertions (or from joint to joint), together with any bone or neurovascular structures within the tissue mass being resected. This is therefore a Grade 4 surgical procedure and may be achieved by either radical local resection or amputation depending upon the structures to be excised.

Malignant bone tumours

There is controversy about the most appropriate surgical treatment of malignant (Stage I and II) primary tumours involving the limb bones. Two general views are expressed. There are those who advocate that only a radical type of surgical procedure should be employed in the treatment of a malignant bone tumour irrespective of its stage. It is noted, however, that some who subscribe to this view refer to operations such as through-bone amputation, a Grade 3 procedure, as 'radical' surgery. The other point of view shared by an increasing number of surgeons is that if it is possible to remove a malignant tumour completely by wide local excision, and then make good the defect by performing a reconstructive procedure, then this may be preferable in selected cases to performing a primary amputation. These surgeons adopt a differential approach to Stage I and Stage II tumours and would consider local resection for Stage II lesions after preoperative adjuvant therapy.

The commonest malignant musculoskeletal tumours of connective-tissue origin are the osteosarcoma and chondrosarcoma. A brief consideration of the characteristics and behaviour of these tumours is helpful in evaluating the surgical techniques used in their treatment to be described below.

Osteosarcoma

This is by far the commonest primary bone tumour of connective-tissue origin. Characteristically, osteosarcoma attacks children and young adults; 80% of patients present before they are 30 years old. Osteosarcoma exhibits a predilection for the metaphyses of the long bones, particularly those around the knee.

It was mentioned earlier that histological examination of an osteosarcoma reveals a heterogeneous picture. Varying amounts of tumour bone formation can usually be seen but the presence of malignant cartilage matrix, fibroblastic differentiation and giant-cell formation may complicate diagnosis (Malcolm, 1987). Diagnosis depends entirely upon finding histological evidence of bone formation by tumour cells and this may only be evident in a small portion of a large tumour.

Osteosarcoma also occurs in the elderly although usually in areas of bone which have been subjected to radiotherapy in the past or in areas of Paget's disease. The prognosis in the elderly is worse than that for osteosarcoma occurring spontaneously in the younger age groups.

Osteosarcomas have been subdivided histologically depending upon the predominance of neoplastic bone, cartilage or fibrous tissue but this has little prognostic significance. However, there is a significant difference in the behaviour and therefore prognosis between the classical high-grade 'central' osteosarcoma which originates within the medullary cavity of a bone and the small percentage of osteosarcomas which occur on the surface of a bone. Two types of the latter tumour are recognized: the parosteal or juxtacortical and the periosteal. These tumours are associated with a much better prognosis than the high-grade central osteosarcomas and behave initially more like locally aggressive tumours. Metastases to the lung occur late and complete excision of the primary tumour is associated with a 5-year survival of 95%.

It is well recognized that osteosarcomas in common with other sarcomas metastasize by the venous route to the lungs. Later in the disease the tumour disseminates from the lungs to multiple sites and to other parts of the skeleton. Secondary bone metastases have been found at post-mortem in 15% of patients who died from disseminated osteosarcoma (Enneking and Kagan, 1975).

It is, however, the controversy surrounding the occurrence of 'skip' lesions from a primary osteosarcoma which has perhaps contributed most to the differences of opinion about surgical management. A skip lesion refers to a deposit of osteosarcoma within a bone at some distance from the primary tumour and separated by apparently normal non-involved bone tissue. Enneking and Kagan (1975) following a prospective study reported the presence of skip lesions in 10 patients from a group of 40 with histologically confirmed osteosarcomas. They found that skip lesions occurred both distally and proximally to the primary tumour and more significantly that half of the lesions occurred in an adjacent bone, therefore demonstrating transarticular spread. However, most specialized pathologists conclude that the occurrence of skip lesions is rare (Malcolm, 1987) and therefore concern about the presence of an unsuspected skip lesion preoperatively should perhaps not contribute significantly to a decision about the most appropriate surgical procedure.

Lymphatic spread to the regional lymph nodes is not common but was estimated to occur in 11% of a group of patients with osteosarcoma treated by Caceres, Zaharia and Tantalean (1969). The possibility of regional lymph node metastases is therefore of more significance in planning definitive surgery.

Chondrosarcoma

The incidence of chondrosarcoma is approximately half that of osteosarcoma (Dahlin and Henderson, 1956), it occurs most frequently in an older age group with a peak incidence in the age range 35–55 years. Chondrosarcomas tend to occur in central sites with a predilection for the pelvis, ribs, scapulae and proximal long bones.

Dahlin and Henderson (1956) observed that chondrosarcomas characteristically grow slowly and bring about a fatal outcome by local enlargement although they may metastasize by the blood stream and through lymphatic channels. Chondrosarcomas, however, may exhibit all grades of malignancy ranging from low-grade slow-growing tumours, very unlikely to metastasize, to high-grade sarcomas which metastasize early (Malcolm, 1987).

Gitelis et al. (1981) reviewed the experience gained with chondrosarcoma at the Rizzoli Institute (Bologna, Italy) and demonstrated a close correlation between the grade of a tumour, estimated by its X-ray experience and histological characteristics, and its prognosis. Three grades of chondrosarcomas were recognized, the lower grades being associated with a better prognosis. Only 9% of Grade 1 lesions metastasized, whereas this occurred in 44% of Grade 3 lesions. This correlated with a 10-year survival rate of 87% in patients with a Grade 1 lesion and only 27% of those with Grade 3 lesions. In particular Gitelis et al. (1981) observed the importance of adequate surgery in preventing recurrences and improving the lengths of survival and disease-free intervals. They stressed that 'adequate' surgery required a chondrosarcoma to be removed with either a wide or a radical margin. Only 6% of adequately treated patients suffered a local recurrence compared with 69% of those treated by inadequate surgery. The earlier findings of Dahlin and Henderson (1956) who commented on the ease with which chondrosarcoma implants locally in surgical wounds, including the biopsy wound, were confirmed.

Gitelis *et al.* (1981) concluded that adequate surgery remains the only effective means for treating chondrosarcoma of bone and mentioned that a trend towards limb-saving procedures had evolved at the Rizzoli Institute in recent years.

Amputation
Until comparatively recently the surgical treatment for the vast majority of patients presenting with a sarcoma of high-grade malignancy in a limb bone involved amputation of the extremity. Dahlin and Coventry (1967) studied the cases of 408 patients with osteosarcoma treated at the Mayo Clinic between 1909 and 1964. The preferred method of treatment was amputation for surgically accessible lesions. Recurrences in the amputation stump, indicating inadequate surgical treatment, developed in only 10 patients but despite this the 5-year survival rate was found to be approximately only 20%.

In an attempt to avoid the tragedy of a patient undergoing an amputation only to die of metastatic disease within a short time, Cade (1955) developed a method of treatment of osteosarcoma by using preoperative radiotherapy to the primary lesion in order to contain the tumour locally for an interval prior to amputation. The patient was observed for a period of 6 months and if metastases did not occur in the lungs within this time only then was amputation of the involved limb performed. Later, Sweetnam, Knowelden and Seddon (1971) retrospectively studied all cases of osteosarcoma of the femur and tibia treated at the major centres in Great Britain between 1952 and 1959 and in whom a combination of radiotherapy and amputation was usually employed. They found that the survival rate for the patients under 20 years of age was 22%. Amputation has therefore been demonstrated to be effective treatment for the local disease in osteosarcoma but when used alone or in combination with radiotherapy it is not curative in the majority of cases.

There is still controversy about the level at which an amputation should be performed. Osteosarcoma most commonly occurs in the metaphysis of the distal femur. Opinion differs about whether amputation should be carried out through the femoral shaft proximal to a tumour (a Grade 3 surgical procedure) or should hip disarticulation be performed in order to obtain radical margins (a Grade 4 surgical procedure). This is an important question as function after an above-knee amputation is considerably better than that following hip disarticulation. Nevertheless, the principal aim of surgery is to ensure complete removal of the primary disease and this must not be compromised by performing an inadequate procedure.

As a result of their large retrospective study, Dahlin and Coventry (1967) concluded that there was no advantage in including a joint between the tumour and the site of amputation. They pointed out, however, that care must be taken to ensure that the level of bone section was above the most proximal extent of the tumour along the medullary cavity. Prior to more sophisticated imaging methods being available, Dahlin and Coventry recommended that the level of bone section should be at least 3 in proximal to the most proximal extent of tumour visible on an X-ray.

Recently, Simon *et al.* (1986) studied retrospectively the results of the treatment of osteosarcoma of the distal end of the femur in a number of major centres. They found no differences either in the lengths of the disease-free interval or survival rates between a group of patients treated by hip disarticulation and a group treated by above-knee amputation. Although local recurrence of tumour was not seen in the patients who had undergone hip disarticulation this occurred in approximately 10% of those who underwent above-knee amputation, but did not adversely effect the overall prognosis of this group. Furthermore, Caceres, Zaharia and Tantalean (1969) reported that despite a trend towards more extensive surgery in their own consecutive series of patients with osteosarcoma no improvement in survival had been noted. In their centre, modified hemipelvectomy had replaced even hip disarticulation for the treatment of bone and soft-tissue sarcomas of the thigh, and interscapulothoracic amputation had become the treatment of choice for tumours of the upper limbs without obvious improvement in results. They concluded that even these extensive procedures did not prove to be 'radical' in terms of the total surgical removal of the tumour in some cases, and they implicated the presence of regional lymph node metastases as a cause of failure of surgical treatment.

Simon *et al.* (1986) found no differences in overall results in three groups of patients treated for osteosarcoma of the distal femur by hip disarticulation, above-knee amputation, or wide local excision followed by a reconstructive procedure. The incidence of local recurrence in the latter two groups was similar and it was felt that this may be explained by the presence of occult skip metastases described by Enneking and Kagan (1975). All but one of these patients who developed a local recurrence died of their disease. Despite this the overall mortality rate in each of the three groups was the same. It was postulated therefore that the patients who developed local recurrence had a more aggressive pattern of the disease with a poorer prognosis and that they would not have been cured by a more extensive surgical procedure.

Amputation should therefore be regarded as one method of removing the primary tumour in patients who develop a bone sarcoma in an extremity. Used alone, or in conjuction with radiotherapy in patients with osteosarcoma, it is curative in 20–25% of cases. If a level of amputation is chosen which provides a wide surgical margin (a Grade 3 surgical procedure) the prognosis is equal to that obtained by radical amputation (a Grade 4 surgical procedure). Unless amputation by disarticulation is required to achieve a wide surgical margin it is therefore better to perform a more conservative through-bone amputation. This offers an equal prospect of cure and provides a superior functional result.

Wide excision and reconstruction
The limitations of even extensive surgery in the treatment of other malignancies, for example carcinoma of the breast, has been recognized for some years. A similar awareness of the limitations of surgery for bone sarcomas together with improved results due to adjuvant therapy has led to an increasing trend towards the use of procedures described as limb 'sparing' or limb 'salvage'. The evidence presented above indicates that this approach is entirely justified provided that the surgical principles described earlier are observed and that it is unequivocally understood that the main aim of surgery is to remove the tumour in its entirety. It is stressed therefore that the minimum surgical treatment for a malignant bone tumour is a Grade 3 surgical procedure.

Improved imaging techniques has led to the more accurate preoperative staging of bone tumours. The local extent of a tumour with particular reference to the degree of muscle involvement and proximity to major neurovascular structures can now be gauged preoperatively with confidence. If it appears that a tumour can be removed by wide excision and yet preserve sufficient muscle function and the neurovascular status of the distal part of the limb, then a limb-saving procedure may now be considered. This surgical approach would in most cases be expected to provide a superior cosmetic result and also maintain function better than an amputation.

Considerable experience in limb-saving techniques has been gained over the past 10–15 years in many centres. Some of the more commonly employed techniques are briefly considered here.

Rotationplasty

This technique originally developed more than fifty years ago to compensate for an abnormally short limb resulting from congenital defects of the femur has more recently been applied to osteosarcoma involving the distal femur (Kotz and Salzer, 1982). The operation is performed by excising a segment of the distal thigh and knee joint to include the tumour by dividing the bones through the proximal femur and proximal tibia and fibula. The excised segment of the thigh is removed leaving a defect between the stump of the proximal thigh and the remainder of the leg below the knee which are then connected only by the sciatic nerve and femoral vessels. The leg is then rotated through 180° and joined to the stump of the thigh by opposing the cut surfaces of the tibia and femur and fixing these, usually with a metal plate and screws. In this way the leg below the knee takes the place of the excised segment of thigh, and the ankle joint, rotated through 180°, serves as a knee joint. By fitting a hinged prosthesis into which the foot and ankle inserts, the functional result is similar to that of a below-knee amputation.

Kotz and Salzer (1982) described the results of this precedure performed on 4 children aged from 4 years to 11 years. Despite initial reservations by both the patients, their parents and some members of hospital staff because of the rather grotesque appearance of the lower extremity postoperatively this was ultimately well accepted and has been justified by the functional results. Furthermore the absence of 'phantom' pains resulting from an amputation neuroma has been an additional benefit. Since then rotationplasty has now virtually replaced above-knee amputation for osteosarcomas of the distal femur in children treated at the University Hospital of Vienna and is now used with increasing frequency in adults with this disease (Kotz, personal communication). Enthusiasm for this procedure is increasing in other European centres, and in Holland above-knee amputation for tumours of the distal femur is now comparatively rare (Taminiau, personal communication).

Resection arthrodesis

The majority of sarcomas involving the limb bones occur towards the end of the bone and therefore a wide local excision usually has to include the adjacent joint. Following resection of a bone tumour and the adjacent joint, the skeletal defect created may then be bridged with struts of autogenous bone graft in order to create an arthrodesis. Although movement at the joint is lost a stable arthrodesis will allow a limb to be used for strenuous activities and this technique helps to restore limb length after bone resection. Unlike a prosthesis an arthrodesis is not subject to wear or loosening with time and vigorous use.

An example of a resection arthrodesis is illustrated in Figure 13.4. The patient was a 21-year-old male who presented with a pathological fracture through the proximal shaft of his left humerus. Staging studies demonstrated the underlying tumour to be a Stage IIB sarcoma and although precise histological diagnosis was difficult in this case the tumour was considered most likely to be a variant of Ewing's sarcoma. There was a good response to chemotherapy demonstrated by radiological evidence of fracture healing and regression of the extraosseous tumour which was visible on the initial CT scan. Extracapsular resection of the shoulder joint and the proximal two-thirds of the humerus was then performed and skeletal continuity restored by using dual parallel fibular grafts secured to the scapula neck proximally and the remnant of the humeral shaft distally. The fibular grafts were reinforced by a strut of iliac crest placed between their proximal ends and the lateral border of the scapula. After the surgical procedure, the patient completed his course of chemotherapy and when last seen 18 months postoperatively was found to be disease free. He demonstrated normal function of his left hand, wrist and elbow and had regained a degree of scapulothoracic movement at the shoulder sufficient for domestic activities.

For tumours around the knee, resection arthrodesis may be similarly performed using dual fibular grafts together with an intramedullary rod. The equivalent procedure at the Mayo Clinic is performed with a stout titanium fibre rod the ends

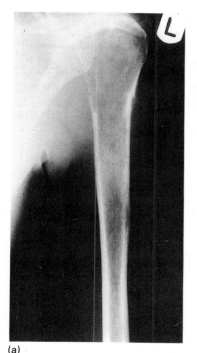
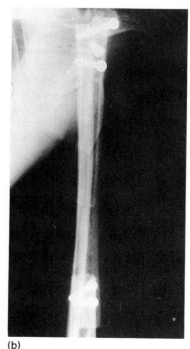

(a)   (b)

Figure 13.4 (a) X-ray of upper humeral shaft which is infiltrated with tumour. There is a fracture through the proximal third. (b) Postoperative X-ray following wide excision and resection arthrodesis. The proximal humerus has been reconstructed with dual fibular grafts reinforced proximally with a segment of iliac crest

of which are inserted into the medullary cavities of the femur and tibia respectively and the body of the rod is surrounded by strips of iliac crest bone graft (Sim, Bowman and Chao, 1983).

Allograft transplantation

There is general agreement that autogenous bone graft is the most satisfactory material for filling skeletal defects. However, the supply of autograft is of course limited and this together with the constraints of shape, lack of strength and the absence of an articular surface limits its use in the management of some types of defects encountered in bone tumour surgery. The advantages of allograft bone is that there is no practical limit to the size, shape, or quantity of bone which may be obtained. The need to sacrifice normal structures is circumvented and there is no donor site morbidity. Furthermore, large sections of allograft bone which include a joint surface may be used for joint reconstruction, and if allograft is removed with the associated ligaments and tendons intact these can be used to stabilize the graft within the recipient site.

Parrish (1973) reported encouraging long-term results following the replacement of all or part of the end of a long bone excised during tumour resection, with the equivalent bone obtained from cadaver donors. More recently Mankin, Doppelt and Tomford (1983) reported the first 10 years experienced with allograft transplantation in 150 patients at the Massachusetts General Hospital. This method of reconstruction is continuing to be developed in this centre. After experimental studies designed to investigate the fate of allograft bone in the recipient's tissues Mankin, Doppelt and Tomford concluded that the bone tissue should be dead and this should be achieved by freezing. It was also concluded that the cells of articular cartilage should be viable. These investigators developed a technique for storing composite allografts by removing these under aseptic conditions and slowly freezing them to $-80°C$ after immersing the articular cartilage in a 10% aqueous glycerol solution, in order to maintain the viability of the chondrocytes. Immediately prior to implantation in the recipient after excision of a bone tumour the allografts are rapidly thawed. By treating allograft material in this way Mankin, Doppelt and Tomford have demonstrated that bones may be stored for long periods prior to implantation. Following implantation new bone formation has been demonstrated to occur on the surface of the allograft cortex and biopsies have revealed viable although abnormal articular cartilage cells to be present.

After evaluating the results of their 10-year experience Mankin, Doppelt and Tomford concluded that allograft transplantation is a successful procedure primarily for the management of lesions of low-grade malignancy. In the absence of complications the functional results were in the main regarded as good or excellent. However, the rate of complications, in particular infection, allograft fracture, and non-union between the graft and the recipient's bone, remained relatively high. They concluded therefore that this procedure must still be regarded as experimental in that further investigation was required into the immune response associated with allograft bone transplantation.

Replacement arthroplasty

In parallel with the recent advances in implant design for the replacement of joints destroyed by degenerative disease, there has been a similar interest in replacing with prosthetic components the bone and joint excised during surgery for bone tumours. Some commercially available ranges of prostheses include 'tumour prostheses' which are made with particularly long stems to compensate for the length of the bone resection, and many implant manufacturers offer a service to provide 'custom-made' implants to replace the segment of a bone intended for resection. The disadvantages of 'custom-made' prostheses are that several weeks are usually required for their manufacture, and the surgeon is then committed to the level of bone section decided upon at the time the implant is requested. Furthermore, once a 'custom-made' prosthesis has been produced for a particular patient there is then perhaps some obligation on the surgeon to insert the prosthesis even though the tumour may have progressed locally during the time required for its manufacture which renders the procedure less safe.

The prosthesis illustrated in Figure 13.5 developed be professor R. Kotz (manufactured by Howmedica) is a 'modular' prosthesis which, by selecting the

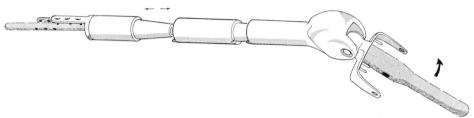

Figure 13.5 The Kotz 'modular' prosthesis. This combination of components is assembled for replacement of the distal femoral shaft and knee joint

appropriate lengths of the components from the range provided, will allow a prosthesis of the required length to be constructed by a surgeon at the time of the surgical procedure. The advantages of this prosthesis are that no delay in manufacture of a specific implant is encountered and the appropriate level of bone section can be decided upon at the time of surgery. This modular system may be used to replace the proximal tibia, proximal and distal femur (a total femoral prosthesis can be constructed) and a modular system for humeral replacement is currently being evaluated.

Figure 13.6a is a radiograph demonstrating a Grade 1 chondrosarcoma involving the proximal femur of a 21-year-old female. This was treated by wide excision and the insertion of a Kotz modular prosthesis (Figure 13.6b) in order to replace the hip joint and proximal femoral shaft. The appearance of the lower limb postoperatively was nearly normal and the range of movement at the prosthetic hip joint satisfactory for domestic activities. The procedure therefore avoided amputation which in this case would necessarily have involved hip disarticulation. Resection arthrodesis could have been attempted but even if successful would represent a significant disability and probably necessitated limb shortening.

An X-ray of the left knee of a 63-year-old female who presented with a 3-month history of pain is shown in Figure 13.7a. The X-ray appearances were unremarkable other than for some irregularity of the cortex of the lateral femoral condyle. Further staging studies were more informative. The CT scan (Figure 13.7b) revealed a tumour within the lateral femoral condyle extending into the adjacent soft tissues and the presence of a lesion was more obviously demonstrated by the isotope bone scan (Figure 13.7c). Biopsy confirmed the presence of a Grade

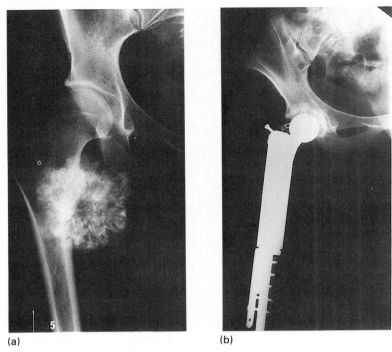

(a)   (b)

Figure 13.6 (a) A Grade I chondrosarcoma involving the proximal femur of a 21-year old female; (b) a wide local excision of the tumour was performed and reconstruction achieved by insertion of the Kotz modular prosthesis shown in this radiograph

2 chondrosarcoma. This was treated by wide excision and reconstruction using a Kotz modular prosthesis to replace the distal femur and the knee joint (Figure 13.7d).

The early functional results of prosthetic replacement following wide excision of a tumour in common with those used for degenerative joint disease are good. However, the complications of loosening and wear of the prosthetic components can be predicted to occur with time particularly in the younger, more active patients. Furthermore, the occurrence of deep infection associated with these prostheses is at present a significant problem particularly in patients receiving chemotherapy before and after their surgery. No long-term results are yet available for evaluation and careful follow-up of all the patients undergoing this type of procedure is required before the indications and value will be determined. However, even if mechanical failure occurs revision of the prosthesis remains a possibility and of course amputation followed by the fitting of an artificial limb is always available.

Chemotherapy and radiotherapy

The prospect of survival for patients with bone and soft-tissue sarcomas remained low (approximately 20–25% for osteosarcoma) until the early 1970s when an

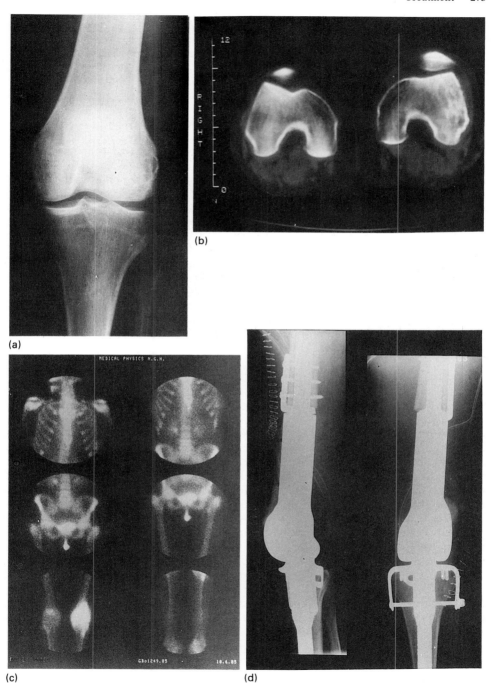

Figure 13.7 (a) A radiograph of the left knee of a 63-year old female who presented with a 3-month history of pain; there is some irregularity of the cortex of the lateral femoral condyle; (b) more obvious changes were visible on a subsequent CT scan; (c) clear evidence of an abnormality was demonstrated as a 'hot' area on an isotope bone scan; (d) biopsy of the lateral femoral condyle confirmed the presence of a Grade 2 chondrosarcoma which was treated by wide local excision and insertion of the Kotz modular prosthesis shown in this radiograph

improvement began to be seen. Now in the 1990s the 5-year survival rate for patients with soft-tissue sarcoma involving the limbs is 70–80% and for osteosarcomas, within the range of 50–60% (Eilber, Eckhardt and Morton, 1984). Some of the improvement can be explained by a better understanding of the pathology and staging of these tumours which in turn has led to an improved surgical approach. The remainder is due to advances in radiotherapy and chemotherapy.

Although radiotherapy or chemotherapy used alone is unlikely to cure a patient with a bone or soft-tissue sarcoma, there is evidence that these treatments used in conjunction with an adequate surgical procedure do improve the prospects of long-term survival.

Radiotherapy is of limited value in the treatment of primary bone tumours although it may be used for palliation in surgically inaccessible lesions. In the treatment of soft-tissue sarcomas, however, radiotherapy is more effective and is often used as an adjunct to surgery. After excision of a liposarcoma, especially a high-grade lesion, postoperative radiotherapy has been shown to significantly reduce the risk of local recurrence (Enneking, 1983). Similarly, in the treatment of fibrosarcomas and malignant fibrous histiocytomas, although radical margins should be achieved if possible during excision, postoperative radiotherapy is useful in supplementing less aggressive surgical procedures especially in the elderly.

The contribution of chemotherapy to the improved prospects of patients with sarcomas, particularly osteosarcoma, remains controversial (Craft, 1984). Sarcomas of bone and soft tissue are undoubtedly sensitive to some cytotoxic drugs, the most effective of which are Adriamycin, methotrexate and cisplatinum, although there is a wide variation in response between tumour types. Some rapidly proliferating sarcomas, for example Ewing's sarcoma, are very sensitive to cytotoxic drugs while most chondrosarcomas are almost totally resistant. Osteosarcomas and fibrosarcomas demonstrate a broad spectrum of responsiveness within these extremes.

Rosen et al. (1982) developed a chemotherapy regimen in which patients received preoperative treatment based on methotrexate. Following excision of the tumour, the patients then either continued on the same treatment or this was changed depending upon the degree of tumour necrosis seen on histological examination of the resected specimen. This treatment pattern is now commonly employed in many centres although the long-term survival of 80–90% achieved by Rosen et al. have not yet been observed by others. Performing the surgical procedure during the middle of the chemotherapy courses has the advantage of allowing the effectiveness of the regimen to be determined directly by histological examination of the resected tumour.

It is because of the variations in results obtained by different groups of investigators that some even question whether chemotherapy has a role in osteosarcoma. Because of an understandable reluctance to withhold potentially beneficial treatment in a lethal disease, no randomized controlled trials of cytotoxic drugs incorporating a 'no treatment arm' have been undertaken. However, many controversies surrounding the management of bone tumours could be settled if a standard method of patient selection and reporting, taking into account all the relevant prognostic factors, could be devised (Craft, 1984). It is in this way that a correct combination of treatments leading to continued improvement in results may be found.

Pulmonary metastases

Despite improved results in the treatment of bone and soft-tissue sarcomas, metastatic spread initially to the lungs still occurs in a distressingly high proportion of patients. At present pulmonary metastases appear in approximately 40% of patients treated for osteosarcoma and unless they are treated their progression leads to death in the majority of patients within eighteen months.

It has been known for the past fifty years that resection of a solitary pulmonary metastasis in patients who had previously undergone nephrectomy for adenocarcinoma of a kidney could result in cure. More recently, Martini, Huvos and Mike (1971) demonstrated that resection of multiple pulmonary metastases could be curative in patients with osteosarcoma, and this procedure is now practised routinely in many centres. Pairolero and Telander (1983) found that 40% of the patients treated surgically for pulmonary metastases at the Mayo Clinic were alive 5 years after thoracotomy. Survival was longest in those patients who had experienced a disease-free interval of greater than 1 year, although even in those patients in whom the disease-free interval was less then 1 year 25% were alive 3 years after their initial thoracotomy. Approximately half of these patients underwent multiple thoracotomies and it was noted that the procedures caused little morbidity and that rapid recovery was the rule. On the basis of this experience Pairolero and Telander concluded that thoracotomy and excision of pulmonary metastases, repeated several times if necessary, was an effective treatment for many patients with advanced disease.

The value of the CT scan in demonstrating the presence of deposits of metastatic sarcoma too small to be seen on the plain X-ray was mentioned earlier. This investigation forms an essential part of the preoperative staging studies. Regular postoperative CT examination of the lungs, initially at 3-monthly intervals, is recommended as the appearance of pulmonary metastases, although of serious prognostic significance, does not necessarily mean that the prospects for cure are hopeless.

Tumour of haematopoietic and reticuloendothelial tissue origin

Although these tumours numerically account for a large proportion of primary malignant bone tumours, surgery does not usually play a major part in their management and they are therefore considered only briefly here.

Plasmacytoma (myeloma)

This neoplasm, which is the single most common primary malignant tumour to involve the skeleton, is composed of abnormal plasma cells. It may occur as a single focus of tumour, at least initially ('solitary' plasmacytoma), but is more usually multicentric (multiple myeloma). It occurs rarely in patients under 40 years of age and because of associated haematological abnormalities these patients are likely to present primarily to a haematologist. The tumours occur in those regions of the skeleton containing haematopoietic marrow – the vertebrae, ribs, skull, pelvis and proximal limb bones. It appears characteristically on X-ray as 'punched out' areas of bone destruction, which appear to excite no surrounding new bone formation.

Of practical importance to the surgeon is the experience of Rubins, Qazi and

Woll (1980) who described the occurrence of massive bleeding after open biopsy of a plasmacytoma in 2 patients. Because of this they recommended that open biopsy should be reserved for those patients in whom the serum and urinary protein studies or bone-marrow aspirate failed to confirm the diagnosis.

Radiotherapy is the treatment of choice for localized disease. Patients with disseminated disease are better treated by chemotherapy combined with radiotherapy if necessary. Despite treatment 5-year survival is of the order of 10% and many patients die within 2 years of diagnosis (Dahlin and Unni, 1986). Death occurs from anaemia, renal failure as a result of tubular blockage by protein casts, or spinal cord involvement. The prognosis for those patients who present with solitary lesions is better, and although many have stressed that the solitary lesion is the forerunner of the disseminated disease Dahlin and Unni conclude that such dissemination may be long delayed and perhaps not inevitable.

Lymphoma

The skeleton is often involved by generalized lymphoma of soft-tissue origin. Occasionally patients present with a lymphoma in bone with no evidence of extraosseous involvement and a diagnosis of primary lymphoma of bone is made.

These tumours occur more commonly in the age groups 20–50 years and demonstrate a predilection for the long bones, in particular the femur. X-ray examination demonstrates extensive involvement of the affected bone or bones and occasionally the changes extend along the entire shaft. The areas of patchy bone destruction produce a mottled appearance and the outline of the bone tends to become blurred. On occasion the X-ray appearances closely resemble those of chronic osteomyelitis.

Lymphoma has the best prognosis of all the primary malignant tumours of bone; following chemotherapy and radiotherapy 60% 5-year survival has been observed (Malcolm, 1987).

Ewing's sarcoma

Ewing's sarcoma is a primary bone tumour composed of round cells which present a rather uniform histological appearance. Although the histogenesis is not known, Ewing's sarcoma is included in this section as the physical characteristics of the tumours and their X-ray appearances are more in keeping with neoplasms of marrow cell origin than of the more 'solid' tumours of connective-tissue origin.

Ewing's sarcoma is a highly malignant tumour which predominantly affects children and young adults. It can involve any bone but it demonstrates a predilection for the pelvis and proximal femur. In the long bones the tumour usually involves the diaphysis. X-ray examination reveals permeative cortical destruction characteristically surrounded by lines of periosteal new bone formation. Extraosseous soft-tissue extension occurs early.

Malcolm (1987) has pointed out the danger of incorrectly diagnosing Ewing's sarcoma as osteomyelitis. Each occurs predominantly in the same age groups, the X-ray appearances may be identical and the physical signs similar. Furthermore, the findings of pyrexia, a raised erythrocyte sedimentation rate and raised white blood cell count are common to both. Biopsy should confirm the diagnosis of Ewing's sarcoma, but it should be noted that the centre of the tumour is often extensively necrotic, and as the cells have no firm supporting stroma they are easily traumatized during biopsy. Careful sampling of the periphery of the soft-tissue extension is therefore recommended.

Until recently Ewing's sarcoma was usually treated by radiotherapy alone and the prognosis was poor with less than 20% of the patients surviving 5 years. A better prognosis was observed in patients with the more peripheral tumours treated surgically and surgery is now being used more commonly for the primary treatment of accessible lesions. With the development of effective chemotherapy regimens, the prognosis for patients with Ewing's sarcoma has improved significantly and by combining radiotherapy or surgery with chemotherapy 50% of patients with this disease now survive 5 years.

Secondary bone tumours

Although this chapter deals mainly with the primary tumours of bone the occurrence of secondary deposits is much commoner. Most skeletal secondary deposits originate from primary malignant tumours of the prostate, breast, kidney, thyroid, or lung and less commonly from the gastrointestinal tract. The commonest sites for the occurrence of bone metastases in descending order of frequency are the vertebrae, pelvis, ribs, femur and skull. Their appearance is usually heralded by pain which is constant and remorselessly increases in severity. As the metastases increase in size vertebral collapse and pathological fractures of the long bones may occur and give rise to increase in pain and disability.

Diagnosis is based initially on clinical suspicion aroused by the onset of skeletal pain in a patient who has previously been treated for a primary malignant tumour. Occasionally a pathological fracture may occur spontaneously through a bone metastasis from a previously unsuspected primary tumour. Diagnosis is usually confirmed by plain X-ray although it should be noted that up to 50% of the bone of a vertebral body may be destroyed before radiological changes become visible (Galasko, 1971). Most bone metastases appear on X-ray as irregular osteolytic lesions with little evidence of new bone formation. Typically, however, bone metastases from carcinoma of a prostate are osteoblastic and appear as areas of increased density on the plain X-ray. A radio-isotope bone scan is much more sensitive than X-ray examination in detecting the presence of bone metastases and will demonstrate in the majority of patients that multiple lesions are present.

Biopsy is essential before definitive treatment is planned and is better performed by a closed 'needle' technique. This technique allows biopsy of the less accessible lesions in the vertebrae and pelvis and when used for lesions in the long bones it is less likely than open biopsy to result in pathological fractures. Although treatment is necessarily palliative, a positive approach is required by all those involved in order to ensure that the remainder of a patient's life, which may span several years, is of the highest quality possible.

The main objectives of treatment are to relieve pain and maintain function. Radiotherapy has an important role and is usually effective, at least initially, in relieving bone pain. In hormone-sensitive tumours, either administration of hormonal agents or appropriate endocrine surgery may also be used.

Surgery is usually reserved for the treatment of pathological fractures or impending fracture of the limb bones. Pathological fractures of the proximal femur are most appropriately treated by excision of the diseased bone and replacement with a prosthetic hemiarthroplasty. Pathological fractures of the shafts of the long bones are better treated by internal fixation. The use of intramedullary rods inserted through the diseased lengths of bone and augmented by insertion of methylmethacrylate into bone defects has been found to be particularly useful. This provides immediate stable fixation and therefore facilitates rapid return to normal function. If internal fixation is performed by using a metal plate and screws the insertion of methylmethacrylate into the bone defect may also improve the strength of the fixation achieved.

The advantages of the team approach to the treatment of patients with primary bone tumours has been stressed throughout this chapter. The team approach is equally important in the management of patients with secondary bone tumours as it is only by combining the expertise of all the disciplines involved that the use of the most appropriate treatment for an individual patient will be ensured.

A hope for the future is that the trend for central referral of patients with tumours of the musculoskeletal system will continue. This will then allow the teams involved in their treatment to increase their experience more rapidly and improve their techniques. The use of internationally accepted classification and staging systems will then allow results of treatment at the various centres to be compared. In this way successful treatment can be expected to be identified more readily.

References

Baker, H. L. Jr, Berquist, T. H., Kispert, D. B. *et al.* (1985) Magnetic resonance imaging in a routine clinical setting. *Mayo Clinic Proceedings*, **60**, 75–90

Caceres, E., Zaharia, M. and Tantalean, E. (1969) Lymph node metastases in osteogenic sarcoma. *Surgery*, **65**, 421–422

Cade, S. (1955) Osteogenic sarcoma: A study based on 133 patients. *Journal of the Royal College of Surgeons Edinburgh*, **1**, 79–111

Craft, A. W. (1984) Controversies in the management of bone tumours. *Cancer Surveys*, **3**, 733–750

Dahlin, D. C. and Coventry, M. B. (1967) Osteogenic sarcoma. *Journal of Bone and Joint Surgery*, **48A**, 101–110

Dahlin, D. C. and Henderson, E. D. (1956) Chondrosarcoma, a surgical and pathological problem. *Journal of Bone and Joint Surgery*, **38A**, 1025–1038

Dahlin, D. C. and Unni, K. K. (1986) *Bone Tumours*, 4th edn, Charles C. Thomas, Springfield, Ill.

Eilber, F. R., Eckhardt, J. and Morton D. L. (1984) Advances in the treatment of sarcomas of the extremity. *Cancer*, **54**, 2695–2701

Enneking, W. F. (1983) *Musculoskeletal Tumor Surgery*, Churchill Livingstone, Edinburgh

Enneking, W. F. (1986) A system of staging musculoskeletal neoplasms. *Clinical Orthopaedics and Related Research*, **204**, 9–24

Enneking, W. F. and Kagan, A. (1975) 'Skip' metastases in osteosarcoma. *Cancer*, **36**, 2192–2205

Enzinger, F. M. and Weiss, S. W. (1983) *Soft Tissue Tumours*, Mosby, St Louis, pp. 6–7

Galasko, C. S. B. (1971) The resection of bone metastatic cancer. *Journal of Bone and Joint Surgery*, **53B**, 554

Gitelis, S., Bertoni, F., Picci, C. P. and Campanacci, M. (1981) Chondrosarcoma of bone. *Journal of Bone and Joint Surgery*, **63A**, 1248–1257

Hudson, T. M., Haas, G., Enneking, W. F. and Hawkins, I. F. (1975) Angiography in the management of musculoskeletal tumours. *Surgery*, **141**, 11–21

Illingworth, C. and Dick, M. B. (1968) *A Textbook of Surgical Pathology*, 10th edn, Churchill, London, p. 103

Kotz, R. and Salzer, M. (1982) Rotationplasty for childhood osteosarcoma of the distal part of the femur. *Journal of Bone and Joint Surgery*, **64A**, 959–969

Lichtenstein, L. (1951) Classification of primary tumours of bone. *Cancer*, **4**, 335–341

Malcolm, A. J. (1987) Pathology of bone tumours. In *Bone Tumour Management* (ed. R. R. H. Coombs and G. E. Friedlaender), Butterworths, London, pp. 3–21

Mankin, H. J., Doppelt, S. and Tomford, W. (1983) Clinical experience with allograft implantation. *Clinical Orthopaedics and Related Research*, **174**, 69–86

Martini, N., Huvos, A. G. and Mike, V. (1971) Multiple pulmonary resections in the treatment of osteogenic sarcoma. *Annals of Thoracic Surgery*, **12**, 271–278

Pairolero, P. C. and Telander, R. L. (1983) Role of thoracotomy in primary malignant bone tumours. In *Diagnosis and Treatment of Bone Tumours: A Team Approach* (ed. F. H. Sim), Slack, Inc., New Jersey, pp. 67–73

Parrish, F. F. (1973) Allograft replacement of all or part of the end of a long bone following excision of a tumour. *Journal of Bone and Joint Surgery*, **55A**, 1–22

Rosen, G., Caparros, B., Huvos, A. G. *et al.* (1982) Preoperative chemotherapy for osteogenic sarcoma. *Cancer*, **49**, 1221–1230

Rubins, J., Qazi, R. and Woll, J. E. (1980) Massive bleeding after biopsy of plasmacytoma. *Journal of Bone and Joint Surgery*, **62A**, 138–140

Rydholm, A. (1983) Management of patients with soft tissue tumours. *Acta Orthopaedica Scandinavia*, Suppl. 203, Vol. 54

Sim, F. H. (ed.) (1983) *Diagnosis and Treatment of Bone Tumours: A Team Approach*. Slack, Inc., New Jersey

Sim, F. H., Bowman, W. E. and Chao, E. Y. S. (1983) Limb salvage and reconstructive techniques. In *Diagnosis and Treatment of Bone Tumours: A Team Approach* (ed. F. H. Sim) Slack, Inc., New Jersey, pp. 77–104

Simon, M. A. (1982) Current concepts review. Biopsy of musculoskeletal tumours. *Journal of Bone and Joint Surgery*, **64A**, 1253–1257

Simon, M. A., Aschliman, M. A., Thomas, N. and Mankin, H. J. (1986) Limb-salvage treatment versus amputation for osteosarcoma of the distal end of the femur. *Journal of Bone and Joint Surgery*, **68A**, 1331–1337

Simon, M. A. and Enneking, W. F. (1976) The management of soft-tissue sarcomas of the extremities. *Journal of Bone and Joint Surgery*, **58A**, 317–327

Sweetnam, R., Knowelden, J. and Seddon, H. (1971) Bone sarcoma. Treatment by irradiation, amputation, or a combination of the two. *British Medical Journal*, **2**, 363–367

Chapter 14

Lymphoma

M. Soukop

Hodgkin's Disease (HD)

The condition was first described by Thomas Hodgkin in 1832, although he was uncertain as to its nature.

In the past twenty years, the prognosis has changed dramatically as a consequence of a greater understanding of the natural history of the disease, the development of effective chemotherapy and a rational approach to treatment.

Incidence and epidemiology

HD occurs worldwide but with widely varying frequency, ranging from 1 to 9.1/100 000 population. Hence, nowhere is it a truly common cancer. A degree of under- or misdiagnosis may occur in certain countries as the pathological diagnosis often requires an expert opinion. This, however, does not explain the worldwide variations (Correa and Connor, 1971).

In Scotland (1980 data), the incidence was 3.75/100 000 for males and 2.10/100 000 for females, and is steadily rising as per most developed countries. The figures also reveal the usual male:female ratio of 1.5:1, found in most countries. The age-related incidence in the UK follows a bimodal distribution, the early peak between 10 and 30 years, and the later peak after 55 years. A similar bimodal pattern is seen for most developed countries. In third world countries, although a bimodal pattern may still be seen, the early peak is larger and at a younger age.

Aetiology

The age distribution, increased risk to other family members (sibs up to six-fold) and cluster cases, e.g. colleges, army, etc., have all suggested an infectious aetiology (Grufferman *et al.*, 1977). The Epstein–Barr virus (EBV) seemed initially a promising candidate as subjects with a past history of glandular fever have an increased risk of HD. The search has been fruitless.

If EBV has any role in the development of the disease, it may be by altering immune responses. More recently, retroviruses have been considered, but all investigations have proved negative to date. Immunological mechanisms clearly are of importance in the development of HD as an increased incidence is found in patients with immunological disorders, either congenital, acquired or iatrogenic. The increased familial risk has also encouraged investigations of genetic factors.

However, little has emerged to date, apart from a minor increase in persons with HLA-A1 and HLA-A12 tissue type.

Pathology

The Reed–Sternberg (RS) cell and its variants, essential in making a diagnosis of HD, is now recognized from experimental work to be the malignant cell of the disease. The cell is characteristically large or with multi, often lobulated, nuclei. The origin of these cells from B or T lymphocytes, dendritic or interdigitating reticulum cells, or macrophages or myelomonocytic precursors, is still uncertain. Some studies have proposed different cells of origin for the different subtypes of HD. The experimental studies have often been hampered by the small number of RS cells present in most tumours.

HD is pathologically classified according to the Lukes and Butler system (Lukes and Butler, 1966). Since the original description, there have been a few additional details and facets. For details of current modified Lukes and Butler classification, see Table 14.1.

Table 14.1 Lukes–Butler classification of Hodgkin's disease

Group	Approximate incidence	Pathological features	Prognosis
Lymphocyte predominant	5–10%	Lymphocytes + + + Reed–Sternberg cells + Diffuse and nodular forms	Very good
Mixed cellularity	30–40%	Lymphocytes + + Reed–Sternberg cells + +	Good
Lymphocyte depleted	10%	Lymphocytes + Reed–Sternberg and often bizarre forms + + +	Poor
Nodular sclerosis	40%	Type I Type II	Very good Poor

The lymphocyte predominant group is not very common, occurring often in relatively younger patients. The salient pathological feature was the marked lymphocyte infiltration with relatively few and often difficult to find Reed–Sternberg cells. Recently, two subtypes of lymphocyte-predominant HD have been recognized, nodular and diffuse. The nodular group in its natural history more resembles the low-grade non-Hodgkin's lymphomas, with cases of late relapse after therapy (Regula, Hoppe and Weiss, 1988). Some cases of diffuse lymphocyte-predominant HD will, if untreated, change histologically with time to more aggressive cell types, mixed cellularity or lymphocyte depleted.

Mixed cellularity HD is more common, representing a half-way stage in the continuum between lymphocyte-predominant and lymphocyte-depleted groups. Reed–Sternberg cells are generally more common than those found in lymphocyte predominant. Patients may quite often have microscopic evidence of wider spread than staging tests suggest, especially in spleen. The prognosis is generally quite good.

Pathological specimens of patients with lymphocyte-depleted HD, as the name suggests, have a paucity of lymphocytes; also often present are numerous and bizarre formed Reed–Sternberg cells. Patients may often be relatively older and the disease outside the reticuloendothelial system. The incidence of B symptoms is also higher than for other groups of HD. The prognosis is poor compared to other HD groups.

Nodular sclerosis HD is quite common representing nearly 40% of all HD incidence. The salient pathological feature seen in this category is the fibrous bands running through and separating involved lymphoid nodules. This is the only group of HD in which the disease is more common in females. Another quite common feature is large mediastinal lymph gland masses at presentation.

A recent development has been the recognition that most patients with nodular sclerosing HD have prominent lymphocytic infiltration and relatively few Reed–Sternberg cells. Simplistically, this could be viewed as a lympho-cyte-predominant version of nodular sclerosing HD and is now termed Type I. It has generally a similar prognosis to that of lymphocyte-predominant HD. The second subtype, Type II, has similar features in terms of lymphocyte and Reed–Sternberg cells to lymphocyte-depleted HD and the prognosis is accordingly much poorer.

It is important to recognize that none of these groupings have rigid criteria and, therefore, a patient with histological features borderline between MC and LD may be classified MC or LD by different pathologists.

Hodgkin's disease and immunity

An unusual feature of HD is the early derangement of cell-mediated immunity. HD is associated with defective T cell function, supporting the view that it is a malignancy of the interdigitating dendritic cell (monocyte series) which present antigens to T cells. It has been recognized for some time that patients, even with early disease, have depressed delayed hypersensitivity reactions to a wide variety of antigens, perhaps resulting from this failure of antigen presentation. In contrast, at least by current testing methods, humoral immunity appears to be little affected. The altered cellular-mediated immunity of patients with HD results in an increased risk to certain infection, including tuberculosis, candida, aspergillus and herpes simplex and zoster. Disease progression as well as therapy will compromise the immune status further and hence a high index of suspicion for opportunistic infections should be maintained in the care of patients with HD.

Clinical presentation

Most commonly, patients present with a painless, enlarged lymph node in the neck (approximately 70% of cases) (Ultman and Moran, 1973), less commonly, an enlarged node in the axilla or inguinal region. It is important to realize that the size of the gland may fluctuate and is hence frequently regarded initially as due to infection. A biopsy is essential to make the diagnosis.

NB. Tissue should always be sent fresh for marker studies. In some cases, frozen sections should be sent before a definitive surgical procedure is carried out. I have known of cases where a radical neck dissection or a mastectomy was performed when only a biopsy was required. However, the biopsy must be adequate. It can be very difficult to make a full and accurate diagnosis of a lymphoma on a trucut or needle biopsy.

A small number of patients present with extranodal sites of disease, such as skin. This is much less common than in the non-Hodgkin's lymphomas. When symptoms occur, they are usually as follows:

1. Fever – especially in the evenings.
   Pel–Ebstein fever, although often mentioned, is rare and only applies to patients with a cyclical pattern of 3–4 days with fever, followed by 3–4 days without fever.
   A source of infection must also be excluded, especially as patients with HD are prone to infection due to altered immune responses.
2. Night sweats – A diagnosis of night sweats should only be made if this is clear cut. It often consists of severe drenching sweats requiring the patient to change the bed clothes.
3. Weight loss – Categorized to be significant if more than 10% of body weight lost in 3–6 months for no other apparent reason.

The three clinical features above are part of the staging of HD and are described as B symptoms when present. They have important prognostic significance as they frequently occur in the presence of extensive underlying disease.
   Other symptoms:

Non-specific
1. Tiredness and lethargy which can sometimes be associated with anaemia. When present, anaemia is also a poor prognostic sign representing possibly a paraneoplastic suppression of marrow function, marrow involvement, or resulting from an autoimmune process (see below).
2. Pruritus. At one time this was included as a B symptom but it is no longer felt to be sufficiently specific. The pathophysiology of the pruritus is uncertain, but has been felt to be related to histamine release. However, it is poorly responsive to antihistamines or other measures other than effective therapy for HD.
3. Skin lesions. Erythematous conditions, including erythroderma, erythema multiforme, erythema nodosum.

Specific
1. Alcohol-related pain. A rare relationship between the consumption of small amounts of alcohol with, within one hour, the development of severe pain, often at the site of underlying HD. The cause is unknown.
2. Autoimmune haemolytic anaemia. Antibody production as a result of the presence of HD, giving a Coombs' positive haemolytic anaemia. Successful therapy of HD is the therapy of the condition.
3. Compression of vital structures secondary to glandular enlargement, e.g. renal failure, superior vena caval obstruction, obstructive jaundice.
4. Infiltration of organs, e.g. pulmonary.
5. Paraneoplastic syndromes, e.g. leucoencephalopathy, subacute cerebellar degeneration.

Staging

The value of staging in HD is several-fold:

1. Identification of sites of disease, hence enabling appropriate therapy.
2. To ensure the disappearance of all sites of identifiable disease with therapy.

3. Correlation with prognosis.
4. To allow comparison of results between centres.

HD generally spreads from one lymph node area to the adjacent areas in a progressive fashion but will eventually spread beyond the reticuloendothelial system and any body tissue can be affected. Rare cases (less than 10%) originate in extranodal sites.

Standard staging techniques:

Method

History   Including B symptoms.

Examination:

1. : CXR   PA
            Lat.
            Penetrated AP view for assessment of mediastinal bulk
    (a) *CT Scan:* Relatively accurate and repeatable but only able to give evaluation of lymph node size, i.e. cannot ensure that a node is not affected if it is within the normal size range. Hence, sequential and follow-up scans often more useful.
    (b) *Lymphangiogram:* As good, if not better, than CT for assessment of inguinal/lower para-aortic chain. May give more data on nodal structure of normal-sized glands. Requires expert hands, otherwise high failure rate for the technique. Poor/impossible evaluation of high para-aortic or coeliac nodes or spleen. Although some dye may remain for weeks or months. Follow-up X-ray films to assess response often less than satisfactory.
    (c) *Ultrasound:* May be of value in combination with the above.
    (d) *Isotope Scanning:* Nodal assessment with gallium – of limited value and accuracy. Useful in some diagnostically difficult situations.
    (e) *Bone:* Imaging only if indicated clinically/biochemically.
2. *Haematology:*
    - Red cell – anaemia if present usually normochromic/normocytic. Occasionally autoimmune haemolytic.
    - White blood count – differential – neutrophilia, sometimes relative leucopenia – poor prognosis.
    - Eosinophilia occasionally – not prognostically significant.
    - Platelet – thrombocytopenia may indicate marrow involvement.
    - ESR – may be a marker of disease activity or extent.
    - Marrow – aspirate and trephine: As the structural relationship between cells is important in establishing a diagnosis of HD in the marrow, a trephine should always be carried out.
        In addition to an aspirate, some centres recommend samples from both iliac crests.
3. *Biochemistry:*
    - Urea and electrolytes.
    - Liver function tests.
    - Serum proteins.
    - LDH – may be a useful indicator of disease extent.
    - Calcium, phosphate.

4. *Laparotomy with splenectomy:*
A laparotomy to assist in staging the disease is now rarely carried out for the following reasons:
- Better understanding of the natural history of the disease.
- Use of CT scan to identify nodal involvement, i.e. coeliac axis and higher para-aortic sites.
- Better salvage therapy for those patients with relapsed HD.
- The delay in initiating therapy and the morbidity of the operation. The increased risk of infection, especially in children, resulting from the splenectomy which was part of the staging procedure.

When a staging laparotomy occurs, it should be performed by an expert to obtain maximal information, including multiple nodal sampling of specified sites (clips should not be used as they interfere with subsequent radiological assessment). Wedge biopsies of liver, splenectomy, possibly oophoropexy and bone biopsy (Rosenberg, 1985a).

The Ann Arbor staging classification was devised and based on prognostic features of clinical disease involvement (Table 14.2) (Carbone *et al.*, 1971).

Table 14.2 Ann Arbor staging classification for Hodgkin's disease

---

Staging classification

Stage I   Involvement of a single lymph node region or of a single extralymphatic site or organ (IE)

Stage II   Involvement of two or more node regions on the same side of the diaphragm, or of a localized extranodal involvement and one or more lymph node regions on the same side of the diaphragm (IIE)

Stage III   Involvement of lymph nodes on both sides of the diaphragm which may include the spleen (IIIS) or a localized extranodal site (IIIE) or both (IIIES)

Stage IV   Diffuse involvement of one or more extralymphatic organs

Additional points

(i)   Symptoms A or B

(ii)   Localized extranodal site implies that it might be treatable with radiotherapy

(iii)   Stage III can be further classified:

Stage III_1 – involvement of spleen, coeliac or portal nodes or any combination of these

Stage III_2 – involvement of para-aortic, iliac, mesenteric with or without upper abdominal disease

---

Clearly, those patients with more advanced involvement tend to have a poor prognosis, although overall prognosis is multifactorial (Haybittle *et al.*, 1985). If disease clearly originated in an extranodal site, i.e. skin, then it is staged as IE providing it is localized. If the disease has increasing lymph node involvement, then staging a patient as having perhaps IIE or IIIE or really Stage IV disease can often be difficult. The relationship of the extranodal disease to nodal sites can sometimes be a guide as can the extent of extranodal involvement.

Category A patients are asymptomatic, contrasting with significant weight loss, night sweats or unexplained pyrexia in Category B (see clinical presentation).

Therapy

The treatment modalities available consists of radiotherapy or chemotherapy.

Radiotherapy

In general, radiotherapy is used for local or early stage disease, although it may be used in selected cases in combination with chemotherapy. It is used in patients with truly local disease. In Stage IA, especially with good histology, local radiotherapy to the involved site will probably be adequate. The use of an extended field technique will depend on the precise individual patient details and is a specialist decision. The use of an upper mantle or inverted Y technique depending on the lymph node site is no more effective and more toxic than local field techniques.

Radiotherapy with an upper mantle (above diaphragm) inverted Y (below diaphragm) can be used for Stage II disease but would only be advisable in asymptomatic patients A or favourable histology. Many clinicians will treat patients with Stage IIA with chemotherapy from the outset, their decision being influenced by the bulk of disease present, the site of primary disease and their confidence in the staging findings.

The radiotherapy dose and schedule will vary with patient and centre (Tubiana *et al.*, 1981) but an adequate dose of minimum 4000 cGy will be required, usually given in 20 fractions over 4 weeks (upper mantle) (Kaplan, 1966). Attention to cord and lung sparing is essential.

Chemotherapy

Chemotherapy will usually be given as first-line therapy for patients with IB, some IIA, IIB, III and IV disease.

It is now some twenty years since the original report of MOPP therapy (mustine, vincristine, procarbazine and prednisolone) (Table 14.3) from De Vita's group at the National Cancer Institute (De Vita, Serpick and Carbone, 1970). This was the first demonstration that the majority of patients could be cured with cyclical combination chemotherapy (Longo *et al.*, 1986). Since that time, progress in therapy has concentrated on several themes:

1. Substitution of one drug for another in the MOPP regime, e.g.
   C-MOPP – cyclophosphamide for mustine
   MVPP – vinblastine for vincristine
   ClVPP – chlorambucil and vinblastine for mustine and vincristine.
   Conclusion: None of the substitutions have improved the response rate compared to MOPP, although this has not been done in a randomized study.
   Reduced toxicity has been reported by some groups C1VPP compared to MOPP.
2. Addition of agents to MOPP, e.g. MOPP-Bleo.
   Conclusion: No additional benefit.
3. Value of maintenance therapy.
   Conclusion: A number of studies have clearly shown no value in maintenance. Although it may occasionally delay relapse in patients who will do so, the disease may be more resistant to salvage therapy. Maintenance therapy gives rise to greater side-effects, both acute and delayed (see toxicity of therapy).
4. Identification of non-cross-resistant regimes to MOPP, e.g. ABVD (Table 14.3).
   In 1974, Bonadonna and Santoro described their results from Milan with ABVD, finding it to be equally effective and non-cross-resistant with MOPP, i.e. useful as a salvage therapy in MOPP-resistant patients.
5. Identification of new agents, e.g. VP16 (Etoposide).
   Originally found to have some activity in patients with resistant disease, now it has become part of first-line and/or salvage regimes.

Table 14.3 Examples of combination chemotherapy regimens in Hodgkin's disease

MOPP Regimen (28-day cycle)	
Mustine	6 mg/m² days 1 and 8 i.v.
Vincristine (Oncovin)	2 mg (max) or 1.4 mg/m² days 1 and 8 i.v.
Procarbazine	100 mg/m² days 1–14 orally
Prednisolone	40 mg/m² days 1–14 orally
ABVD Regimen (28-day cycle)	
Doxorubicin (Adriamycin)	25 mg/m² days 1 and 15 i.v.
Bleomycin	10 mg/m² days 1 and 15 i.v.
Vinblastine	10 mg/m² days 1 and 15 i.v.
DTIC	375 mg/m² days 1 and 15 i.v.
Hybrid MOPP/EVAP (28-day cycle)	
Mustine	6 mg/m² day 1 i.v.
Vincristine (Oncovin)	1.4 mg/m² (max. 2 mg) day 1 i.v.
Doxorubicin (Adriamycin)	25 mg/m² day 8 i.v.
Etoposide (VP16)	150 mg/m² days 8, 9 i.v.
Vincristine	6 mg/m² day 8 i.v.
Prednisolone	25 mg/m² days 1–14 orally
Procarbazine	100 mg/m² days 1–7 orally

6. Alternating and hybrid regimes.

   With the recognition of poor prognostic groups histologically, or with bulky disease, changes in first-line management strategy were made to use:

   (a) Alternating MOPP/ABVD (one cycle of MOPP followed by one cycle of ABVD) in an attempt to prevent the development of resistant disease (Goldie and Coldman, 1985; Bonadonna, Valagussa and Santoro, 1986)

   (b) Hybrid MOPP/EVAP (Table 14.3)

   Studies of these approaches are still in progress, compared to MOPP. Already some studies indicate that this may be a superior approach; however, therapy of patients relapsing following such multidrug combinations is difficult as multidrug resistance is often present.

7. Role of intensive approaches, e.g. bone marrow transplantation.

   This experimental approach is beginning to find a place in the management of some patients with relapsed HD (Jagannath et al., 1986). In general the patients are relatively young, the disease should be still somewhat responsive to conventional treatment, although the likelihood of cure from standard therapy be very poor.

   Therapy consists usually of intensive combination chemotherapy including drugs, if possible, that the patient may not have been exposed to previously. However, this is perhaps less important than the dose which aims to eradicate partially resistant disease. In general, the technique uses reinfusion of autologous marrow and hence marrow free from demonstrable disease is probably advisable.

   In poor prognosis patients, initial or remission marrow harvest is increasingly recommended so that it would be available in the future if required. The risk of not doing so at that stage may be to risk marrow involvement or chemotherapy/radiotherapy compromised marrow, with poor rescue potential.

Toxicity

Radiotherapy

Acute – Maximal usually towards or at the end of a course of therapy. Toxicity depends on the site, extent and dose therapy.

Delayed – e.g. pulmonary fibrosis, spinal cord damage, can largely be avoided by careful planning, but individual patients will rarely develop problems. Marrow damage from extensive primary radiotherapy, i.e. upper mantle and inverted Y, may compromise adequate chemotherapy if the patient relapses.

In combination with MOPP chemotherapy, an increased incidence of second malignancies is reported (Tucker *et al.*, 1988). The risk from an upper mantle or inverted Y alone is probably no greater than the background risk for a similar population.

Chemotherapy

Non specific – Side-effects such as nausea and vomiting are of major importance to the patient and correct attempts to provide adequate antiemetic cover are essential and will reduce the risk of reflex vomiting (Morrow, 1984).

Many drugs will cause alopecia, e.g. Adriamycin, cyclophosphamide.

The individual drugs can also cause specific side-effects, e.g. neuropathy with vincristine, cardiomegaly with Adriamycin.

A review of this subject is outside the scope of this article. The use of these complex regimes should only be undertaken by those expert in the field, otherwise cure will be compromised or toxicity excessive.

Prognosis

Cure is a retrospective diagnosis but is likely to be so for the vast majority of patients achieving and remaining in complete remission 5 years from the conclusion of their therapy. A 'cure' therefore would be expected in greater than 65% of all patients, with cure more likely in those with favourable histology and lesser extents of disease (up to 95%) and lower rates (50%) for those with unfavourable histology, more extensive disease (Table 14.4) (Rosenberg and Kaplan, 1985).

Table 14.4 Poor prognostic features in Hodgkin's disease

Histology	Lymphocyte depleted Nodular sclerosing type II
Stage	Extensive disease IV
Symptoms	B symptoms i.e. especially IIIB, IVB
Bulk disease	Disease measuring greater than 7 cm diameter, especially if at multiple sites
Age	Older patients
Additional prognostic factors	High lactate dehydrogenase Anaemia Neutropenia or thrombocytopenia at presentation

Non-Hodgkin's lymphomas (NHLs)

The NHLs are a diverse group of diseases affecting individuals of all ages. These conditions have aroused considerable interest as greater understanding of their biology has paralleled progress in our knowledge of the normal immune system. The diversity of lymphomas occurs as there is a representative tumour for each stage in the development of normal lymphocytes. During the past 20 years the 5-year survival rate overall for the NHLs has improved dramatically.

Incidence and aetiology

The NHLs occur three to four times more commonly than HD. The incidence for the USA and the UK being about 8/100 000 for men and 5–6/100 000 for women. The incidence rises steadily from childhood with age.

Some types of NHL occur much more frequently in certain geographical areas, e.g. Burkitt's lymphoma in Africa.

A number of conditions predispose to the development of lymphoma, e.g.:

- congenital conditions – ataxia, telangiectasia, Klinefelter's, coeliac disease and X-linked lymphoproliferative disease.
- acquired conditions – renal and cardiac transplantation, Sjögren's syndrome, rheumatoid arthritis, acquired immune deficiency syndrome (AIDS).

In animals there is convincing evidence of virally-induced lymphomas, e.g. Marek's disease in chickens caused by a herpes-type DNA virus, also lymphomas in cows by a C-type retrovirus. Additionally, lymphomas of viral origin also occur in rodents, birds and cats.

In man, a strong association exists between Epstein–Barr virus (EBV) and African Burkitt's lymphoma; however, a true causal relationship has yet to be established. Furthermore, this strong relationship is only rarely present for Burkitt's lymphoma outside Africa. The only established link between virus and human lymphoma is that of the retrovirus, human T cell leukaemia/lymphoma virus (HTLV-1) and a rare but aggressive T cell lymphoma found principally but not exclusively in Japan and the Caribbean (Broder *et al.*, 1984).

Radiation is also of aetiological importance in the potential development of NHL. Data for this follows the atomic bombing of Hiroshima and Nagasaki and irradiation of the spine of patients with ankylosing spondylitis.

Pathology

The wide variety of NHL and the profusion of different terminologies to describe them have led to considerable confusion. All classifications have been based on morphological appearances, although some with variations and refinements attempting to incorporate estimation of the immunological function of the cells from their appearance. No classification exists yet that integrates morphology with immunological function; although developing fast the immunological criteria are still far from perfect.

The value of a classification is based upon its ability to predict appropriate treatment strategies and prognosis. An early classification with merit was described by Rappaport (1966). This classification is purely morphological; it recognizes the prognostic importance of follicular (nodular) as opposed to diffuse infiltrative NHL and the relative 'maturity' or 'primitiveness' of the tumour cell of origin which is given by its appearance, including size.

An error in the nomenclature of the classification is the use of the term histiocyte for large primitive looking cells, now recognized as only rarely being true histiocytes, usually being centroblasts or lymphoblasts (B or T). The Kiel classification (Lennert, Stein and Kaiserling, 1975) attempted on morphological grounds to make immunological conclusions but clearly errors can occur, as lymphomas morphologically appearing to be of T cell origin may in fact be B cell on immunological testing or vice versa. Although clearly important in terms of accurate categorization, the real value of such additional immunological information with regard to natural history and prognosis will only become available in the future.

As numerous other classifications also existed in the late 1970s, the National Cancer Institute sponsored a collaborative international study to evaluate existing classifications using biopsy material and clinical data from 1175 cases of NHL. Out of this study developed the International Working Formulation (The Non-Hodgkin's Lymphoma Pathologic Classification Project, 1982) which allows cross-referencing with other classifications and hence a means of comparing data from different countries and studies (Table 14.5).

Broadly speaking, the Working Formulation from a simplistic and practical point of view separates lymphomas into low, intermediate and high grade. This is based more on natural history and survival characteristics rather than microscopic differentiation. Low-grade lymphomas represent the most indolent group with the best untreated survival, the high grade with the most aggressive course and the intermediate, as its name suggests, between these extremes. Even within the groups, however, natural history characteristics vary so that overall follicular mixed histologies (both small, centrocytic and large cell, centroblastic) are less indolent than follicular small cleaved (predominantly small cell or centrocytic) lymphoma. Additionally, patients may have disease which is 'in between' two categories, e.g. variations in interpretation amongst pathologists exist as to what percentage of small to large cells represents the transition from mixed to predominantly large cell disease (from 20 to 50% of large cell within the tumour).

On examination of sections of nodal material, it also becomes apparent that the number of centroblasts to centrocytes often varies with the high power field. Some attempts at standardization of the number of cells counted has been made, although the value of such an approach is uncertain.

Low-grade lymphoma
A. Small lymphocytic lymphoma has cells indistinguishable from those of chronic lymphocytic leukaemia. The difference between the two being clinical, the lymphoma having nodal disease often with marrow involvement, the leukaemia purely having marrow involvement and a peripheral blood lymphocyte count greater than 4000/mm^3. Small cell lymphocytic lymphoma often presents with widespread involvement with 70–80% of patients having Stage IV disease.

The lymphocytes are of B cell origin with appropriate surface immunoglobulins on testing; additionally some patients may have a monoclonal gammopathy.
B. Follicular, predominantly small cleaved cell. This is the common type of low-grade lymphoma. Cells are slightly larger than normal lymphocytes and are slightly irregular in shape, the nuclei are also irregular and indented.

Table 14.5 Classification of non-Hodgkin's lymphomas (malignant lymphomas, ML)

Working formulation	Kiel equivalent (Lennert)	Rappaport equivalent
Low-grade		
A ML, Small lymphocytic; consistent with CLL plasmacytoid	ML, Lymphocytic, CLL lymphoplasmacytic/oid	Diffuse, well differentiated lymphocytic
B ML, Follicular predominantly small cleaved cell; diffuse areas, sclerosis	ML, Centroblastic-centrocytic (small cell) follicular ± diffuse	Nodular, poorly differentiated lymphocytic
C ML, Follicular, mixed, small cleaved and large cell; diffuse areas, sclerosis		Nodular, mixed lymphocytic/ histiocytic
Intermediate-grade		
D ML, Follicular, predominantly large cell; diffuse areas, sclerosis	ML, Centroblastic-centrocytic (large cell), follicular or diffuse	Nodular, histiocytic
E ML, Diffuse, small cleaved cell; sclerosis	ML, Centrocytic (small cell)	Diffuse, poorly differentiated lymphocytic
F ML, Diffuse, mixed, small and large cell; sclerosis, epithelioid cell component	ML, Centroblastic-centrocytic (small cell) diffuse; lymphoplasmacytic/oid, polymorphous	Diffuse, mixed lymphocytic/ histiocytic
G ML, Diffuse, large cell; cleaved cell; non-cleaved cell, sclerosis	ML, Centroblastic-centrocytic (large cell) diffuse, centrocytic (large cell), centroblastic	Diffuse, histiocytic
High-grade		
H ML, Large cell; immunoblastic, plasmacytoid, clear cell, polymorphous, epithelioid cell component	ML, Immunoblastic	Diffuse, histiocytic
Polymorphous Epithelioid cell component	T-Zone lymphoma ML, lymphoepithelioid	
I ML, Lymphoblastic; convoluted cell, non-convuluted cell	ML, Lymphoblastic, convoluted cell type, unclassifiable	Diffuse, histiocytic
J ML, Small non-cleaved cell; Burkitt's lymphoma, follicular areas	ML, Lymphoblastic, Burkitt's type and other B-lymphoblastic lymphomas	Diffuse, undifferentiated
Miscellaneous		

Composite
    Mycosis fungoides
    Histiocytic extramedullary plasmacytoma
	Mycosis fungoides	

Unclassifiable Other	ML, Plasmacytic	

C. Follicular, mixed small cleaved and large cell. As the percentage of large cells within the population of lymphoma cells increases the condition becomes generally less indolent in behaviour. The term mixed is often used subjectively for tumours containing 30–50% large cells. As the disease becomes more aggressive, the follicular appearance may become progressively more effaced with a few areas of diffuse tumour cell infiltration.

Intermediate-grade lymphoma
D. Follicular, predominantly large cell. Although still basically follicular in appearance, the predominant tumour cell is large cell (centroblastic). The natural history is more aggressive and the necessity for treatment being more urgent. More than half the patients present with advanced disease and also extranodal sites of involvement such as skin, gut and the nodes of Waldeyer's ring are not uncommon. Once again, this lymphoma is of B cell origin.
E. Diffuse small cleaved cell. A lymphoma of small cell type (centrocytic) but there is effacement, destruction and infiltration of the normal nodal or follicular appearance, implying a more aggressive natural history.
F. Diffuse mixed small and large cell. A heterogeneous group morphologically. Cell surface and immunological marker studies confirm this heterogeneity with some lymphoma marking for B and others for T cell origin. Because of this heterogeneity and the relative rarity of the category, the exact natural history of the subsets of this group is uncertain.
G. Diffuse large cell. Both this and category (H) (see Table 14.5) would have been described in the Rappaport classification as diffuse 'histiocytic' lymphoma. Those patients with tumours of category (G) are of B cell origin and have a more favourable outcome. This group is, however, at the aggressive end of intermediate lymphomas and many clinicians would manage these patients similarly to those of high-grade type.

High-grade lymphoma
H. Large cell immunoblastic. This category includes a number of specific subtypes, such as the polymorphic which includes the $HTLV_1$, associated Japanese T cell lymphoma, peripheral T cell lymphoma, T zone lymphoma and immunoblastic T cell sarcoma. The epithelioid subtype is termed Lennert's lymphoma. Its polymorphism can make distinction from some cases of Hodgkin's disease a diagnostic pitfall.

In addition, the polymorphism with considerable size difference in cells can lead to some cases being classified as diffuse, mixed, small and large cell lymphoma.

The Japanese T cell variant has a very aggressive natural history; that of the peripheral T cell lymphoma is much more variable as also is the tumour cell size. Some cases may in fact have tumour cells resembling those of small cleaved type.
I. Lymphoblastic lymphoma. This is almost always a T cell tumour frequently presenting in young males with mediastinal node enlargement. Bone marrow and subsequent brain involvement are common. The cells are similar to those of lymphoblastic leukaemia and the intensity of the therapeutic approach is also similar.
J. Small non-cleaved. Lymphomas of this category comprise Burkitt's lymphoma and non-Burkitt's types. The cell size is intermediate between small cleaved

and large non-cleaved cells. These are extremely aggressive lymphomas with very rapid tumour doubling times. The tumours are of B cell origin and both types may be associated with characteristic cytogenetic translocations. These affect the immunoglobulin gene loci on the chromosomes 2, 14 and 22 and chromosome 8 at a site near to the c-myc cellular oncogene.

Other types
About 5% of lymphomas in most reported series are unclassifiable. There are, however, some additional types worth mentioning, including mycosis fungoides (MF) which is a cutaneous lymphoma of T-helper cell origin.

Immunological phenotyping and gene rearrangement

Recent techniques following the identification and production of monoclonal antibodies have improved the determination of the cell of origin of many lymphomas (Martin *et al.*, 1984); however, many pitfalls remain in identification.

Firstly, although tests have been devised to examine fixed material immunologically, the accuracy is uncertain as fixation interferes with the cell surface immunoglobulin. It is therefore preferable, wherever possible, to examine fresh frozen material. As many cells within a node are not in fact tumour cells, it is usual to find some cells marking with either T or B monoclonal markers. An experienced pathologist is required to help assess whether the morphological appearance of the immunologically marking cells and their position within the lymph node seems abnormal.

Clearly a tumour is 'more' monoclonal than one would expect for a reactive node. More recently, newer techniques for assessing monoclonality have been developed. Molecular genetic analysis can detect immunoglobulin gene rearrangements in lymphomas of B cell origin (Arnold *et al.*, 1983). Similar techniques for T cell gene rearrangement are also becoming available (Bertness *et al.*, 1985). Such methods will perhaps help to reduce the incidence of unclassifiable lymphomas and also aid the assessment of small sample biopsy material, needle aspirate and bone marrow involvement.

Clinical presentation

Like HD, the most common presentation is a painless lump in the neck. Interestingly, this node may fluctuate in size although it is generally progressive and this may lead to delay in diagnosis.

NHLs are more commonly widespread at presentation than HD, and unusual lymph node sites are more commonly involved or are primary sites of disease, e.g. Waldeyer's ring. Equally, skip areas of nodal involvement are more likely to occur, as also are primary or metastatic sites of extranodal disease. The classical B symptoms – fever, night sweats and weight loss are probably less frequent that in HD.

Staging techniques for detection of sites of involvement are similar to those for HD and equally the Ann Arbor classification is used, although it is less reliable and of more prognostic variability when applied to the NHLs. However, it is of value in helping to plan and assess response to therapy.

Therapy

The two main methods of therapy are radiotherapy and chemotherapy. Because of the variability in histological classification, it is perhaps best and simplest to consider therapy in the categories of low-, intermediate- and high-grade disease.

Low-grade disease

All the NHLs of this grouping are extremely sensitive to radiation. However, as most of the patients have widespread disease at presentation, a distinction must be drawn between control and cure (Rosenberg, 1985b). Clearly, however, if a patient appears, following all available staging tests, to have truly local disease, local radiotherapy may have a 70–80% chance of confirming 5-year disease free survival. Studies of Horning and Rosenberg (1984) have suggested that early chemotherapy for those patients with more advanced disease at presentation or with disease relapse following initial radiotherapy is not necessary or beneficial for those who do not have:

1. rapidly progressive clinical disease;
2. evidence of marrow failure due to tumour infiltration;
3. bulky nodal disease, especially if painful, unsightly or compressing vital strictures, e.g. ureters.
4. bulky or painful spleen or liver.

A subset of patients has been identified in whom the disease may fluctuate or even spontaneously regress. This policy of observation without therapy must be carefully supervised in order not to miss early warning signs or change in the pace of the disease including transformation of histological appearance from low to high-grade type. It is wise to recommend re-biopsy in patients with a sudden disease progression. Providing that an urgent or rapid response to therapy is not essential, therapy, when necessary, can be kept simple (oral) and largely non-toxic. Many patients would receive single alkylating agents often with prednisolone. Responses to such therapy, although likely to take some weeks, are generally quite high and may lead to good control but never cure. Even in patients apparently in complete remission, new immunological and molecular techniques can identify persisting tumour cells in the peripheral circulation and bone marrow. Subsequent relapses can be further treated with single or combination chemotherapy with a variety of drugs. Sometimes, unfortunately, previous exposure to alkylating agents leads to multidrug resistance. However, the use of earlier combination chemotherapy does not at present appear to improve long-term survival although it may increase response rates or duration of remissions and certainly does increase treatment-related toxicity. The median survival for patients with low-grade NHLs Stage III or Stage IV at presentation is about 5 years. Studies are under way examining aggressive combination chemotherapy with a conservative approach.

In younger patients with these low-grade NHLs, studies are under way to explore the use of biological response modifiers as initial therapy or as maintenance treatment to extend remission times. Trials are also in progress examining the use of autologous bone marrow transplantation with high-dose chemotherapy with or without irradiation and also the policy of more aggressive induction chemotherapy protocols.

Intermediate-grade lymphoma

This group comprises approximately 40–45% of cases. It includes follicular large cell, diffuse small cleaved cell, diffuse mixed (small and large cell) and diffuse large cell.

Many clinicians would, however, consider that only follicular mixed (small and large cell) (Longo *et al.*, 1984) classified by the Working Formulation as low grade and the first group in the intermediate category, follicular large cell, have anything like a 'semi-indolent' clinical behaviour. Hence, although some clinicans may treat patients with these two histological types rather less intensively than the high grade classification below, many others would use identical regimes.

The other groups in the intermediate grade should always, where clinically appropriate, be treated with regimes similar to those for high grade lymphomas.

Early, Stage I disease is rather more common in intermediate than the low-grade lymphomas. Following the staging procedures already described, patients with Stage I and some patients with Stage II, if contiguous nodes are present, can be treated by radiotherapy. This might be particularly so for elderly patients or those not fit for chemotherapy.

Other patients with Stage II disease, and all those with Stage III or IV intermediate-grade lymphoma, should be treated with combination chemotherapy. The initial alkylating-based regimes were replaced in the 1970s by the anthracycline-based CHOP regimen (cyclophosphamide, doxorubicin, vincristine and prednisolone) (Coltman *et al.*, 1986). This, in turn, has been replaced in many centres by more intensive combinations, e.g. M-BACOD, MACOP-B (Klimo and Connors, 1987) PROMACE-MOPP, COPBLAM. All these are anthracycline-containing regimes, some with the addition of etoposide and an alkylating agent. The regimens all use multidrugs to reduce the development of tumour resistance and use frequent therapy every week or ten days to prevent tumour regrowth between treatments.

The intensification of such therapies has led to improved results being reported from specialist centres, approximately 80% complete remission rates with 60–70% long-term survival. Bias in some of these results may arise by patient selection, i.e. entering patients on study who are often younger, and perhaps fitter and, therefore, more able to tolerate the intensive treatment.

Trials are at present underway comparing CHOP to these more intensive schedules.

Generally, patients achieving complete remission can be regarded as probably cured 3 years after therapy for diffuse large-cell lymphoma. This is much less certain for patients with follicular large-cell and diffuse small-cleaved lymphomas where, unfortunately, relapses may still occur 8–10 years after therapy.

Patients who relapsed after therapy traditionally did very badly. In younger patients with disease still relatively sensitive to chemotherapy, a policy of high-dose chemotherapy (with or without radiotherapy) and autologous bone marrow transplantation, has been adopted by many centres (Philip *et al.*, 1987; Takvorian *et al.*, 1987). This is particularly appropriate in those patients with marrow free from involvement; in those with marrow infiltration, techniques for purging the marrow before it is reinfused are being tried.

The intermediate lymphomas are frequently of B cell origin but may be of T cell origin. This latter group, especially if marrow involvement is present, has a propensity for metastasis to the central nervous system. Patients felt to be at particular risk may receive prophylactic cranial irradiation and intrathecal methotrexate (Mackintosh *et al.*, 1982).

Particular problems exist in the therapy of lymphomas in those patients in whom the disease is secondary to immunosuppressive drugs, e.g. post-transplant, or in those with AIDS or other immunosuppressive problems. In addition, therapy may be poorly tolerated in the elderly. It is well known that reduction in therapeutic dose intensity significantly reduces complete remission rates and hence survival.

High-grade lymphomas

The high-grade lymphomas include large-cell immunoblastic and lymphoblastic types and Burkitt's lymphomas. They represent about 15–20% of all NHLs.

The immunoblastic sub-type can be regarded as similar to, but more aggressive than, the diffuse large cell of intermediate grade.

Lymphoblastic lymphoma is usually of T cell origin, generally presents in young adults, especially men, and characteristically with a large mediastinal mass. As bone marrow involvement and central nervous system spread are common, intensive combination chemotherapy, similar to that for T cell, ALL with central nervous system prophylaxis, is necessary. About half the patients can be cured with such therapy (Coleman *et al.*, 1986). Burkitt's lymphoma was first recognized in Africa and is an extremely rapidly progressive B cell lymphoma of small non-cleaved type. The tumour is often exquisitively sensitive to chemotherapy which, because of the rate of progression of the disease, is given as a matter of urgency. Patients should be protected, however, by pretreatment with allopurinol as a tumour lysis syndrome may cause hyperuricaemia, hyperphosphataemia – leading to renal failure and death.

A problem of hyperkalaemia must also be monitored carefully. Central nervous system prophylaxis and therapy is essential. The disease is eminently curable providing the disease is diagnosed early and treated promptly.

A European or American form with similarities to Burkitt's is also recognized. Although relatively rare, its behaviour and management has similarities and differences with the above (Miliauskas *et al.*, 1982).

Other lymphomas

Primary gastrointestinal lymphomas   Primary gastrointestinal lymphomas, while comprising only a small percentage of all gastrointestinal tumours, need to be distinguished from the adenocarcinomas as they have different management and prognosis (Haber and Meyer, 1988). They represent 1–4% of the tumours of stomach, small bowel and colon; however, they are amongst the most common extranodal sites for non-Hodgkin's lymphomas.

These tumours occur most frequently in the stomach and small bowel and only rarely in the large bowel. The cell of origin is sometimes a true histiocyte, although dispute still exists, with some groups suggesting a T cell origin for the 'histiocytic' tumours. This 'histiocytic' lymphoma is often associated with underlying coeliac disease and may frequently have associated involvement of the Waldeyer's ring.

For the surgeon, such a patient may present as an acute emergency with a small bowel perforation. Awareness of the possibility of an underlying small bowel lymphoma will allow for a careful intra-abdominal assessment of disease and staging, which will be of considerable assistance in planning therapy and prognosis. At operation, fresh tissue for immunological markers should be obtained. Other lymphomas of the gastrointestinal tract are of B cell origin (50–60% of the total). These are usually of intermediate- or high-grade type and are treated accordingly.

Adult T cell leukaemia/lymphoma   This is a rare T cell lymphoma described a few years ago, especially in the Caribbean and Japan. It is of special interest as it is associated with human T cell lymphotrophic virus type I (HTLV1 – retrovirus). It has now been reported from centres in many countries but is always rare.

Cutaneous T cell lymphoma/mycosis fungoides   A lymphoma of helper T cell origin affecting skin at least in the early stages of disease, although later can be widely systematized. A feature in the later stages is the characteristic Sézary cell in the peripheral blood. Early control of the disease involves topical chemotherapy, photochemotherapy with psoralens and ultraviolet light (PUVA) and electron beam irradiation. When the disease is systematized, combination chemotherapy may be of palliative benefit; alpha-interferon has been reported to be sometimes of benefit.

References

Arnold, A., Cossman, J., Bakhshi, A. *et al.* (1983) Immunoglobulin gene rearrangements as unique clonal markers in human lymphoid neoplasms. *New England Journal of Medicine,* **309**, 1593–1599

Bertness, V., Kirsch, I., Hollis, G. *et al.* (1985) T-cell receptor gene rearrangements as clinical markers of human T-cell lymphomas. *New England Journal of Medicine,* **313**, 534–538

Bonadonna, G., Valagussa, P. and Santoro, A. (1986) Alternating non-cross-resistant combination chemotherapy or MOPP in stage IV Hodgkin's disease. *Annals of Internal Medicine,* **104**, 739–746

Broder, S., Bunn, P. A., Jaffe, E. S. *et al.* (1984) NIH Conference. T cell lymphoproliferative syndrome associated with human T-cell leukaemia/lymphoma virus. *Annals of Internal Medicine,* **100**, 543–557

Carbone, P. P., Kaplan, H. S., Musshoff, K. *et al.* (1971) Report of the Committee on Hodgkin's disease staging. *Cancer Research,* **31**, 1860–1861

Coleman, C. N., Picozzi, V. J., Cox, R. S. *et al.* Treatment of lymphoblastic lymphoma in adults. *Journal of Clinical Oncology,* **4**, 1628–1637

Coltman, C. A., Dahlberg, S., Jones, S. E. *et al.* (1986) CHOP is curative in thirty per cent of patients with large cell lymphoma: A twelve-year South-West Oncology Group follow-up. In *Advances in Chemotherapy* (ed. A. T. Skarin): Update on treatment for diffuse large cell lymphoma. Wiley, New York, pp. 71–77

Correa, P. and O'Connor, G. T. (1971) Epidemiologic patterns of Hodgkin's disease. *International Journal of Cancer,* **8**, 192–201

DeVita, V. T., Serpick A. and Carbone, P. P. (1970) Combination chemotherapy in the treatment of advanced Hodgkin's disease. *Annals of Internal Medicine,* **73**, 881–795

Goldie, J. H. and Coldman, A. J. (1985) Genetic instability in the development of resistance. *Seminars in Oncology,* **15**, 222–230

Grufferman, S. G., Cole, P., Smith, P. G. and Lukes, R. J. (1977) Hodgkin's disease in siblings. *New England Journal of Medicine,* **296**, 248

Haber, D. A. and Mayer, R. J. (1988) Primary gastrointestinal lymphoma. *Seminars in Oncology,* **15**, 154–169

Haybittle, J. L., Hayhoe, F. G., Easterling, M. J. *et al.* (1985) Review of British National Lymphoma Investigation studies of Hodgkin's disease and development of a prognostic index. *Lancet,* **i**, 967–972

Horning, S. J. and Rosenberg, S. A. (1984) The natural history of initially untreated low-grade non-Hodgkin's lymphomas. *New England Journal of Medicine,* **311**, 1471–1475

Jagannath, S., Dicke, K. A., Armitage, J. O. *et al.* (1981) High dose cyclophosphamide, carmustine and etoposide and autologous bone marrow transplantation for relapsed Hodgkin's disease. *Annals of Internal Medicine,* **104**, 163–168

Kaplan, H. S. (1966) Evidence for a tumoricidal dose level in the radiotherapy of Hodgkin's disease. *Cancer Research,* **26**, 1221–1224

Klimo, P. and Connors, J. M. (1987) Updated clinical experience with MACOP-B. *Seminars in Haematology,* **24** (Suppl. 1), 26–34

Lennert, K., Stein, H. and Kaiserling, E. (1975) Cytological and functional criteria for the classification of malignant lymphomata. *British Journal of Cancer,* **31** (Suppl. 2), 29–43

Longo, D. L., Young, R. C., Hubbard, S. M. *et al.* (1984) Prolonged initial remission in patients with nodular mixed lymphoma. *Annals of Internal Medicine,* **100**, 651–656

Longo, D. L., Young, R. C., Wesley, M. *et al.* (1986) Twenty years of MOPP therapy for Hodgkin's disease. *Journal of Clinical Oncology,* **4**, 1295–1306

Lukes, R. J. and Butler, J. J. (1966) The pathology and nomenclature of Hodgkin's disease. *Cancer Research,* **26**, 1063–1081

Mackintosh, F. R., Colby, T. V., Podolsky, W. J. *et al.* (1982) Central nervous system involvement in non-Hodgkin's lymphoma: An analysis of 105 cases. *Cancer,* **49**, 586–595

Martin, S. E., Zhang, H. Z., Magyarosy, E. *et al.* (1984) Immunologic methods in cytology: Definitive diagnosis of non-Hodgkin's lymphomas using immunologic markers for T- and B-cells. *American Journal of Clinical Pathology,* **82**, 666–673

Miliauskas, J. R., Berard, C. W., Young, R. C. *et al.* (1982) Undifferentiated non-Hodgkin's lymphomas (Burkitt's and non-Burkitt's types): The relevance of making this histologic distinction. *Cancer,* **50**, 2115–2121

Morrow, G. R. (1984) Clinical characteristics associated with the development of anticipatory nausea and vomiting in cancer patients undergoing chemotherapy treatment. *Journal of Clinical Oncology,* **2**, 1170–1176

Philip, T., Armitage, J. O., Spitzer, G. *et al.* (1987) High-dose therapy and autologous bone marrow transplantation after failure of conventional chemotherapy in adults with intermediate-grade or high-grade non-Hodgkin's lymphoma. *New England Journal of Medicine,* **316**, 1493–1498

Rappaport, H. (1966) Tumours of the haematopoietic system. In *Atlas of Tumour Pathology,* Section 3, Fascicle 8. Washington DC Armed Forces Institute of Pathology

Regula, D. P., Hoppe, R. T. and Weiss, L. M. (1988) Nodular and diffuse types of lymphocyte predominant Hodgkin's disease. *New England Journal of Medicine,* **318**, 214–215

Rosenberg, S. A. (1985a) Laparotomy and splenectomy in Hodgkin's disease: A reappraisal after twenty years. *Scandinavian Journal of Haematology,* **34**, 289–292

Rosenberg, S. A. (1985b) The low-grade non-Hodgkin's lymphomas: Challenges and opportunities. *Journal of Clinical Oncology,* **3**, 299–310

Rosenberg, S. A. and Kaplan, H. S. (1985) The evolution and summary results of the Stanford randomised clinical trials of the management of Hodgkin's disease. *International Journal of Radiation Oncology, Biology and Physics,* **ii**, 5–15

Takvorian, T., Canellos, G. P., Ritz, J. *et al.* (1987) Prolonged disease-free survival after autologous bone marrow transplantation in patients with non-Hodgkin's lymphoma with a poor prognosis. *New England Journal of Medicine,* **316**, 1499–1505

The Non-Hodgkin's lymphoma Pathologic Classification Project (1982) National Cancer Institute sponsored study of classifications on non-Hodgkin's lymphomas: Summary and description of a working formulation of clinical usage. *Cancer,* **49**, 2112–2135

Tubiana, M., Hayat, M., Henry-Amar, A. *et al.* (1981) Five year results EORTC randomised study of splenectomy and spleen irradiation in clinical trials I and II of Hodgkin's disease. *European Journal of Cancer and Clinical Oncology,* **17**, 355–363

Tucker, M. A., Coleman, C. N., Cox, R. S. *et al.* (1988) Risk of second cancers after treatment for Hodgkin's disease. *New England Journal of Medicine,* **318**, 76–81

Ultman, J. E. and Moran, E. M. (1973) Clinical course and complications in Hodgkin's disease. *Archives of Internal Medicine,* **131**, 311–353

Chapter 15

Principles of cancer chemotherapy

M. A. Cornbleet

Introduction

The idea that many cancers are systemic diseases requiring a systemic approach if therapy is to be effective is not a new one. As early as the 1860s, potassium arsenite was used in attempts to treat leukaemia, without noticeable success, and observations of the side-effects of mustard gas poisoning in the trenches during World War I also provoked some therapeutic experiments in those diseases characterized by myelo- and lymphoproliferation. Leukaemia is an obviously disseminated disease at presentation, but it has become increasingly clear that some apparently localized tumours may be incurable by purely local treatment if occult dissemination has occurred. The concept of 'micrometastatic' disease has been extremely important in the evolution of 'adjuvant' and 'neoadjuvant' systemic treatment.

During the early 1940s, the observations of Huggins and others of the hormone sensitivity of prostate and breast cancer encouraged the search for medical means of altering the behaviour of cancer, and the search was rewarded by the response of childhood lymphoblastic leukaemia to antifolates and the development of the alkylating agents during the 1950s. Initial expectations were only of slowing tumour growth, so the therapeutic strategy tended towards the use of single agents in sequence as resistance developed. Because of the toxicity in normal tissues, chronic continuous administration slowly gave way to higher dose intermittent use with time intervals to allow normal tissue recovery. It was assumed that to use more than one cytotoxic drug would be unacceptably toxic and it was some time before this assumption was challenged. Since the early studies in Hodgkin's disease and testicular teratoma, the use of two or more agents in combination has become the norm, so that the identification of active new agents has required the development of different strategies.

Although the early successes in the treatment of some clearly chemosensitive tumours encouraged the belief that chemotherapy could be curative, it has become very clear that the degree of chemosensitivity varies considerably, and that many of the common epithelial tumours are at present only amenable to palliation if treated in an advanced stage. In animal tumour models, early treatment may be curative when the same treatment in more advanced tumours can be no more than palliative. This observation has led to the development of initial chemotherapy prior to definitive local therapy and is sometimes referred to as 'neoadjuvant' therapy by analogy with the prophylactic treatment of micrometastatic disease after local treatment – adjuvant therapy. The former being actively investigated in some tumour types, for example bladder and breast cancers, and is widely employed in the treatment of osteosarcoma.

The decision to recommend chemotherapy must therefore be based on a careful appraisal of the potential benefits as well as the costs (in terms of toxicity and discomfort) and the particular circumstances and wishes of the patient. The therapeutic index is often very narrow, but patients may have many reasons for seeking some form of active treatment, and the clinician has a responsibility to remain fully informed as therapeutic options change over time so that the advantages and disadvantages of different approaches can be discussed and a properly informed decision reached.

Many large textbooks and learned journals are devoted to the drug treatment of cancer, and it would be inappropriate in a brief chapter to attempt to do more than outline some of the basic principles that govern the appropriate use of these agents, and to discuss some of the results which can be expected from the use of currently available drugs as well as the side-effects which have to be anticipated from their use.

Biological principles

If all malignant cells remained confined to the site (or originating organ) of the initial malignant transformation, the solution of the 'cancer problem' would be expected in the development of increasingly efficient forms of local therapy. In fact, it has been evident that the ability to cure cancer with local means alone is hindered by the presence of viable metastases outside the treatment field (whether it be surgical or radiotherapeutic). Thus, the role of chemotherapy (and other systemic approaches to treatment such as hormone therapy) is essentially that of the treatment of metastatic disease, either clinically manifest or occult (the so-called micrometastases). As it grows, a cancer with the capacity to invade and cross basement membranes will shed cells into lymphatic or vascular channels which have the potential to establish metastatic clones perhaps long before the primary tumour reaches a sufficient size to present as a clinical tumour. Early experiments by Skipper (Skipper et al., 1950; Skipper, Schabel and Wilcox, 1964; Skipper, 1978), using the mouse leukaemia L1210 as a model tumour system, established a number of principles which have continued to influence the way in which chemotherapy is used. Unfortunately, the L1210 leukaemia differs in several critical respects from any human cancer with the possible exception of Burkitt's lymphoma: it has a growth fraction (that proportion of cells in a tumour engaged in active proliferation) which approaches 100%, is a rapidly growing tumour with nearly 60% of cells engaged in DNA synthesis at any time, and its life cycle is consistent and predictable. It has become clear that human solid tumours have cell cycle times which are inconsistent and usually long, the growth fraction is small and many cells contributing to the tumour bulk are not clonogenic, i.e. are not themselves giving rise to new tumour cells or capable of growing as metastases. Despite these differences, Skipper was able to define some important guiding principles (Skipper, Schabel and Wilcox, 1964), for example that injection of a single clonogenic malignant cell is sufficient to lead to the death of the animal.

Because of the homogeneity of the L1210 tumour cell population, these early experiments allowed the number of cells remaining after chemotherapy to be calculated by observing the survival time after treatment. In this way, it was possible to establish that tumour cell kill followed first-order kinetics rather than the widely assumed zero-order kinetics. In the latter, a fixed dose of drug will result in the death of a fixed number of cells (regardless of total number of cells present), whereas the former implies that a fixed dose will kill a constant fraction of a population regardless of its size. Thus, with a first-order reaction, a dose of drug that reduces a population from 1000 cells to 10 will reduce a population of 100 cells to 1 if the populations have equivalent growth fractions and sensitivity. It follows that the smaller the population of cancer cells, the greater the chances of eradicating it. This is particularly so as other data suggests that the growth fraction decreases as tumour size increases (Mendelsohn, 1960; Simpson-Herren, Sanford and Holmquist, 1974).

The importance of tumour size in determining curability has been reinforced by the hypothesis advanced by Goldie and Coldman (1979). Drawing on the principles worked out in bacterial genetic studies by Luria and Delbruck in the early 1940s (that resistance to antibiotics emerged not as a result of surviving exposure but as a result of expansion of a resistant clone that arose as a result of spontaneous mutation) (Luria and Delbruck, 1943), Goldie and Coldman related the likelihood of resistance to cytotoxic drugs emerging to the number of tumour cells. With rates of spontaneous mutation in the range of 10^{-6} or higher they concluded that the probability of at least one resistant cell being present was very high by the time the population size reached 10^6 cells, well below the size of a clinically detectable tumour. Among other implications, this hypothesis has provided the theoretical basis for much current clinical research into the use of combination chemotherapy and, in particular, alternating 'non-cross-resistant' combinations of cytotoxic drugs. Also, since the number of resistant cells is related to the tumour burden it is apparent that the number of resistant cell lines is likely to be considerable when the patient presents with widespread metastases. The mathematical model predicts that resistance can develop over as few as 2 logs of growth, equivalent to only six doublings or about 2–4 weeks for a typical tumour. Thus, delays in starting treatment may assume considerable significance as far as potential for cure is concerned without influencing the evident initial response to chemotherapy. For human cancers which comprise a variety of normal and malignant cell populations, the apparent doubling time of the tumour may be misleading, since it depends on the rate of cell loss as well as tumour and normal cell divisions. When the rate of cell loss is high, the number of tumour cell doublings required to achieve a detectable tumour mass (10^9 cells or $1\,cm^3$) is considerably increased, and the opportunities for resistance-conferring mutations to occur are concomitantly increased.

Although tumour cells do not, by and large, differ from their normal counterparts in the time taken to divide, the growth fraction of tumours is generally higher. In normal tissues which are rapidly self-renewing, such as bone marrow or gastrointestinal mucosa, a proportion of the stem cell fraction remains in the resting phase of the cell cycle unless disturbed by chemotherapy. This differential effect has been quantified by Bruce and co-workers in normal murine bone marrow and murine lymphoma following exposure to different chemotherapeutic agents. The killing ability varied considerably depending on whether the drugs acted only during a specific phase of the cell cycle (cell-cycle phase specific), affected cells in the resting phase of the cycle as well (cell-cycle nonspecific) or were active regardless of whether cells were dividing, a distinction which forms the basis of one of the classifications of cytotoxic drugs (Table 15.1).

Other classifications of cytotoxic drugs have been proposed, the most commonly

Table 15.1 Classification of chemotherapeutic agents according to dose-survival curves for lymphoma and marrow colony-forming cells (modified from Bruce, Meeker and Valeriote, 1966)

Class	Type	Differential sensitivity between marrow and lymphoma	Examples
I	Non-selective, phase non-specific	None	Gamma radiation possibly nitrosoureas and nitrogen mustard
II	Specific to particular phase of the cell cycle	500-fold greater kill of lymphoma colony-forming cells	Vincristine, methotrexate, etoposide
III	Cell cycle specific, phase non-specific	10 000-fold greater cell kill of lymphoma colony-forming cells	Adriamycin, cyclophosphamide

used being based on the supposed mechanism of action. This classification divides drugs into four general categories: alkylating agents, antimetabolites, hormonal agents and plant alkaloids (Table 15.2).

Alkylating agents are reactive chemicals which bind covalently to many cellular constituents. Of the many thousands of compounds which have this property several chemically diverse agents are in frequent clinical use. They appear to share a common mechanism of action in which DNA appears to be the most significant but not exclusive target. DNA synthesis is inhibited fairly rapidly at concentrations

Table 15.2 Classification of cytotoxic drugs by mechanism of action

1. Alkylating agents
   (a) Classic alkylating agents
       (i)   Bis (chloroethyl) amines, e.g. chlorambucil, cyclophosphamide ifosfamide, mechlorethamine, melphalen
       (ii) Ethyleneimines, e.g. thio-TEPA
       (iii) Alkyl sulfonates, busulfan
   (b) Nitrosoureas, e.g. carmustine (BCNU), estramustine, lomustine (CCNU), semustine (Me-CCNU), streptozotocin, chlorozotocin
   (c) Antitumour antibiotics
       (i)   Anthracyclines, e.g. daunorubicin, doxorubicin (Adriamycin), rubidazone
       (ii) Other antitumour antibiotics, e.g. actinomycin D, mithramycin, mitomycin C, bleomycin
   (d) Miscellaneous alkylator-like agents, e.g. cisplatinum, dacarbazine, hexamethylmelamine

2. Antimetabolites
   (a) Folate antagonists, e.g. methotrexate, dichloromethotrexate, amethopterin
   (b) Purine antagonists, e.g. azathioprine, 6-mercaptopurine, thioguanine
   (c) Pyrimidine antagonists, e.g. 5-azacytidine, cytosine arabinoside, 5-fluorouracil

3. Hormonal agents
   (a) Oestrogens
   (b) Progestogens
   (c) Androgens
   (d) Corticosteroids
   (e) Antihormonal agents, e.g. tamoxifen

4. Plant alkaloids
   (a) Vinca alkaloids, e.g. vincristine, vinblastine, vindesine
   (b) Podophyllotoxins, e.g. etoposide (VP-16), teniposide (VM-26)

which have little or no effect on protein or RNA synthesis. Most alkylating agents form positively charged carbonium ions in aqueous solution, and this charged group attacks nucleophilic (electron-rich) sites on the nucleic acids, proteins and small molecules such as sulphydrils and amino-acids. The favoured sites of attack in the DNA molecule are the N^7 position of guanine (which accounts for about 90% of the alkylated sites), the 1 position of guanine, the 1,3 and 7 positions of adenine and the N^3 position of cytosine. The consequences of base alkylation include not only misreading of the DNA code but also cross-linking of DNA and single- and double-stranded breaks. In addition, synthesis of DNA, RNA and protein is inhibited. Alkylating agents with two active groups (bifunctional) leads to cross-linkage of DNA. Despite their common mechanism, alkylating agents differ widely in their pharmacokinetic, transport and solubility characteristics, and are not uniformly cross-resistant (Bergsagel, 1975).

The antimetabolites are compounds which interfere with the utilization of a natural metabolite by virtue of a chemically similar structure. Of the vast number of such compounds, the only antimetabolites in clinical use at present are analogues of folic acid or nucleic acid precursors, either purine or pyrimidine bases. The first antimetabolite used in clinical cancer chemotherapy was an analogue of folic acid, following observations that children with acute leukaemia had low plasma folate levels. Providing folate supplementation led to an abrupt worsening of their condition, and an analogue of folic acid (aminopterin) was synthesized and used for the first time to treat leukaemia in 1948.

Many products of natural, usually plant, origin have been screened for antitumour activity, and several classes of useful drugs have emerged. The mitotic inhibitors include the vinca alkaloids (vincristine, vinblastine and the synthetic agent vindesine) derived from the Periwinkle plant; they cause metaphase arrest, probably by damaging the spindle apparatus. The podophyllotoxins (VP-16 – etoposide and VM-26 – teniposide) which were derived from the American Mandrake or May Apple (*Podophyllum pelatum*) are also spindle poisons which cause metaphase arrest. Etoposide is the more widely used and has considerable activity against malignant lymphomas, small-cell lung cancer and testicular tumours. The antitumour antibiotics include bleomycin, Adriamycin, actinomycin D and mitomycin C. Bleomycin is the name of a group of antibiotics derived from *Streptomyces verticulis*, which inhibit incorporation of thymidine into DNA. The anthracycline antibiotics, Adriamycin and daunorubicin, are structurally similar derivatives of the fungus *Streptomyces peucetius* var. *caesius* which have a wide spectrum of clinical activity. Both inhibit nucleic acid synthesis and are believed to intercalate into the double helical structure of DNA by virtue of their planar anthraquinone nucleus attached to an amino sugar. Other possible mechanisms of action, for example, free radical generation causing superoxide generation have been invoked to explain both the clinical activity as well as the dose-limiting cardiotoxicity.

Hormonal therapy for cancer originated in 1895 when an oophorectomy was performed for breast cancer, but it was not until the 1950s that orchidectomy and oestrogens were shown to be effective in the management of advanced prostate cancer (Huggins and Bergenstal, 1952). The specificity of hormone action depends on the presence of specific receptors in the target tumour tissue. The translocation of the hormone/receptor complex to the nucleus leads to interaction with DNA and subsequent modulation of gene activity. Corticosteroids are of value in the treatment of breast cancer, prostate cancer, haematological malignancies (lymphoma, leukaemia and myeloma), as well as the supportive care of patients with anorexia, hypercalcaemia, raised intracranial pressure or adrenal failure.

Pharmacological principles

Almost all anticancer drugs in current use share two properties: they work by altering DNA synthesis or function and they do not kill resting cells unless such cells are destined to divide soon after exposure to the drug. We currently lack sufficient understanding of the fundamental differences between the normal and malignant cell to be able to design pharmacological agents capable of exploiting these differences selectively. It follows from these considerations that both the therapeutic and toxic consequences of exposure to cytotoxic drugs are related to the concentration of drug to which the cell is exposed and the duration of that exposure (concentration–time relationship). Since this relationship generally holds across species if metabolism and excretion follow similar pathways, doses of drugs administered to animals can be used to guide the initial doses administered to patients (Schabel and Simpson-Herren, 1978; Skipper, 1978). Cross-species comparisons for some agents are more appropriately made if the doses are expressed in mg/m^2, as surface area is closely related to cardiac output which in turn is related to renal and hepatic blood flow (the major organs of detoxification and excretion) (Brockman, 1975).

The considerable potential for causing side-effects when prescribing cytotoxic drugs has led to increasing attention being given to the dose and schedule of administration which optimizes the therapeutic index. While it is often tempting to reduce the dose to minimize toxicity, all the principles on which current treatment is premised argue against this for the 'conventional' agents (different considerations may apply to some of the 'biological response modifiers' such as the interferons). For almost all drugs in common use there is a steep dose–response relationship in experimental systems, though controversy remains about the benefits to be expected from pushing the doses of agents such as the alkylating agents and cisplatinum to the limit in clinical practice (Cornbleet, Leonard and Smyth, 1984). Some studies have shown that if doses which result in high complete remission rates are reduced by even 20%, a significant reduction in cure rate may occur (Schabel and Simpson-Herren, 1978). Similar observations have been made in clinical practice, for example in the treatment of malignant lymphoma and small-cell carcinoma of the lung. In this difficult area, the clinical situation must override such theoretical considerations on occasion, and the patient's condition and wishes are paramount. The amount of a drug and the time period over which it is administered have been combined in the concept of 'dose intensity' which is reported increasingly frequently, and a reduction in dose intensity has been invoked as a cause of treatment failure. Thus, in the adjuvant (postsurgical) treatment of early breast cancer, relapse-free survival has been reported to be significantly improved for those receiving more than 75% of the doses prescribed by the protocol (Bonadonna and Valagussa, 1981). However, a variety of factors contribute to the dose and frequency of chemotherapy which a patient is able to tolerate, and these may interact to confound interpretation of patterns of treatment failure. The utility of maintenance chemotherapy is called into question by the concept of 'dose intensity' as usually dose and frequency are both reduced over time. It may be significant that the only malignant disease in which maintenance chemotherapy is still routinely employed is childhood lymphoblastic leukaemia in which doses are constantly adjusted to the maximum tolerated.

During the early years of the systematic study of cancer chemotherapy it was appreciated that the available drugs were too toxic to be used more than one at a time. The early studies were therefore performed with single agents used continuously in low dose until either toxicity or disease progression required treatment to stop. At that point an alternative agent might have been considered. As understanding of the mechanism of action of some of these drugs began to increase, it became apparent that higher doses used intermittently might allow for improved normal tissue recovery and effectiveness. The most vulnerable tissue was the bone marrow, and it emerged empirically that an interval of 3 weeks between courses of treatment usually allowed the peripheral blood count to return to pretreatment levels. Although such regimens were modestly effective, it became apparent that this was also a method of selectively encouraging the emergence of drug-resistant clones of tumour cells.

The first attempts to combat this problem by using a number of cytotoxic drugs at the same time ('combination chemotherapy') were made in the treatment of malignant lymphomas and Hodgkin's disease, largely because there were a number of active agents already available (DeVita, Serpick and Carbone, 1970). The success of this approach has been such that it is now difficult to carry out studies to identify active new agents for some cancers because of the ethical difficulty of using such an agent in a patient who has not previously been treated with the best available combination (see below – Cancer Drug Development). The logic of combination chemotherapy received a powerful boost with the publication of the Goldie–Coldman hypothesis (see above), with its suggestion that extensive metastatic tumours (likely to contain a number of *de novo* resistant cell lines) might be more effectively treated with a variety of active drugs. Another implication of the hypothesis is that as many of the active agents as possible should be introduced at the outset of treatment in order to minimize the chances of a resistant clone emerging. This has provoked much clinical research into the use of alternating different combinations of agents which are believed to be non-cross-resistant. In practice this usually means combinations of agents with different mechanisms of action, since it is difficult to verify 'non-cross-resistance' unless previous studies have demonstrated activity of one combination of drugs in patients who have been identified as refractory to a second combination. Such studies are always difficult to interpret, because of the heterogeneity of the patient populations.

The general principles upon which most combination chemotherapy regimens are based can be summed up as follows:

1. Only drugs with known activity against the particular tumour type should be included in the combination, and the most active agents should be preferred.
2. Agents should be selected as far as possible to have non-overlapping second organ toxicities. Thus, two agents which are cardiotoxic are not ideally combined. (This rule is not absolute if sufficient is known about the metabolism and excretion of the agents. For example, both methotrexate and cisplatinum are potentially nephrotoxic, but they can be safely combined in the treatment of bladder cancer if care is taken to monitor methotrexate excretion and to ensure that folinic acid rescue is maintained for an adequate length of time.)
3. All the agents employed should be used in their optimal dose and schedule.

4. Combinations of drugs should be given at consistent intervals, and as frequently as normal tissue recovery will permit.
5. Drugs are included that enhance or act synergistically with (and do not antagonize) the activities of other agents in the combination, either by sequential scheduling or by pharmaocological mechanisms.

Exceptions to these guidelines that have proven successful can be cited from a variety of tumour types, but the general principles remain valid.

Complications of cancer chemotherapy

The two consequences of cytotoxic chemotherapy most frequently identified by patients in discussion prior to starting treatment are alopecia and vomiting. If asked about the effects of chemotherapy patients will frequently respond that 'it makes you very sick and makes your hair fall out'. While both these preconceptions are true to some extent, increasing sophistication in the use of anti-emetic drugs (and the development of new agents such as the 5-hydroxytryptamine antagonists) has allowed many patients to complete their chemotherapy with no (or only minimal) nausea and vomiting. Alopecia remains a significant problem with some, but by no means all drugs. Unfortunately, some of the most active agents, for example Adriamycin and etoposide, will inevitably cause hair loss which can usually be only partly mitigated by manoeuvres such as scalp cooling (Dean, Salmon and Griffith, 1979) or the application of a tourniquet (Soukop et al., 1978). Alopecia has a significance far beyond the merely cosmetic. It is a constant reminder to the patient (and their family and friends) of the nature of their illness and its implications. Patients can be reassured that regrowth of hair on completion of treatment is inevitable (at least in areas where time had not already taken its toll!).

Because we currently lack sufficient understanding of the fundamental differences between a malignant cell and its normal counterpart, cancer chemotherapy has developed largely empirically. All the currently used agents have some capacity to damage normal cells as well as cancer cells, and the decision to prescribe chemotherapy must always follow a careful appraisal of the risks and benefits, as well as demanding scrupulous attention to the details of safe and effective administration of these highly active drugs. Among the organs which may be damaged as a consequence of cytotoxic chemotherapy are the following:

Bone marrow Almost all presently used drugs have the capacity to produce significant anaemia, neutropenia and thrombocytopenia as a result of bone marrow suppression. Prior extensive radiotherapy may enhance the risk of serious myelosuppression which is cumulative with some agents (e.g. alkylating agents). The nadir of the blood count is usually between 10 and 14 days, although some drugs may cause a later fall in the blood count that requires a reduced frequency of administration, e.g. the nitrosoureas and mitomycin C. The blood count has normally recovered by 21 days and this is the interval most frequently chosen for repeat administration. A blood count must be performed prior to each treatment, and failure to have recovered to satisfactory, levels should lead to either a delay in treatment or a dose reduction, or both. Premature retreatment may provoke severe myelosuppression with the consequent risks of infection, haemorrhage, etc.

Gastrointestinal   Considerable research efforts have recently been directed at the mechanisms of chemotherapy-mediated nausea and vomiting, which may be due either to central nervous system effects or to effects on the gastrointestinal tract itself. Intensive anti-emetic therapy with agents such as metoclopramide (in high dose) and dexamethasone should minimize the frequency of vomiting (Allan *et al.*, 1984), though the distressing nausea may persist for several days after the most emetic of treatments, e.g. those that include cisplatinum. Some drugs, such as vincristine, also interfere with gastrointestinal motility via an effect on the autonomic nervous system, which may cause constipation and/or pain, and in severe cases may cause an ileus. Mucositis may be severe in neutropenic patients, and may also be a specific side-effect of drugs such as methotrexate or 5-fluorouracil.

Lungs   Although pulmonary toxicity is rare, busulfan, chlorambucil and bleomycin can cause diffuse pulmonary infiltration which may result in fibrosis. The risks are usually cumulative and dose-related, though with bleomycin the first indications may occur shortly after treatment is initiated.

Heart   The anthracycline antibiotics, Adriamycin and daunorubicin, can cause both acute and cumulative cardiotoxicity which may ultimately progress to a fatal congestive cardiomyopathy. The risks are not clinically significant below cumulative doses of $550\,mg/m^2$, although myocardial biopsies reveal evidence of damage at lower doses. Previous mediastinal irradiation, and possibly concurrent cyclophosphamide treatment, exacerbate the risks, and in such circumstances the total dose given should be restricted to $450\,mg/m^2$. Acute ECG changes related to anthracycline therapy are not associated with later development of cardiomyopathy. Newer analogues of Adriamycin, such as epirubicin or dihydroxy-anthracenedione (mitoxantrone), may prove to be significantly less damaging to the myocardium. In very high doses ($>7\,g/m^2$), cyclophosphamide has been reported to cause an acute haemorrhagic cardiomyopathy (Buckner *et al.*, 1972), but conventional doses have been associated with neither acute nor chronic cardiac damage.

Nervous system   Vincristine is the most frequently used cytotoxic neurotoxin. Loss of tendon reflexes may be followed by paraesthesiae, and an autonomic neuropathy may develop. Sensory changes usually precede a motor weakness which is symmetrical. These changes may be reversible on stopping treatment, but usually only very slowly. The syndrome of inappropriate antidiuretic hormone (ADH) secretion may also occur, resulting in water intoxication. Other agents associated with neurotoxicity include 5-fluorouracil (cerebellar ataxia), cisplatinum (tinnitus, deafness and peripheral neuropathy) and methotrexate (fits, arachnoiditis, necrotizing encephalopathy).

Liver   Prolonged treatment with methotrexate can cause severe hepatocellular damage leading to cirrhosis, though this is most commonly seen following the protracted low-dose therapy employed in treating psoriasis. Other agents, for example mithramycin and asparaginase, may cause transient liver injury.

Infertility   Azoospermia is very frequent following combination chemotherapy and the prepubertal testis is not immune to damage, particularly by alkylating agents

(Aubier *et al.*, 1989). Although spermatogenesis may recover after chemotherapy in adult life, there is a strong case for recommending sperm banking for young men (if not already azoospermic) who wish to preserve fertility. Alkylating agents are also the most frequently implicated in chemotherapy-assisted amenorrhoea, 40–50% of women experiencing permanent ovarian failure (Miller, Williams and Leissring, 1971). The likelihood of menstruation returning diminishes the closer the woman is to the probable menopause at the time she receives treatment (Koyama *et al.*, 1977).

Alopecia   Hair loss is a frequent but not inevitable consequence of chemotherapy, the vinca alkaloids, anthracyclines and podophyllotoxins being most frequently incriminated. Procedures such as scalp cooling may reduce or prevent hair loss, and should be offered to particularly concerned patients (see above). Although occasionally all body hair may be lost, eyebrows and axillary and pubic hair are less commonly affected. Hair may start to regrow while treatment continues, but this does not appear to be related to development of resistance by the tumour cells.

Urinary tract   A wide variety of agents are uro- or nephrotoxic, either as a direct effect or as a consequence of the excretion of metabolites. Cisplatinum and methotrexate (both highly active against bladder cancer which may have already prejudiced renal function) cause renal toxicity which may be minimized by maintaining a high flow rate of alkaline urine. Following treatment with high-dose cyclosphosphamide or ifosfamide, excretion of the metabolite acrolein may cause a severe haemorrhagic cystitis unless adequate hydration and the chelating agent mercapto-ethane sulphonate (MESNA) are employed (Shaw and Graham, 1987). The dosage of those drugs primarily eliminated via the kidneys, for example methotrexate, may require modification in patients with renal failure. Where a specific antidote is available, as with folinic acid for methotrexate prolonged administration may be indicated in such circumstances.

Second tumours   The risk of developing a second malignancy following chemotherapy is small, but may be higher than previously appreciated as more patients are surviving longer. Alkylating agents are usually incriminated, and their use in patients with a likely long survival (such as children and patients with lymphomas) is diminishing as less carcinogenic alternatives are emerging. The risks appear to be higher in patients who have received both alkylating agents and radiotherapy. The most frequent second tumour is acute myeloid leukaemia, which may be preceded by characteristic changes in the karyotype, and which is commonly refractory to chemotherapy (Perlman and Walker, 1973).

Teratogenicity   In experimental animals many cytotoxic drugs are teratogenic and there is an increased incidence of miscarriage among women receiving anti-cancer treatment during the first 3 months of pregnancy. During the later part of pregnancy the risks to the foetus are relatively small (Stutzman and Sokal, 1968), and must be set against the risks to the mother of delaying the initiation of therapy. Early delivery by caesarean section as soon as fetal viability permits should be considered, and close collaboration with the obstetrician is essential. During the first trimester, fetal death or miscarriage is the most likely consequence of chemotherapy, although severe congenital malformations have been reported.

Cancer drug development

The thirty or so drugs in current use in cancer chemotherapy have been developed by many different routes, but in the past 20 years the process of evaluating potentially useful compounds has been greatly refined in an effort to reduce the risks of missing an active agent. Many thousands of compounds are screened for activity each year, and those that warranted further investigation might reasonably be selected for one of four main reasons: (1) random screening of chemical compounds; (2) synthesis of analogues of existing anti-cancer drugs; (3) the chance observation of growth-inhibitory properties, or (4) the rational design of new drugs on the basis of known biochemical pathways to exploit. While the last of these is the most satisfying, it is only slowly beginning to bear fruit. The random process gained credibility as a result of its success in the development of anti-malarial therapy in the early 1940s. The major screening programme is carried out by the National Cancer Institute (NCI) in America, and many thousands of compounds have been assessed in this programme since its inception in 1955 (40 000 compounds were screened in 1975 alone). The success of any such enterprise depends in large part on the relevance of the screening method to the eventual activity of the drug against human cancers. The mainstay of the NCI's programme was the murine leukaemia L1210 (see above) and activity against this experimental tumour was a prerequisite for further evaluation against other experimental tumours. In 1975 the screening methods were changed to allow the inclusion of a panel of more representative animal tumours, including human tumours growing as xenografts in immune-suppressed animals, and pre-screening is performed in the sensitive P388 mouse leukaemia. To date, no currently useful anti-cancer agent has been without identifiable activity in such a preclinical screen.

An ideal animal screening system would be: (1) relatively simple to use so that many compounds could be screened at reasonable cost; (2) capable of selecting compounds with a reasonable likelihood of clinical activity in man; (3) capable of discriminating against inactive compounds; (4) sufficiently sensitive not to reject active compounds.

Once an agent has been identified (Figure 15.1) as active against the tumours in the screening panel, the preclinical evaluation moves to address the problems of formulation and toxicology, and these may present considerable difficulties for the pharmaceutical chemist. Preclinical toxicology used to involve elaborate (and expensive) testing in rodents, dogs and monkeys, but has now been refined to a system that relies on mice, following the accumulation of data that allow comparisons to be made across species. These studies allow determination of a dose-response curve from which the lethal dose (LD) in 10% (LD_{10}), 50% (LD_{50}) and 90% (LD_{90}) of experimental animals can be derived. The LD_{10} is the basis on which the dose for initial clinical study is established. To further enhance safety, the practice has been to initiate studies in patients at 10% of the LD_{10} in dogs.

These compounds that survive this extensive preclinical evaluation have still to go through four phases of clinical testing before they are accepted into general clinical practice. This process is time consuming, expensive and ethically challenging, particularly in the early stages before clinical activity has been demonstrated. In phase I studies the objective is to determine the maximally tolerated dose, most acceptable schedule and to identify the dose-limiting toxicities and their reversibility. Parallel studies will determine the pharmacokinetic profile, metabolism and pathways of elimination of the compound. Because the initial dose

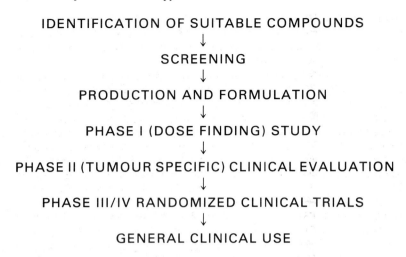

IDENTIFICATION OF SUITABLE COMPOUNDS
↓
SCREENING
↓
PRODUCTION AND FORMULATION
↓
PHASE I (DOSE FINDING) STUDY
↓
PHASE II (TUMOUR SPECIFIC) CLINICAL EVALUATION
↓
PHASE III/IV RANDOMIZED CLINICAL TRIALS
↓
GENERAL CLINICAL USE

Figure 15.1 Steps in cancer drug development

chosen is based on the LD_{10} in mice, the patients initially treated are not likely to gain a therapeutic benefit, and indeed this is only a subsidiary purpose of a phase I study. The burden of careful and frank explanation to the patient of the expectations of the 'treatment' is considerable, and both time and sensitive consideration of the patient's wishes are mandatory. Patients considered for participation in Phase I studies are those with histologically confirmed advanced malignancy no longer amenable to conventional therapy who appreciate that a potentially valuable new treatment is under evaluation but that they may not personally benefit from it. It is perhaps surprising how frequently patients are willing to participate on this basis. A typical study requires three patients to be completely evaluated at each dose level before the dose is increased, usually according to a modified Fibonacci schedule. The first escalation is usually a doubling of the dose, then an increase in fractions of 66%, 50% and then in further steps of 33% until toxicity is identified. This requires very frequent and careful patient evaluation, with monitoring of as many clinical, haematological and biochemical parameters as possible.

Once a practicable dose and schedule have been determined, a Phase II study will normally be initiated unless an unacceptable toxicity has been identified. Phase II studies are disease-specific, and are conducted for the purpose of identifying the spectrum of clinical antitumour activity, and to determine the toxicity in relation to the therapeutic effect (the therapeutic index). The number of patients required in a Phase II study is determined by the anticipated response rate. The usual requirement is a response rate of 20%, and, under ideal circumstances, a drug may be regarded as inactive at this level if there are no responses in the first 14 fully evaluable patients treated, i.e. there is a 95% probability that the true response rate is <20% under these circumstances. One or two responses in the initial 14 would indicate the need to treat 10–15 more patients in order to truly assess response rate. In reporting the results of a Phase II study, the response rate should be accompanied by the confidence interval (usually expressed as the range within which the true response has a 95% probability of being found). The clinical heterogeneity of malignant disease is such that usually more than the minimum number of patients are treated before a potentially promising agent is discarded. Also, it may be necessary to perform separate Phase II studies investigating different schedules or routes of administration.

Once the spectrum of clinical activity has been determined, Phase III and IV studies are concerned with establishing the place of the new agent in the therapeutic armamentarium. In Phase III studies the new drug is compared with the current standard treatment. This is ideally done as a prospective randomized trial of the new drug against the best available single agent in previously untreated patients, but the success of combination chemotherapy in many cancers has made it difficult for such studies to be performed in some circumstances. For example, the activity of etoposide in testicular teratoma had first to be demonstrated in patients with recurrent disease resistant to 'conventional' treatment (Fitzharris *et al.*, 1980). It is easy to envisage situations in which active drugs will be discarded for failing to demonstrate activity or having excessive toxicity if evaluation is confined to such heavily pretreated patients. In other circumstances, for example advanced breast cancer, chemotherapy is widely regarded as at best palliative and the need to identify active new agents is pressing. Under these conditions, it is less ethically challenging to consider a trial of a new drug before proceeding with 'conventional' treatment, and the new drug certainly receives a fairer evaluation in this way. Many trials are now performed in which the new drug replaces one agent in an active combination, and the two combinations randomly assigned to different treatment groups. Evaluations that rely exclusively on non-randomized comparisons are always less satisfactory however scrupulously the historical controls are chosen. The potential sources of bias can never be completely eliminated from non-randomized comparisons because they may not be identifiable unless patients are investigated uniformly and treated concurrently with the only variable being the form of treatment.

Phase IV studies are concerned with the integration of a new drug into the complete therapeutic strategy in conjunction with other therapeutic modalities, for example radiotherapy or surgery. Again, this usually requires prospective randomized clinical comparisons involving large numbers of patients, and so often require to be carried out by several centres and, increasingly, national or even international collaboration.

Conclusions

The role of chemotherapy has expanded rapidly in the past 20 years, but there is clearly considerable room for improvement. Given the lack of sophistication of our understanding of the basic biology of cancer, it is perhaps more surprising that chemotherapy is ever effective at all than that it is not more so. Some ten cancers are currently curable with chemotherapy, either alone or in combination with other treatment modalities (Table 15.3). Although these tumours account for only about 10% of cancers diagnosed, they tend to be those occurring in children and young adults so that the number of patient-years saved by successful treatment is greatly out of proportion to their frequency. On the other hand, many of the common solid tumours of adults such as non-small-cell lung cancer, colorectal cancer and malignant melanoma are effectively refractory to chemotherapy when advanced and new ideas and new drugs are urgently required. Many patients with these

Table 15.3 Current response status of major tumour types

Cancers curable with currently available chemotherapy

Gestational trophoblastic tumours	Childhood acute lymphoblastic leukaemia
Testicular tumours	Hodgkin's disease
Wilms' tumour	Ewing's sarcoma
Acute myeloid leukaemia	Burkitt's lymphoma
High-grade non-Hodgkin's lymphoma	Embryonal rhabdomyosarcoma

Tumours highly sensitive to chemotherapy, response prolongs life

Small-cell lung cancer	Ovarian cancer
Neuroblastoma	Breast cancer
Other non-Hodgkin's lymphomas	Adult acute leukaemias
Multiple myeloma	

Chemosensitive tumours

Chronic myeloid leukaemia	Chronic lymphocytic leukaemia
Soft-tissue sarcomas	
Stomach cancer	Squamous carcinomas of head and neck
Bladder cancer	Cervical cancer

Cancers refractory to currently available chemotherapy

Non-small-cell lung cancer	Renal cancer
Colorectal cancer	Thyroid cancer
Malignant melanoma	Pancreatic cancer
Hepatocellular cancer	
Squamous carcinoma of oesophagus	

---

tumour types will wish to explore the newer approaches and drugs, even though they fully understand the limited nature of our expectations. We owe it to them to ensure that these ideas are properly evaluated as quickly as possible, so that at the very least other patients can be spared the false hopes generated by overenthusiasm. At some point in the future, it is perhaps possible to see 'conventional' cytotoxic chemotherapy replaced by cocktails of biological response modifiers (e.g. interferon, tumour necrosis factor and/or interleukin 2) and monoclonal antibodies to specific oncogene products that will have complete antitumour selectivity and no normal tissue toxicity. However, until that time, the current agents are the best available, and major efforts need to be directed at ensuring that they are deployed as effectively as possible.

References

Allan, S. G., Cornbleet, M. A., Warrington, P. S. *et al.* (1984) Dexamethasone and high-dose metoclopramide: efficacy in controlling cisplatin-induced nausea and vomiting. *British Medical Journal,* **289**, 878–879

Aubier, F., Flamant, F., Brauner, R. *et al.* (1989) Male gonadal function after chemotherapy for solid tumours in childhood. *Journal of Clinical Oncology,* **7**, 304–309

Bergsagel, D. E. (1975) Treatment of plasma cell myeloma with cytotoxic agents. *Archives of Internal Medicine,* **135**, 172–176

Bonadonna, G. and Valagussa, P. (1981) Dose-response of adjuvant chemotherapy in breast cancer. *New England Journal of Medicine,* **304**, 10–15

Brockman, R. W. (1975) Circumvention of resistance: Pharmacologic basis of cancer chemotherapy. In *27th Annual Symposium on Fundamental Research.* University of Texas, M. D. Anderson Hospital and Tumor Institute, Williams and Wilkins, Baltimore, pp. 691–711

Bruce, W. R., Meeker, B. E. and Valeriote, F. A. (1966) Comparison of the sensitivity of normal hematopoietic and transplanted lymphoma colony-forming cells to chemotherapeutic agents administered *in vivo*. *Journal of the National Cancer Institute,* **37**, 233–245

Buckner, C. D., Rudolph, R. H., Fefer, A. *et al.* (1972) High-dose cyclophosphamide therapy for malignant disease; toxicity, tumor response, and the effects of stored autologous marrow. *Cancer,* **29**, 357–365

Cornbleet, M. A., Leonard, R. C. F. and Smyth, J. F. (1984) High-dose alkylating agent therapy: a review of clinical experiences. *Cancer Drug Delivery* **1**, 227–238

Dean, J. C., Salmon, S. E. and Griffith, K. S. (1979) Prevention of doxorubicin-induced hair loss with scalp hypothermia. *New England Journal of Medicine,* **301**, 1427–1429

DeVita, V. T., Serpick, A. A. and Carbone, P. P. (1970) Combination chemotherapy in the treatment of advanced Hodgkin's Disease. *Annals of Internal Medicine,* **73**, 891–895

Fitzharris, B. M., Kaye, S. B., Saverymuttu, S. *et al.* (1980) VP-16213 as a single agent in advanced testicular tumours. *European Journal of Cancer,* **16**, 1193–1197

Goldie, J. H. and Coldman, A. J. (1979) A mathematic model for relating the drug sensitivity of tumours to the spontaneous mutation rate. *Cancer Treatment Reports,* **63**, 1727–1733

Huggins, C. and Bergenstal, D. M. (1952) Inhibition of human mammary and prostatic cancer by adrenalectomy. *Cancer Research,* **12**, 134–141

Hutchison, D. J. and Schmid, F. A. (1973) Cross-resistance and collateral sensitivity. In *Drug-Resistance and Selectivity: Biochemical and Cellular Basis* (ed. E. Mihich). Academic Press, New York, pp. 73–126

Koyama, H., Wada, T., Nishizawa, Y. *et al.* (1977) Cyclophosphamide-induced ovarian failure and its therapeutic significance in patients with advanced breast cancer.

Luria, S. E. and Delbruck, M. (1943) Mutations of bacteria from virus sensitivity to virus resistance. *Genetics,* **28**, 491–511

Mendelsohn, M. L. (1960) The growth fraction: a new concept applied to tumors. *Science,* **132**, 1496

Miller, J. J., Williams, G. F. and Leissring, J. C. (1971) Multiple late complications of therapy with cyclophosphamide including ovarian destruction. *American Journal of Medicine,* **50**, 530–535

Perlman, M. and Walker, R. (1973) Acute leukemia following cytotoxic chemotherapy. *Archives of Internal Medicine,* **224**, 250

Schabel, F. M. and Simpson-Herren, L. (1978) Some variables in experimental tumour systems which complicate interpretation of data from *in vivo* kinetic and pharmacologic studies with anticancer drugs. *Antibiotic Chemotherapy,* **23**, 113–127

Shaw, J. C. and Graham, M. I. (1987) Mesna – a short review. *Cancer Treatment Reviews,* **14**, 67–86

Simpson-Herren, L. Sanford, A. H. and Holmquist, J. P. (1974) Cell population kinetics of transplanted Lewis lung carcinoma. *Cell Tissue Kinetics,* **7**, 349–361

Skipper, H. E. (1978) Reasons for success and failure in treatment of murine leukemias with the drugs now employed in treating human leukemias. In *Cancer Chemotherapy* (Vol. I). Ann Arbor, Michigan, University Microfilms International, pp. 1–166

Skipper H. E., Schabel, F. M., Mellet, L. B. *et al.* (1950) Implications of biochemical, cytokinetic, pharmacologic and toxicologic relationships in the design of optimal therapeutic schedules. *Cancer Chemotherapy Reports,* **54**, 431–450

Skipper, H. E., Schabel, F. M. and Wilcox, W. S. (1964) Experimental evaluation of potential anticancer agents XII. On the criteria and kinetics associated with 'curability' of experimental leukemia. *Cancer Chemotherapy Reports,* **35**, 1–111

Soukop, M., Campbell, A., Gray, M. M. and Calman, K. C. (1978) Adriamycin, alopecia and the scalp tourniquet. *Cancer Treatment Reports,* **62**, 489–490

Stutzman, L. and Sokal, J. E. (1968) Use of anticancer drugs during pregnancy. *Clinical Obstetrics and Gynaecology,* **11**, 416–427.

Chapter 16

Recent advances in cancer research

David J. Kerr

Introduction

Traditional surgical approaches to cancer were based on the hypothesis that most solid tumours were amenable to adequate local treatment. This concept has been tempered in recent times by the realization that combined therapy administered by surgeons, radiotherapists and medical oncologists yields improved results.

Advances in medical oncology over the past two decades have meant that a number of tumours (embryonal carcinoma of the testis, Hodgkin's disease, acute lymphoblastic leukemia, Burkitt's lymphoma, Wilms' tumour, choriocarcinoma, etc.) can now be cured, depending on the stage of presentation. Unfortunately, the majority of solid tumours seen in common surgical practice (gastric, colorectal, pancreas, kidney, bladder, prostate, gynaecological cancers) remain on the whole, resistant to chemotherapy. Useful palliation can be achieved, notably with breast cancer, but significant prolongation of survival following chemotherapy is rare.

Given the paucity of objective responses of these tumours to conventional cytotoxic agents, both singly and in combination, the search for novel active agents continues. There are four main sources of new antineoplastic drugs:

1. Chemical modification of pre-existing drugs following definition of structure-activity relationships.
2. Screening of random synthetics, usually supplied by the pharmaceutical industry.
3. Rational design of drugs based on known biochemical differences between tumour and host cells. Although this would seem the most fruitful source of active compounds, in practice it has proved difficult to determine exploitable metabolic or structural differences in tumour cells.
4. Serendipity. Chance played a significant part in the discovery of cisplatinum and asparaginase.

The National Cancer Institute (NCI, Maryland, USA) has undertaken a vast screening procedure in an attempt to find new agents which might be of clinical use. The preclinical new drug research programme has been responsible for the discovery of eight of the sixteen commercially available drugs introduced into clinical use between 1955 and 1984. This required screening of approximately 10 000 compounds per year. It is apparent that the appearance of new drugs of clinical utility is infrequent.

The purpose of this chapter is to describe recent advances, in both clinical and laboratory cancer research, which may contribute to future management of neoplasia. The specific areas which will be discussed include:

1. Optimization of cytotoxic drug delivery by loco-regional routes.
2. Conjugation of cytotoxic drugs to macromolecular carriers.
3. Biological response modifiers.
4. Tumour drug resistance.
5. Oncogenes and growth factors.

Regional chemotherapy

A number of common solid tumours have a propensity for confinement to specific organs or compartments within the body. The regional tumour frequently gives rise to morbidity rather than widespread metastases.

Regional chemotherapy is based on the premise that many cytotoxic drugs have steep toxic and therapeutic dose-response curves. The maximum amount of drug which can be administered systemically is governed by the side-effects consequent upon systemic exposure, e.g. myelosuppression, alopecia, nausea and vomiting, nephrotoxicity and neurotoxicity. Local administration of chemotherapy, by the intra-arterial or intraperitoneal route, allows generation of greater local drug exposures (high concentrations with prolonged maintenance at the tumour site) with reduced systemic absorption and hence a decrease in associated side-effects. The ideal situation would be one in which the local drug concentration generated was far in excess of that required to kill the clonogenic cells of the tumour, whereas the concentration in the systemic compartment was below the threshold needed for host cell toxicity.

Recent advances in two fields have been made which have contributed greatly to rational drug use of loco-regional routes; understanding of the theoretical pharmacokinetic basis underlying the selectivity of regional drug administration; improved surgical placement of permanent indwelling catheters for intra-arterial and intraperitoneal use.

Pharmacokinetic modelling for drug delivery by intra-arterial infusions has been carried out by Chen and Gross (1980). For instance they have shown that drugs with a high total body clearance such as 5-fluorouracil and fluorodeoxyuridine would tend to have high regional advantages, especially as both drugs have a fairly high hepatic extraction ratio. Any attempts to decrease hepatic arterial blood flow would also tend to enhance regional drug delivery. Similar types of equations have been identified for intraperitoneal drug administration for ovarian carcinoma where the regional advantage varies directly with total body clearance (as above) and inversely with peritoneal drug clearance. Therefore drugs which have a limited rate of egress from the peritoneal cavity tend to have high regional advantages, i.e. the tumour-containing compartment is exposed to significantly higher drug concentrations than the systemic circulation, therefore the therapeutic ratio would be increased. The regional advantages of several drugs which have been tested by the intra-arterial and intraperitoneal routes are summarized in Table 16.1.

The second impetus to regional chemotherapy has been the development of catheters and pumps for the controlled delivery of drug solutions via the arterial or peritoneal route. Regional chemotherapy initially had a rather poor reputation owing to catheter and pump-related side-effects – sepsis, gastrointestinal

Table 16.1 Regional advantage of cytotoxic drugs administered by the intra-arterial or intraperitoneal routes

Drug	Estimated increased tumour exposure of hepatic-arterial infusion	Peritoneal regional advantage (peritoneal peak conc. systemic peak conc.)
5-Fluorouracil	500–100	100
Fluoro-deoxyuridine	100–400	–
BCNU	7–13	–
Mitomycin	3–5	–
Cisplatinum	2–4	25
Methotrexate	3–6	20
Doxorubicin	–	430
Iproplatinum	–	30
Carboplatinum	–	20
Melphalan	–	50

haemorrhage, occlusion and arterial thrombosis, etc. – but these can be circumvented if the catheters are inserted at a single centre with expertise and maintained by dedicated nursing staff. Totally implantable, programmable pumps (Infusaid 400 pumps) are available and have now been implanted in several thousand patients across the world. For drugs which are given by bolus, rather than prolonged infusion, small implanted injection ports attached to silastic catheters can provide convenient access.

Most trials of intrahepatic arterial chemotherapy so far have been relatively small and non-randomized; however, preliminary results have been promising. Hepatic tumour responses as high as 80% have been recorded, with response durations of 8–9 months (Balch, Urist and McGregor, 1983) which are higher than typical response rates of approximately 20% seen in historical controls treated with intravenous 5-fluorouracil. The final result of a large, prospective randomized trial undertaken by the Memorial Sloan-Kettering group comparing intra-arterial with intravenous therapy is awaited with interest. One potential disadvantage of this therapeutic modality is disease recurrence at distant sites, such as lung, despite good local control.

Similarly with intraperitoneal therapy, promising Phase II responses have been reported in ovarian cancer with cisplatinum (Howell, Chu and Wang, 1982), but the results of large, prospective randomized phase III trials are required to demonstrate whether pharmacological sleight of hand can lead to useful improvements in tumour responses and prolong patient survival.

Several lines of research are being pursued currently in an attempt to increase the selectivity and tumoural uptake of cytotoxic drugs administered via the hepatic artery. Ensminger et al. (1985) have recently performed a Phase I clinical and pharmacokinetic trial of intrahepatic arterial biodegradable starch microspheres and mitomycin C. The starch microspheres (40 μm in diameter) have a half-life of approximately 30 minutes in the circulation and temporarily decrease hepatic arterial flow or even totally block it for up to 1 hour in about 25% of patients. As explained, reduction in hepatic blood flow, with a 'damming back effect', will increase organ extraction of the cytotoxic agent.

Concomitant infusion of vasoactive agents, either vasodilators such as verapamil or vasoconstrictors such as vasopressin have been shown to increase tumour blood flow relative to normal tissue. Sasaki *et al.* (1985) have shown that a brief intrahepatic arterial infusion of angiotensin II (10 μg/min over 4 mintues) increases hepatic metastatic blood flow by 2–3-fold relative to normal tissue.

We have synthesized Adriamycin-loaded albumin microspheres (1% Adriamycin w/w) approximately 20–40 μm in diameter (Willmott *et al.*, 1985). The disposition and kinetics of the Adriamycin-loaded microspheres following intra-renal arterial administration to rabbits differ from injection of free Adriamycin, with lower systemic and higher intra-renal Adriamycin concentrations being achieved (Lewi *et al.*, 1986). We are currently conducting a Phase I clinical trial of intrahepatic arterial chemotherapy for patients with hepatic metastases from colorectal carcinoma. The Adriamycin-loaded microspheres are administered with 5-fluorouracil and a short infusion of AII in an attempt to increase cytotoxic drug delivery to the metastatic tumour.

Cytotoxic drug carriers

As previously mentioned cytotoxic drugs have steep toxic-dose response curves and their use is clinically limited by their inability to distinguish neoplastic from normal tissue. Numerous attempts have been made to increase the selectivity of antineoplastic agents by linking them to macromolecular carriers which have a targeting component. Carrier moieties used include proteins, DNA, hormone-drug complexes which bind to tumour-associated hormone cell surface receptors, phospholipid vesicles called liposomes and inert microspheres made of ethylcellulose. Hitherto, these carrier systems have not had a great clinical impact. They certainly alter the pharmacokinetics of the drug delivered and usually provide a slow release-type preparation. This could be important for agents such as doxorubicin in which high peak plasma levels of the drug can be associated with the development of a chronic cardiomyopathy.

A number of general problems remain to be overcome before drug carriers can be used optimally in a clinical setting:

1. The specificity of the targetting component of the drug carrier complex.
2. Stability of the drug carrier complex *in vivo*.
3. Release of the active agent from the carrier at its site of pharmacological action.
4. Non-specific uptake of drug carrier complexes by the reticulo-endothelial system.
5. Immune reactions to the macromolecular carriers.

One method of circumventing some of these problems would be to use an endogenous carrier. Low-density lipoprotein (LDL) is the major cholesterol-carrying nanosphere in human plasma. It is a spherical particle (20 nm in diameter) with a lipid core surrounded by a polar shell comprising cholesterol, phospholipids and protein. A number of previous studies have shown both *in vitro* and *in vivo* that cancer cells show a greater LDL receptor activity than normal tissue (Ginsberg *et al.*, 1982), presumably reflecting an increased requirement for cholesterol for membrane synthesis.

We have demonstrated large numbers of high-affinity LDL receptors on the cell surface of human lung tumour cells in culture and have shown that the daunomycin–LDL complex is cytotoxic in monolayer and spheroid culture systems (Kerr *et al.*, 1986; Kerr and Kaye, 1987).

The concept of Ehrlich's 'magic bullet' is most closely approached by the notion of linking tumoricidal agents to antibodies directed against tumour-specific antigens. The techniques of genetic engineering and mass cell culture have allowed the production of a large number of monoclonal antibodies directed against nominally tumour-specific antigens.

Early clinical trials undertaken with monoclonal antibodies have shown that their administration is feasible and have delineated the expected pattern of toxicity (fever, chills and urticaria are quite common but not dose limiting although immune complex-mediated disturbances of hepatic and renal function have been reported).

Antibodies have two potential roles in cancer therapy, namely directing the immune response to antibody-labelled tumour cells, or by using the antibody as a carrier to deliver some tumoricidal agent to the cancer cell.

It has been demonstrated that monoclonal antibodies bind with relative selectivity to tumour cells, both *in vivo* and *in vitro*. However, there is wide variation in the dose required to saturate all available antibody binding sites which is related to tumour burden, antigen expression, antibody affinity and half-life and tissue penetration by the monoclonal antibody. Initial reports of clinical trials of unlabelled monoclonal antibodies have shown objective responses but these have been of short duration and limited clinical use (B cell lymphoma, T cell lymphoma, melanoma, leukaemia and colon cancer). In addition to the general problems outlined with use of macromolecular drug carriers, a few problems specific to antibody use have been noted, e.g. antigenic modulation (loss of antigen following antibody binding), heterogeneity of antigen expression, development of human anti-mouse antibodies, exfoliated antigens which are shed into the systemic circulation and therefore block antibody binding to the tumour and inability of the host immune system to recognize tumour cells with surface-bound antibodies.

As the antitumour effects of antibodies alone are clinically relatively disappointing, attempts have been made to conjugate toxins, cytotoxic drugs and radio-isotopes to monoclonal antibodies. A number of chemical techniques have been used to bind the cytotoxic agent to the antibody. It is important to maintain stability of the conjugate in the circulation, yet it must be labile enough to release the toxin at its site of cell binding.

A number of antineoplastic drugs have been attached to antibodies, including doxorubicin, daunomycin, vinblastine, methotrexate, chlorambucil, mitomycin and cisplatinum. Some of these conjugates are active *in vivo* in murine tumour models and human studies have been initiated.

Natural toxins, especially ricin, have been used because of their ability to kill tumour cells at very low doses. Ricin consists of two chains, the A chain is an inhibitor of protein synthesis whereas the B chain is responsible for toxin binding to galactose residues, present on the surface of most cell types. Ingeniously, the ricin A chain has been linked to a number of monoclonal antibodies and good antitumoural activity has been shown in animal tumours (Seto *et al.*, 1982). Phase I studies with immunoconjugates of ricin A have been undertaken in melanoma, colorectal cancer and T cell lymphoma.

Radiolabelled monoclonal antibodies have also been used for imaging and therapy. A number of clinical trials using monoclonal antibodies in a variety of solid and haematological tumours have shown that myelosuppression is the dose-limiting toxicity. This may not represent such a problem in the haematological malignancies in which high-dose chemoradiotherapy followed by marrow transplantation is a well-established form of chemotherapy. Further studies in this area may well include use of a wider range of radiopharmaceuticals, use of antibody fragments rather than the whole molecule and perhaps techniques aimed at altering the permeability of the tumour vascular barrier.

Biological response modifiers

The place of surgery, radiotherapy and chemotherapy has been established in combined modality treatment of cancer. Immunotherapy has been considered a fourth extension to treatment, but despite promising laboratory results, clinical experience in the 1970s was rather disappointing.

Advances in molecular biology, especially in the field of genomic cloning, have allowed the production of large quantities of pure proteins which have a number of biological and antitumour activities. These so-called biological response modifiers are agents whose mechanism of action, at least in part, implies alteration of the host's biological responses towards the tumour.

The interferons are a family of three antigenically distinct proteins, α (at least eight species), β (at least two species) and γ (number of species unknown) which are produced by cells in response to viral infection. The interferons have numerous activities *in vitro* and *in vivo*, including direct antiproliferative effects and profound effects on a number of components of the immune system, such as B, T and natural killer cells and macrophages. The interferons also enhance Class II surface antigen expression by tumour cells. This could provide a useful clinical interaction if monoclonal antibody therapy was being directed against tumours expressing Class II antigens.

The clinical responses seen in some Phase II trials of recombinant and natural α-interferon are summarized in Table 16.2. Responses to β- and γ-interferon have

Table 16.2 Clinical activity of α-interferon

Proven activity	Hairy-cell leukaemia
	Non-Hodgkin's lymphoma
	Kaposi's sarcoma
	Multiple myeloma
	Malignant melanoma
	Chronic myelogenous leukaemia
	Cutaneous T-cell lymphomas
Preliminary evidence of activity which requires confirmation	Osteogenic sarcoma
	Renal carcinoma
	Small-cell lung cancer
	Hodgkin's disease
	Astrocytoma
	Chronic lymphocytic leukaemia
	Acute lymphocytic leukaemia
Inactive	Colorectal carcinoma
	Breast cancer
	Non-small-cell lung cancer
	Prostatic carcinoma
	Acute myelogenous leukaemia

been noted, especially in renal-cell carcinoma but clinical experience with these interferons is limited. There is associated toxicity such as chills, myalgia, asthenia and a 'flu-like' syndrome. The highest response rates have been seen in hairy-cell leukaemia, a rare form of leukaemia for which α-interferon has revolutionized its treatment. The interferons are currently being tested in combination with conventional cytotoxic agents and some promising synergistic responses have been noted *in vivo* in tumour xenograft-bearing mice.

Interleukin-2 (IL-2) is a T-cell growth factor which is produced by stimulated T-cells and mediates its effects by binding to an external T-cell surface receptor (the TAc receptor). IL-2 treatment increases the cytotoxic activity of natural killer (NK) cells against a range of tumours. It has also been shown to induce the development of lymphokine-activated killer (LAK) cells from a population of non-T precursor cells.

Two clinical approaches have been developed to use IL-2, either alone in high dose or by the transfer of adoptive immunity. Mononuclear cells harvested from patients after IL-2 treatment can be stimulated to become cytotoxic LAK cells following continued exposure to IL-2 *in vitro*. The lymphocytes are then washed, tested for cytotoxicity *in vitro* against cultured fresh human tumour cells and transfused into the donor patients during IL-2 infusion some 2 weeks later.

The most recent clinical update of results following treatment with IL-2 and LAK cells showed an overall response rate (complete and partial responses) of about 20%, with the majority of responses being seen in renal carcinoma patients (12 of 36 patients responded). The response rate to high dose IL-2 alone was around 12%. Side-effects are, however, serious and include fever, chills, hypotension, fluid accumulation, pulmonary oedema, hepatic and renal failure and arthritis.

Recombinant tumour necrosis factor (TNF) is a 17 kilodalton monokine which has cytotoxic, vascular endothelial and immunoregulatory effects in murine tumour systems. A number of Phase I clinical trials testing various schedules and modes of administration are underway. Significant toxicity has been seen, and usually comprises of rigors, fatigue and malaise. Other toxicities seen include hypotension, confusion, pulmonary toxicity and myelosuppression.

Taken as a group, the biological response modifiers represent treatments early in their evolution, and their true place in cancer treatment, whether alone or in combination, remains to be determined.

Cytotoxic drug resistance

Increasing clinical awareness of the problem of cytotoxic drug resistance has led to a range of laboratory and clinical studies aimed at identifying the underlying mechanism. Traditionally, drug resistance has been divided into two broad groups: intrinsic drug resistance, in which the tumour cells are resistant to cytotoxic therapy *de novo* and is typified by the general unresponsiveness of solid gastrointestinal tumours; acquired drug resistance is seen characteristically in small-cell lung cancer, in which the complete remission rate to initial chemotherapy is high in limited stage disease. However, relapse is almost universal and recurrent tumour is resistant to the initial anticancer drug regimen. On the assumption that there is a direct relationship between cytotoxic drug efficacy and the amount of drug in equilibrium with its site of molecular action, a number of pharmacological postulates which could partially explain drug resistance have been made:

1. Inadequate drug dose or duration of treatment.
2. Wrong drug schedule.
3. Pharmacological sanctuary sites, e.g. the blood–brain barrier excludes most cytotoxic drugs from penetrating to intracerebral tumours.
4. Pharmacokinetic interactions between concomitantly administered cytotoxic drugs.
5. Bioavailability. A number of cytotoxic drugs are administered orally, but their absorption from the gastrointestinal tract and extent of hepatic first-pass metabolism can vary from patient to patient according to tumour burden.

Most of these hypotheses can be tested in clinical and pharmacokinetic studies. *In vitro*, a number of different biochemical mechanisms have been elucidated which account for cellular resistance to specific antineoplastic agents, e.g. cells resistant to methotrexate, a widely used antimetabolite, have been shown to have decreased drug uptake and alterations in the enzyme to which methotrexate binds and inhibits to produce its cytotoxic effect. Resistant cells have been demonstrated with greatly elevated enzyme concentrations, or greatly reduced binding affinity for methotrexate. One aspect of drug resistance which is particularly fascinating is that of the multidrug resistance (MDR) phenotype, whose predominant feature is resistance to a wide range of structurally unrelated cytotoxic agents, many of which are anticancer drugs in current clinical use (e.g. anthracyclines, VP-16, vincristine, vinblastine, actinomycin D). Of the biochemical changes detected in MDR cell lines, the most consistent finding is of increased expression of a plasma membrane glycoprotein gp170 (Kartner *et al.*, 1985). Following a variety of experiments, including single gene transfection studies into sensitive cells, it is apparent that there is a correlation between gp170 expression and the degree of resistance. Sequence analysis of the gp170 gene has shown striking homology with bacterial haemolysin transport proteins. This implies that gp170 has been conserved through evolution and hypotheses have been advanced that it acts as an ATP-dependent export pump which reduces intracellular levels of cytotoxic drugs. Significant levels of P-glycoprotein have been detected in some biopsy specimens from patients with sarcomas and ovarian carcinomas; however, in a recent study Merkel *et al.* (1987) failed to show amplification or increased transcription of the gp170 gene in a study of approximately 300 breast tumour specimens. The clinical relevance of gp170 therefore remains to be determined.

Is there any clinical potential for overcoming drug resistance? A number of *in vitro* studies have shown that it is possible to partially overcome drug resistance using modifying agents such as verapamil (Kaye and Merry, 1985). The mode of action of verapamil in reversing the MDR phenotype is unknown but it may act by inhibiting the pump effect of the gp170 glycoprotein. There are clinical studies currently under way looking at combinations of verapamil with conventional cytotoxic therapy, with some promising initial results.

Oncogenes and growth factors

Diverse exogenous factors (UV irradiation, ionizing radiation, viruses, smoking, chemical carcinogenic exposure) have been associated with the process of carcinogenesis. The mode of action of these various agents was unknown but was assumed to be mediated by a DNA interaction. The mitogenic potential of carcinogenic stimuli was recognized more than three decades ago, and numerous observations of alterations in chromosomal structure in tumour tissue have since been described. The Philadelphia chromosome in chronic myeloid leukaemia is probably the best known of these.

Retroviruses (viruses capable of synthesizing DNA from an RNA template) can cause cancer in many species. Utilizing modern molecular biological techniques it has been possible to identify the retroviral genes responsible for tumorigenesis. These genes are called oncogenes and are responsible for encoding proteins which contribute to the malignant phenotype. The next major step in our understanding of carcinogenesis came with the demonstration that there are genes in the normal human genome (proto-oncogenes) which correspond to the viral-oncogenes. Proto-oncogenes have been demonstrated in eukaryotic and prokaryotic cells, implying evolutionary genetic conservation and therefore that the encoded proteins are functionally important for the cell's economy. A number of oncogenes have been identified by introduction of DNA fragments from human tumour cells into non-malignant NIH-3T3 cells (the process of transfection) and demonstration of consequent transformation into tumour cells. The function of a number of oncogenes is now known (Table 16.3).

Table 16.3 General summary of oncogenes

Retroviral oncogene	Tumour type	Function
v-src	Sarcoma	Kinase
v-abl	Lymphoma	Kinase
v-fes/fps	Sarcoma	Kinase
v-erb B	Sarcoma	EGF-R
v-fms	Sarcoma	CSF1-R
v-ras	Sarcoma/leukaemia	GTPase
v-ros	Sarcoma	Kinase
v-yes	Sarcoma	Kinase
v-raf	Sarcoma	Kinase
v-mos	Sarcoma	Kinase
v-erb A	Leukaemia	?
v-rel	Leukaemia	?
v-myc	Lymphoma/sarcoma Carcinoma	?
v-myb	Leukaemia	?
v-fos	Sarcoma	?
v-sis	Sarcoma	PDGF-2/B

EGF-R = epidermal growth factor receptor;
CSF1-R = colony, stimulating factor 1 receptor;
GTPase = guanosine triphosphatase;
PDGF-2/B = B chain of platelet derived growth factor.

There are three mechanisms which can explain how a protein essential to normal cellular function can lead to malignant transformation. The encoding oncogene may be amplified, i.e. the number of gene copies present in the normal genome may be greatly increased in number, leading to excessive production of the protein. Overexpression of the oncogene with elevated messenger RNA levels and increased protein translation has been described, as have point mutations in the oncogene leading to the production of the protein with altered activity.

Interest has focused on the relationship between proto-oncogenes and growth factors. Growth factors have been defined as polypeptides that stimulate cell proliferation through binding to specific high-affinity membrane receptors. As shown in Table 16.3, a number of oncogene products have been shown to be growth factors themselves or, in the case of the erb-B oncogene, a truncated form of the epidermal growth factor (EGF) receptor (which appears to function independently on exogenous EGF binding). There is no doubt that growth factors play a part in the economy of the normal cell, in control of proliferation and embryogenesis, but it is possible in certain instances to demonstrate that regulation of these potent factors is lost leading to permanent autostimulation and continued growth characteristic of tumour cells. Dickson, McManaway and Lippman (1986) have shown the importance of both growth-stimulatory (transforming growth factor-α, insulin-like growth factor I) and growth-inhibitory (transforming growth factor-β) factors in oestrogen-regulated control of proliferation of oestrogen-receptor (ER) positive breast cancer cells. Oestrogen-induced proliferation of ER+ve cells is associated with synthesis and release of TGF-α and IGF-I. The breast cancer cells have cell surface receptors for these growth factors, therefore an autocrine growth regulatory mechanism has been proposed, i.e. the breast cancer cells produce factors which bind to their own cell membranes and cause stimulation of growth. Conversely, treatment of ER+ve breast cancer cells with the anti-oestrogen tamoxifen decreases the rate of cell proliferation and is associated with secretion by the breast cancer cells of TGF-β, a growth inhibitory factor for epithelial cells.

There are no applications of oncogene research in routine clinical practice. However, as the complex cascade of growth factors and their role in controlling neoplastic proliferation is further understood it may be possible to intervene therapeutically and interrupt the positive feedback loops involved in uncontrolled proliferation.

It is possible, also, that molecular biological research might produce useful markers of disease prognosis. There is an apparent correlation between the degree of N-myc oncogene amplification and prognosis and stage of presentation of the paediatric tumour, neuroblastoma.

It has been possible only to briefly sketch certain areas of current interest in clinical and laboratory research. Clearly the objectives of optimizing tumour drug delivery by taking account of variables such as drug dose, drug intensity, drug schedule, drug timing and the route of drug administration are clinically testable at the moment. However, the concepts which have arisen from oncogene research have far-reaching implications which could translate into patient benefit over the next few decades.

References

Balch, C. M., Urist, M. M. and McGregor, M. L. (1983) Continuous regional chemotherapy for metastatic colorectal cancer using a totally implantable infusion pump. *American Journal of Surgery,* **145**, 285–290

Chen, H-S. G. and Gross, J. F. (1980) Intra-arterial infusion of anticancer drugs: therapeutic aspects of drug delivery and review of responses. *Cancer Treatment Reports,* **64**, 21–40

Dickson, R. B., McManaway, M. E. and Lippman, M. E. (1986) Estrogen-induced factors of breast cancer cells partially replace oestrogen to promote tumor growth. *Science,* **23**, 1540–1543

Ensminger, W. D., Gyves, J. W., Stevson, P. and Walker-Andrews, S. (1985) Phase I study of hepatic arterial degradable starch microspheres and mitomycin. *Cancer Research,* **45**, 4464–4467

Ginsberg, H., Gilbert, H. S., Gibson, J. C. *et al.* (1982) Increased low density lipoprotein catabolism in myeloproliferative disorders. *Annals of Internal Medicine,* **96**, 311–317

Howell, S. B., Chu, B. B. F. and Wung, W. E. (1982) Intraperitoneal cisplatin with systemic thiosulfate protection. *Annals of Internal Medicine,* **97**, 845–851

Kartner, N. Evernden-Porelle, D., Bradley, G. and Ling, V. (1985) Monoclonal antibodies detecting P-glycoprotein in multidrug-resistant cell lines. *Nature (Lond.),* **316**, 820–823

Kaye, S. and Merry, S. (1985) Tumour cell resistance to anthracyclines – a review. *Cancer Chemotherapy and Pharmacology,* **14**, 96–103

Kerr, D. J. and Kaye, S. B. (1987) Aspects of cytotoxic drug penetration with particular reference to anthrocyclines. *Cancer Chemotherapy and Pharmacology,* **19**, 1–5

Kerr, D. J., Kaye, S. B., Look, J. *et al.* (1986) Lipophilic anthrocydine analogues can partially overcome drug penetration barriers in human lung tumour spheroids. *Proceedings of the American Association for Cancer Research,* **27**, 1576

Lewi, H., Willmott, N., Kerr, D. J. and McArdle, C. S. (1986) Adriamycin-loaded albumin microspheres: a new method of delivering cytotoxic therapy. *British Journal of Surgery,* **73**, 612

Merkel, D., Hill, S., Fugua, S. *et al.* (1987) Multiple drug resistance P-glycoprotein gene amplification in human primary breast cancer. *Proceedings of the American Society of Clinical Oncology,* **57**, 221

Sasaki, Y., Shingi, I., Yoshinhisa, H. *et al.* (1985) Changes in distribution of hepatic blood flow induced by intra-arterial infusion of angiotensin II in human hepatic cancer. *Cancer* **55**, 311–316

Seto, M., Umemoto, N., Saito, M. *et al.* (1982) Monoclonal antibody anti-MM46: Ricin A chain conjügate: *In vitro* and *in vivo* antitumour activity. *Cancer Research,* **42**, 5209–5214

Willmott, N., Cummings, J., Stuart, J. F. B. and Florence, A. T. (1985) Adriamycin-loaded albumin microspheres: preparation, *in vivo* distribution and release in the rat. *Biopharm. and Drug Disp.,* **6**, 91–104

Index